THE GREAT HANOI
RAT HUNT

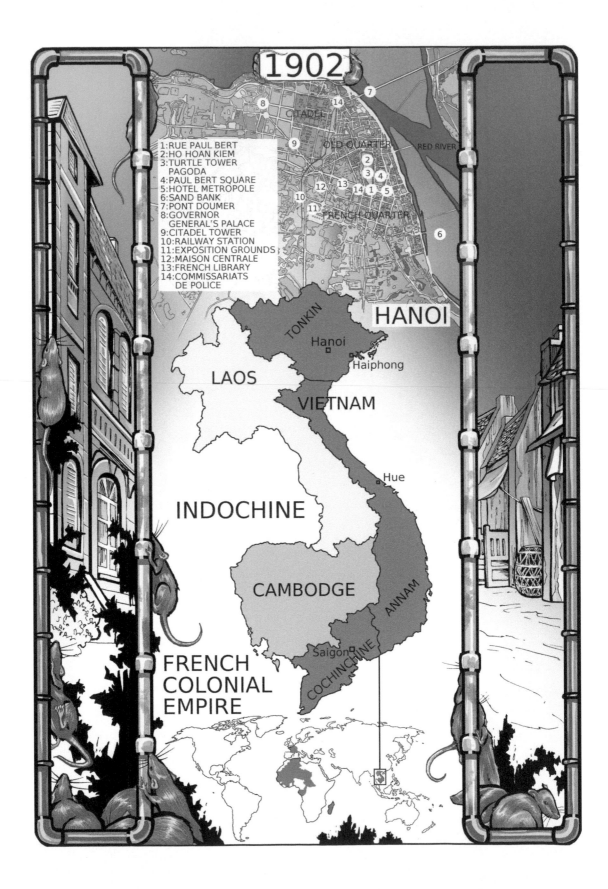

THE GREAT HANOI RAT HUNT

EMPIRE, DISEASE, AND MODERNITY IN FRENCH COLONIAL VIETNAM

MICHAEL G. VANN

LIZ CLARKE

New York   Oxford
OXFORD UNIVERSITY PRESS

To the People of Hanoi

Oxford University Press is a department of the University of Oxford.
It furthers the University's objective of excellence in research, scholarship,
and education by publishing worldwide. Oxford is a registered trade mark of
Oxford University Press in the UK and certain other countries.

Published in the United States of America by Oxford University Press
198 Madison Avenue, New York, NY 10016, United States of America.
© 2019 by Oxford University Press

Library of Congress Cataloging-in-Publication Data

Names: Vann, Michael G., author. | Clarke, Liz, 1982- illustrator.
Title: The great Hanoi rat hunt : empire, disease, and modernity in
    French colonial Vietnam / Michael G. Vann, Liz Clarke.
Description: New York: Oxford University Press, [2018] |
    Series: Graphic history series; 7 | Includes bibliographical references.
Identifiers: LCCN 2018006197 (print) | LCCN 2018007245 (ebook) |
    ISBN 9780190602703 (E-Book) | ISBN 9780190602697 | ISBN 9780190602697 (pbk.)
Subjects: LCSH: Hanoi (Vietnam)—History. | Plague—Vietnam—Hanoi—History. |
    Rats—Control—Vietnam—Hanoi—History. | Vietnam—History—1858–1945. |
    Vietnam—Colonization. | Vietnam—Civilization—French influences.
Classification: LCC DS559.93.H36 (ebook) | LCC DS559.93.H36 V38 2018 (print) |
    DDC 959.7/3—dc23
LC record available at https://lccn.loc.gov/2018006197

9 8 7 6 5
Printed by LSC Communications, Inc., United States of America

"Each new colonial expansion is accompanied, as a matter of course, by a relentless battle of capital against the social and economic ties of the natives, who are also forcibly robbed of their means of production and labor power."

Rosa Luxemburg, *The Accumulation of Capital* (1913)

"History shows again and again
How nature points out the folly of men."

Blue Öyster Cult, "Godzilla" (1977)

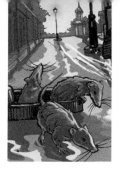

CONTENTS

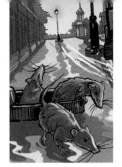

LIST OF MAPS

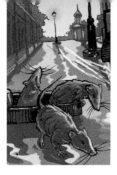

LETTER TO THE READER

Dear reader, this is going to be fun. Trust me. This book is going to be a lot of fun . . . and you just might learn something about some pretty important topics ranging from the history of disease and urban planning to Sinophobia and the political economy of empire.

With the help of the incredibly talented Liz Clarke, I've put together a graphic history that, despite a few creepy and disgusting moments, is as entertaining as it is educational. Over the past twenty years, I have had a wonderful experience researching the material for what I call "The Great Hanoi Rat Hunt"; the French colonial state's quixotic campaign to eliminate plague-bearing rats from the city's sewers. I've traveled to archives in France and Vietnam and read thousands of pages of century-old documents in a quest to find a few elusive references to colonial sewer rats. I've even come face-to-face with the descendants of some of the rodents in question. I have enjoyed sharing this story of empire, modernity, and disease in academic conferences, journal articles, and radio interviews. Time and time again, when I tell this story of a modernization project gone awry, my audience has suggested new ways of looking at the story and alternate interpretations of the events. I hope you will come to your own conclusions and draw your own lessons from the book. I am excited to be sharing this story in a graphic format.

For students of Vietnamese history, this book will add to your knowledge of the nation's capital. Hanoi, with its 1,000-year history, is home to overlapping layers of Vietnamese, Chinese, and French cultural influences. Hanoi is a stunningly beautiful city, and its residents are justly proud of its hybrid post-Colonial charm. This book will also show some of the ways in which various Vietnamese individuals expressed their historical agency, that is to say acted on their own rather than just being acted upon by French colonizers. We will explore the ways in which Vietnamese people resisted the empire.

Students of French history will see how the colonial project, the so-called "civilizing mission," was exported to a far corner of the empire. French Hanoi's history embodies the troubling paradox of France's best traits (the legacy of the Enlightenment and the faith in scientific progress) coexisting with the nation's worst practices (systems of colonial exploitation and racist disdain for the non-white Other). I hope my book expresses the ambiguity and nuance many felt toward colonial modernization projects. Liz Clarke's beautiful illustrations capture and convey the complexity of the colonial encounter, where two cultures lived together within a city but never really understood each other.

Those of you interested in the history of disease and humanity's relationship with the environment will find a fascinating case study that illustrates the ironic and tragic ways in which modernization projects can have unintended consequences. While claiming to make life better for people, Western industrial-capitalism and imperialism disrupted the lives of millions and inadvertently spread a number of deadly diseases around the world. Furthermore, the history of the Third Bubonic Plague Pandemic (1855–1959) surprises us with important insights into the symbiotic relationship between humans and other life forms, be they rodents, insects, or bacteria. Many have argued that modernity was the story of humanity's conquest over nature, but in this story nature seems to have escaped defeat.

My discussion of these various themes is framed within a world historical perspective that takes into account the ways in which cultures and economies have become increasingly intertwined in the modern era. For at least three generations, colonialism tied France and Vietnam together, with each country influencing the other. This story of globalization notes the important role of China as both a lure to the West and the source of a massive global diaspora. Sadly, Sinophobia was a frequent reaction to the world's complicated relationship with China.

Finally, I want you to think about the process of writing history. Ask yourself questions about how historians put their stories together. Where do we find our sources? What kind of evidence do we use? What kind of information makes its way into an archive or a library? What might be silenced and left out of the historical record?

I hope you enjoy this story of rats and men that has captivated me since I found its first traces in the archives many years ago.

–Michael G. Vann

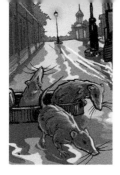

ACKNOWLEDGMENTS

Considering that I have been chasing Hanoi's sewer rats since 1995, I should be thanking just about everyone in my professional and personal life that has had to deal with me for the past two decades. My wife Briana and my daughter MaaNagala put up with years of my chatter about colonial sewer rats and musings about doing history with cartoons. Briana helped with translations and MaaNagala drew some great sketches of grumpy Frenchmen chasing crafty rodents.

I owe the greatest debt to Tyler Stovall, once my doctoral advisor and now my friend, who always encouraged me to do my best and always pushes me to do more. At the University of California, Santa Cruz, Terry Burke and Marc Cioc taught me to think about empire, environment, and labor in a world historical context. My many friends from the French and Vietnamese archives include David Del Testa, Eric Jennings, Penny Edwards, Erica Peters, Christophe Garonne, Sophie Reig, and Claire Edington. The members of the French Colonial Historical Society, who not only survived my 2008–2010 tenure as president but then agreed to follow me to Cambodia in 2014, have been a constant source of camaraderie, vibrant intellectual exchange, and professional networking. Sue Peabody, Ruth Ginio, Ken Orosz, Liz Foster, Bob DuPlessis, and Caroline Herbelin were delightful to work with. I first presented the story of the Great Hanoi Rat Hunt at the 2002 meeting of the FCHS hosted by Yale University. The Western Society for French History, the World History Association, the California affiliate of the World History Association, and the History of Medicine in Southeast Asia group have been important audiences for developing my ideas about empire, disease, and creative ways of investigating cultural history.

Like any good work of world history, I have to thank people around the globe. In France, Jean François-Klein, a.k.a. "Jeff," deserves a special *merci* for his years of encouragement and good will. His enthusiasm for history is rivaled by few. Marie and Lionel Cailloux opened their Parisian home to me, treated me like family, and fed me like royalty. My *ohana* extends from Honolulu to Boston and from Shanghai to London: Rick

Warner, Matthew Berry, Micheline Lessard, Kim Wagner, Marc Gilbert, Alyssa Sepinwall, Christina Firpo, Patricia Bishop-Goldsworthy, Katie Edwards, Martin Thomas, Pierre Singaravélou, Hans Pols, Tran Tuan Anh, Vu Anh, Tran Doan Linh, Le Hong Phong, Troy Crowder, Heather Streets-Salter, Eric Jones, Melissa Pashigian, Keith McPartland, Ben Donaldson, Adrian Saldana, Andy Hill, Tim Yates, Ben Ignacio, Jeff Chang, Garth Taylor, Sam Radetsky, Joey Thomas, Ross Dunn, Tim Keirn, Kim Drieux, Chris "Scuzz" Scurrah, Bung Bintang, Nyoman Ben Sukerta, Krisna Uk, Uji, and Sri Margono have been supportive in many different ways. Even though he insists on telling people that I'm the C.I.A. Station Chief, Bonnie Triyana is my man in Jakarta. His undergraduate research project is a brave piece of historical research, and his *Historia* magazine continues to boldly break new ground. In Yogyakarta, thanks go to my colleagues and students at Universitas Gadjah Mada who listened to a revised version of my research in 2013 and continue to post items about my *sejarah tikus* on social media. In Hanoi, Hoang Anh Tuan (who I first met on a memorable night in Paris) helped with access to the archives, secured a research assistant for me, and hosted Pierre Asselin, Grace Cheng, and me for a delightful evening in Hanoi.

Closer to home, Jeff Dym, Aaron Cohen, Becky Kluchin, Mona Siegel, Mitch Numark, Jeff Wilson, and the rest of my colleagues at Sacramento State have been kind enough to let me bounce ideas off them. Almost two decades of students at U.C. Santa Cruz, Santa Clara University, the U.S. Naval Postgraduate School, Universitas Gadjah Mada, East China Normal University, and Sacramento State have politely listened to me as I tried to convince them that the tragic fate of thousands of sewer rats had relevance to the larger issues of empire, modernity, and disease . . . and yes, this will be on the test. All of these institutions allowed me to develop courses that approached Vietnam, France, and Southeast Asia from a world historical perspective. The faculty of Santa Clara University, where I taught when the first version of "The Great Hanoi Rat Hunt" was published as a journal article, taught me an important lesson on history as a career choice. Dean Sheree Meyers of Sacramento State's College of Arts and Letters approved grants that funded recent rat research. Travel awards from Sacramento State's University Enterprises Inc. further assisted this far-flung endeavor. Special thanks go to David Earwicker, Associate Vice President for the Office of Research Affairs at California State University, Sacramento.

In the 1990s a generous Fulbright grant for doctoral research in France allowed me to first discover Hanoi's sewer rats. More recently, as a Fulbright Senior Scholar in Indonesia I was able to refine my ideas about this micro-history. I hope that the American government continues to fund Fulbright in the future. Such programs of international intellectual exchange are essential for building the kind of world in which I want my child to live. A Senior Fellowship from the Center for Khmer Studies to make a film on French colonial urbanism in Phnom Penh inspired my initial idea to tell the story of *The Great Hanoi Rat Hunt* in this non-traditional format.

At Oxford University Press, the incredibly talented Liz Clarke brought my vision to life. Since I pitched my idea for the rat hunt as a graphic history, Charles Cavaliere has been a wonderful editor. The anonymous and semi-anonymous reviewers provided important suggestions and criticisms.

While I am tempted to dedicate *The Great Hanoi Rat Hunt* to all coffee baristas who helped get me going in the mornings and make it through the long afternoons in the archives and the bartenders who helped me wind down after long days of research, I know that this book must honor the people of Hanoi. They have endured so much yet remain gracious and generous hosts. In particular, I want to single out my friend's grandparents, Nguyen Khac Thu and Nguyen Thi Toan. Both of them fought for their nation's independence and welcomed me into their home.

–Michael G. Vann

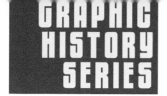

GRAPHIC HISTORY SERIES

Widely acclaimed by educators, the award-winning Graphic History Series introduces students to the ways that historians construct the past. Going beyond simply depicting events in the past, each title in the Graphic History Series combines the power of imagery with primary sources, historical essays, and cutting-edge historiography to offer a powerful tool for teaching history and teaching *about* history.

PUBLISHED

Trevor R. Getz and Liz Clarke, *Abina and the Important Men*

Ronald Schechter and Liz Clarke, *Mendoza the Jew: Boxing, Manliness, and Nationalism*

Rafe Blaufarb and Liz Clarke, *Inhuman Traffick: The International Struggle Against the Transatlantic Slave Trade*

Nina Caputo and Liz Clarke, *Debating Truth: The Barcelona Disputation of 1263*

Andrew Kirk and Kristian Purcell, *Doom Towns: The People and Landscapes of Atomic Testing*

Jennifer A. Rea and Liz Clarke, *Perpetua's Journey: Faith, Gender, & Power in the Roman Empire*

FORTHCOMING

Bryan McCann and Gilmar Fraga, *The Black Lancers and the Ragamuffin Revolt*

Maura Elizabeth Cunningham and Liz Clarke, *Wandering Lives: Art and Politics in Twentieth-Century China*

Karlos K. Hill and Dave Dodson, *The Murder of Emmett Till*

THE GREAT HANOI RAT HUNT

PART I
THE GRAPHIC HISTORY

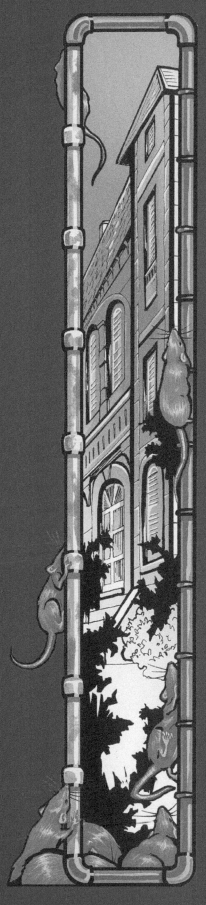

PROLOGUE

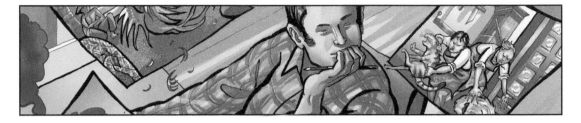

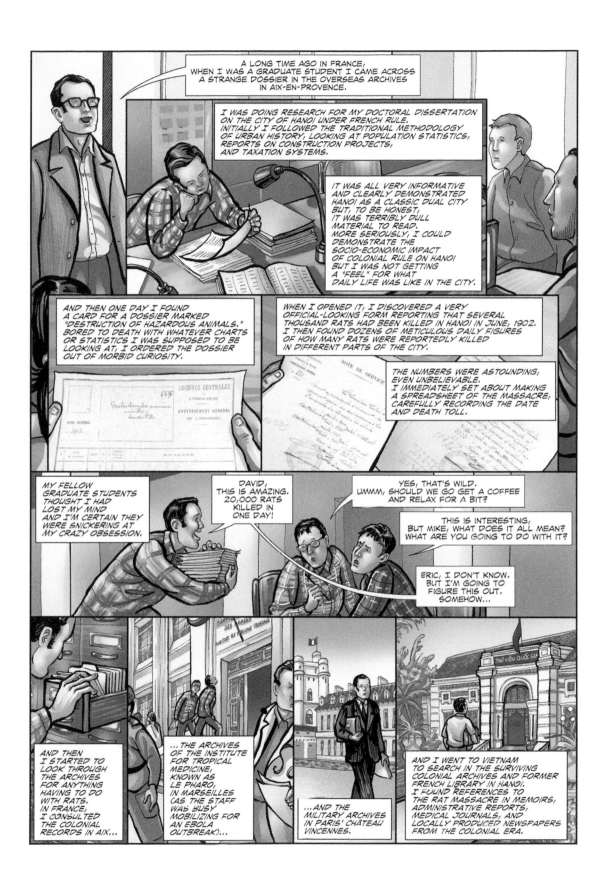

A LONG TIME AGO IN FRANCE, WHEN I WAS A GRADUATE STUDENT I CAME ACROSS A STRANGE DOSSIER IN THE OVERSEAS ARCHIVES IN AIX-EN-PROVENCE.

I WAS DOING RESEARCH FOR MY DOCTORAL DISSERTATION ON THE CITY OF HANOI UNDER FRENCH RULE. INITIALLY I FOLLOWED THE TRADITIONAL METHODOLOGY OF URBAN HISTORY, LOOKING AT POPULATION STATISTICS, REPORTS ON CONSTRUCTION PROJECTS, AND TAXATION SYSTEMS.

IT WAS ALL VERY INFORMATIVE AND CLEARLY DEMONSTRATED HANOI AS A CLASSIC DUAL CITY BUT, TO BE HONEST, IT WAS TERRIBLY DULL MATERIAL TO READ. MORE SERIOUSLY, I COULD DEMONSTRATE THE SOCIO-ECONOMIC IMPACT OF COLONIAL RULE ON HANOI BUT I WAS NOT GETTING A "FEEL" FOR WHAT DAILY LIFE WAS LIKE IN THE CITY.

AND THEN ONE DAY I FOUND A CARD FOR A DOSSIER MARKED "DESTRUCTION OF HAZARDOUS ANIMALS." BORED TO DEATH WITH WHATEVER CHARTS OR STATISTICS I WAS SUPPOSED TO BE LOOKING AT, I ORDERED THE DOSSIER OUT OF MORBID CURIOSITY.

WHEN I OPENED IT, I DISCOVERED A VERY OFFICIAL-LOOKING FORM REPORTING THAT SEVERAL THOUSAND RATS HAD BEEN KILLED IN HANOI IN JUNE, 1902. I THEN FOUND DOZENS OF METICULOUS DAILY FIGURES OF HOW MANY RATS WERE REPORTEDLY KILLED IN DIFFERENT PARTS OF THE CITY.

THE NUMBERS WERE ASTOUNDING, EVEN UNBELIEVABLE. I IMMEDIATELY SET ABOUT MAKING A SPREADSHEET OF THE MASSACRE, CAREFULLY RECORDING THE DATE AND DEATH TOLL.

MY FELLOW GRADUATE STUDENTS THOUGHT I HAD LOST MY MIND AND I'M CERTAIN THEY WERE SNICKERING AT MY CRAZY OBSESSION.

DAVID, THIS IS AMAZING. 20,000 RATS KILLED IN ONE DAY!

YES, THAT'S WILD. UMMM, SHOULD WE GO GET A COFFEE AND RELAX FOR A BIT?

THIS IS INTERESTING, BUT MIKE, WHAT DOES IT ALL MEAN? WHAT ARE YOU GOING TO DO WITH IT?

ERIC, I DON'T KNOW. BUT I'M GOING TO FIGURE THIS OUT. SOMEHOW...

AND THEN I STARTED TO LOOK THROUGH THE ARCHIVES FOR ANYTHING HAVING TO DO WITH RATS. IN FRANCE, I CONSULTED THE COLONIAL RECORDS IN AIX...

...THE ARCHIVES OF THE INSTITUTE FOR TROPICAL MEDICINE, KNOWN AS LE PHARO, IN MARSEILLES (AS THE STAFF WAS BUSY MOBILIZING FOR AN EBOLA OUTBREAK)...

...AND THE MILITARY ARCHIVES IN PARIS' CHÂTEAU VINCENNES.

AND I WENT TO VIETNAM TO SEARCH IN THE SURVIVING COLONIAL ARCHIVES AND FORMER FRENCH LIBRARY IN HANOI. I FOUND REFERENCES TO THE RAT MASSACRE IN MEMOIRS, ADMINISTRATIVE REPORTS, MEDICAL JOURNALS, AND LOCALLY PRODUCED NEWSPAPERS FROM THE COLONIAL ERA.

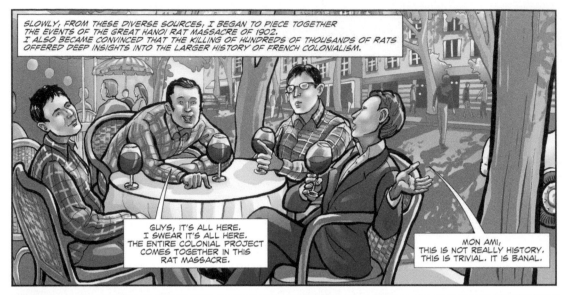

SLOWLY, FROM THESE DIVERSE SOURCES, I BEGAN TO PIECE TOGETHER THE EVENTS OF THE GREAT HANOI RAT MASSACRE OF 1902. I ALSO BECAME CONVINCED THAT THE KILLING OF HUNDREDS OF THOUSANDS OF RATS OFFERED DEEP INSIGHTS INTO THE LARGER HISTORY OF FRENCH COLONIALISM.

GUYS, IT'S ALL HERE. I SWEAR IT'S ALL HERE. THE ENTIRE COLONIAL PROJECT COMES TOGETHER IN THIS RAT MASSACRE.

MON AMI, THIS IS NOT REALLY HISTORY. THIS IS TRIVIAL. IT IS BANAL.

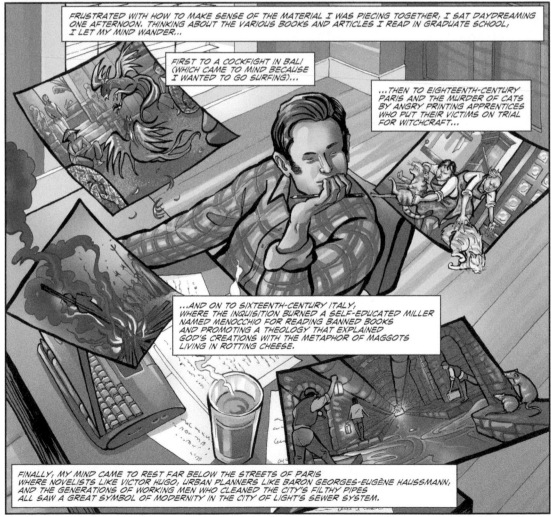

FRUSTRATED WITH HOW TO MAKE SENSE OF THE MATERIAL I WAS PIECING TOGETHER, I SAT DAYDREAMING ONE AFTERNOON. THINKING ABOUT THE VARIOUS BOOKS AND ARTICLES I READ IN GRADUATE SCHOOL, I LET MY MIND WANDER...

FIRST TO A COCKFIGHT IN BALI (WHICH CAME TO MIND BECAUSE I WANTED TO GO SURFING)...

...THEN TO EIGHTEENTH-CENTURY PARIS AND THE MURDER OF CATS BY ANGRY PRINTING APPRENTICES WHO PUT THEIR VICTIMS ON TRIAL FOR WITCHCRAFT...

...AND ON TO SIXTEENTH-CENTURY ITALY, WHERE THE INQUISITION BURNED A SELF-EDUCATED MILLER NAMED MENOCCHIO FOR READING BANNED BOOKS AND PROMOTING A THEOLOGY THAT EXPLAINED GOD'S CREATIONS WITH THE METAPHOR OF MAGGOTS LIVING IN ROTTING CHEESE.

FINALLY, MY MIND CAME TO REST FAR BELOW THE STREETS OF PARIS WHERE NOVELISTS LIKE VICTOR HUGO, URBAN PLANNERS LIKE BARON GEORGES-EUGÈNE HAUSSMANN, AND THE GENERATIONS OF WORKING MEN WHO CLEANED THE CITY'S FILTHY PIPES ALL SAW A GREAT SYMBOL OF MODERNITY IN THE CITY OF LIGHT'S SEWER SYSTEM.

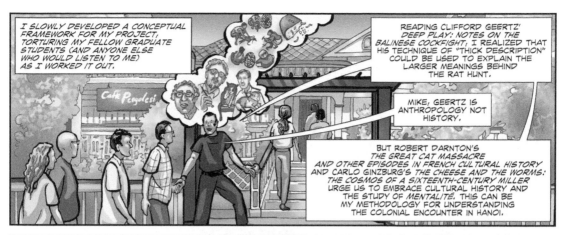

I SLOWLY DEVELOPED A CONCEPTUAL FRAMEWORK FOR MY PROJECT, TORTURING MY FELLOW GRADUATE STUDENTS (AND ANYONE ELSE WHO WOULD LISTEN TO ME) AS I WORKED IT OUT.

READING CLIFFORD GEERTZ' *DEEP PLAY: NOTES ON THE BALINESE COCKFIGHT*, I REALIZED THAT HIS TECHNIQUE OF "THICK DESCRIPTION" COULD BE USED TO EXPLAIN THE LARGER MEANINGS BEHIND THE RAT HUNT.

MIKE, GEERTZ IS ANTHROPOLOGY NOT HISTORY.

BUT ROBERT DARNTON'S *THE GREAT CAT MASSACRE AND OTHER EPISODES IN FRENCH CULTURAL HISTORY* AND CARLO GINZBURG'S *THE CHEESE AND THE WORMS: THE COSMOS OF A SIXTEENTH-CENTURY MILLER* URGE US TO EMBRACE CULTURAL HISTORY AND THE STUDY OF *MENTALITÉ*. THIS CAN BE MY METHODOLOGY FOR UNDERSTANDING THE COLONIAL ENCOUNTER IN HANOI.

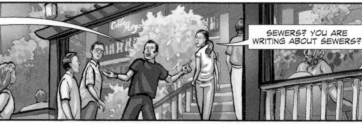

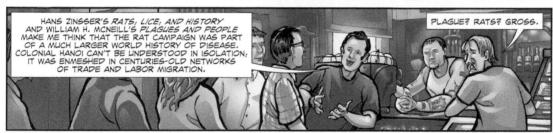

AND GET THIS, DONALD REID'S *PARIS SEWERS AND SEWERMEN: REALITIES AND REPRESENTATIONS* AND ALAIN CORBIN'S *THE FOUL AND THE FRAGRANT: ODOR AND THE FRENCH SOCIAL IMAGINATION* DEMONSTRATE THE IMPORTANCE OF THE FEAR OF FILTH IN THE FRENCH CONSTRUCTION OF MODERNITY.

SEWERS? YOU ARE WRITING ABOUT SEWERS?

HANS ZINSSER'S *RATS, LICE, AND HISTORY* AND WILLIAM H. MCNEILL'S *PLAGUES AND PEOPLE* MAKE ME THINK THAT THE RAT CAMPAIGN WAS PART OF A MUCH LARGER WORLD HISTORY OF DISEASE. COLONIAL HANOI CAN'T BE UNDERSTOOD IN ISOLATION; IT WAS ENMESHED IN CENTURIES-OLD NETWORKS OF TRADE AND LABOR MIGRATION.

PLAGUE? RATS? GROSS.

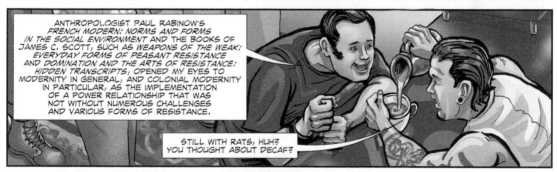

ANTHROPOLOGIST PAUL RABINOW'S *FRENCH MODERN: NORMS AND FORMS IN THE SOCIAL ENVIRONMENT* AND THE BOOKS OF JAMES C. SCOTT, SUCH AS *WEAPONS OF THE WEAK: EVERYDAY FORMS OF PEASANT RESISTANCE* AND *DOMINATION AND THE ARTS OF RESISTANCE: HIDDEN TRANSCRIPTS*, OPENED MY EYES TO MODERNITY IN GENERAL, AND COLONIAL MODERNITY IN PARTICULAR, AS THE IMPLEMENTATION OF A POWER RELATIONSHIP THAT WAS NOT WITHOUT NUMEROUS CHALLENGES AND VARIOUS FORMS OF RESISTANCE.

STILL WITH RATS, HUH? YOU THOUGHT ABOUT DECAF?

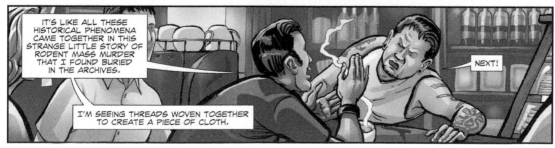

IT'S LIKE ALL THESE HISTORICAL PHENOMENA CAME TOGETHER IN THIS STRANGE LITTLE STORY OF RODENT MASS MURDER THAT I FOUND BURIED IN THE ARCHIVES.

NEXT!

I'M SEEING THREADS WOVEN TOGETHER TO CREATE A PIECE OF CLOTH.

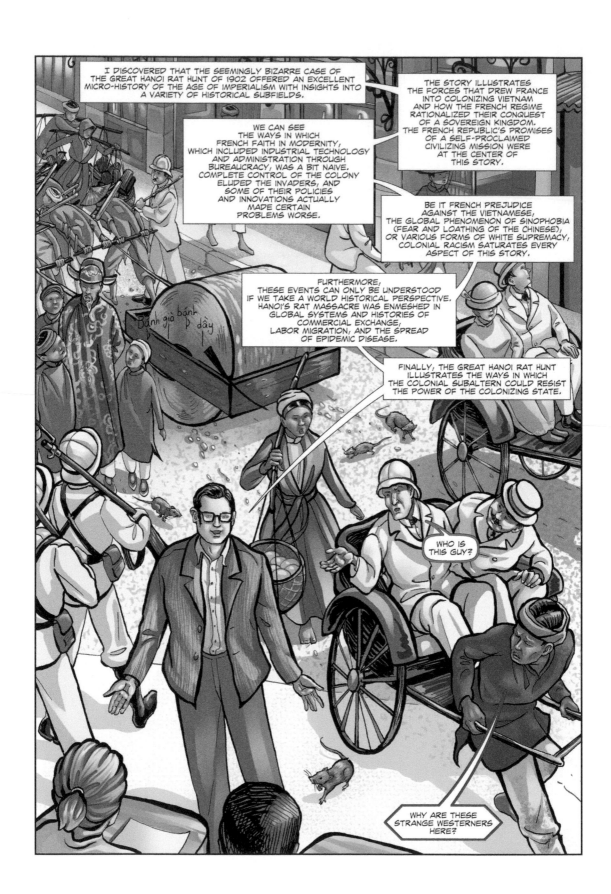

CHAPTER 1
A TAIL OF TWO CITIES

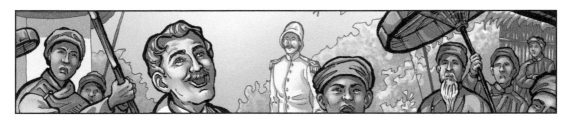

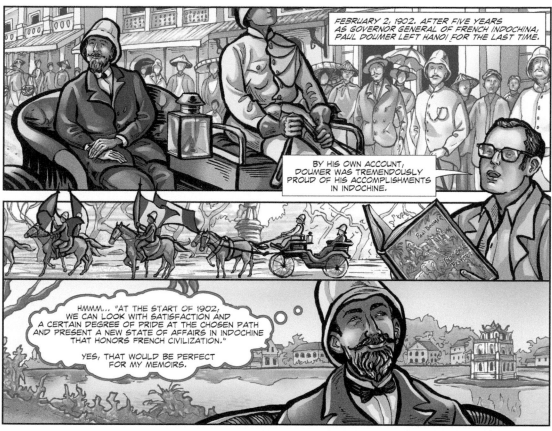

FEBRUARY 2, 1902. AFTER FIVE YEARS AS GOVERNOR GENERAL OF FRENCH INDOCHINA, PAUL DOUMER LEFT HANOI FOR THE LAST TIME.

BY HIS OWN ACCOUNT, DOUMER WAS TREMENDOUSLY PROUD OF HIS ACCOMPLISHMENTS IN INDOCHINE.

HMMM... "AT THE START OF 1902, WE CAN LOOK WITH SATISFACTION AND A CERTAIN DEGREE OF PRIDE AT THE CHOSEN PATH AND PRESENT A NEW STATE OF AFFAIRS IN INDOCHINE THAT HONORS FRENCH CIVILIZATION."

YES, THAT WOULD BE PERFECT FOR MY MEMOIRS.

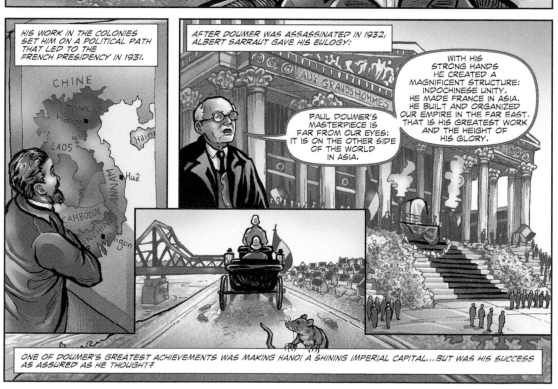

HIS WORK IN THE COLONIES SET HIM ON A POLITICAL PATH THAT LED TO THE FRENCH PRESIDENCY IN 1931.

CHINE
TONKIN
Hanoi
Hainan
LAOS
Huê
ANNAM
CAMBODGE
COCHINCHINE
Saigon

AFTER DOUMER WAS ASSASSINATED IN 1932, ALBERT SARRAUT GAVE HIS EULOGY:

PAUL DOUMER'S MASTERPIECE IS FAR FROM OUR EYES: IT IS ON THE OTHER SIDE OF THE WORLD IN ASIA.

WITH HIS STRONG HANDS HE CREATED A MAGNIFICENT STRUCTURE: INDOCHINESE UNITY. HE MADE FRANCE IN ASIA. HE BUILT AND ORGANIZED OUR EMPIRE IN THE FAR EAST. THAT IS HIS GREATEST WORK AND THE HEIGHT OF HIS GLORY.

AUX GRANDS HOMMES

ONE OF DOUMER'S GREATEST ACHIEVEMENTS WAS MAKING HANOI A SHINING IMPERIAL CAPITAL...BUT WAS HIS SUCCESS AS ASSURED AS HE THOUGHT?

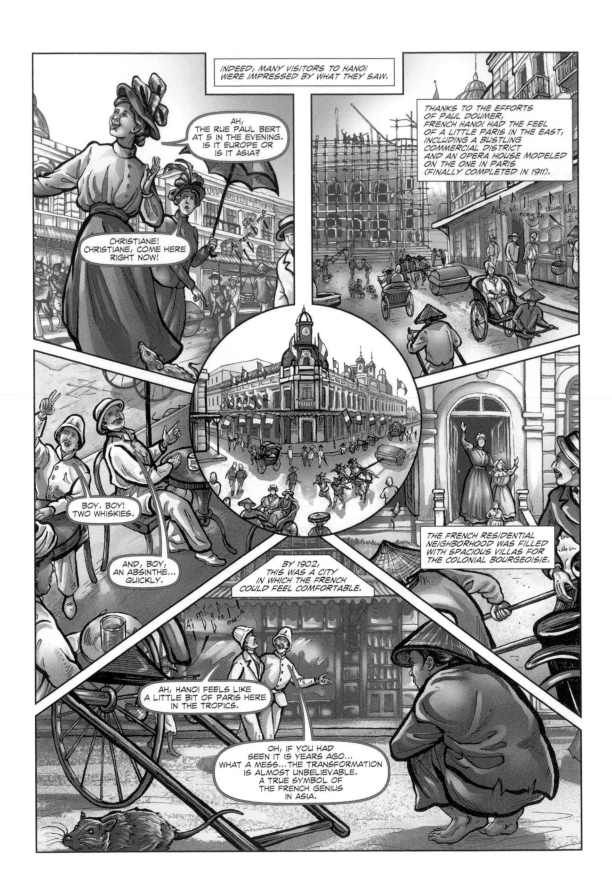

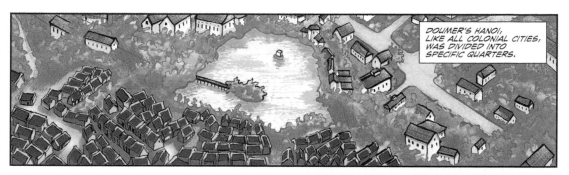

DOUMER'S HANOI, LIKE ALL COLONIAL CITIES, WAS DIVIDED INTO SPECIFIC QUARTERS.

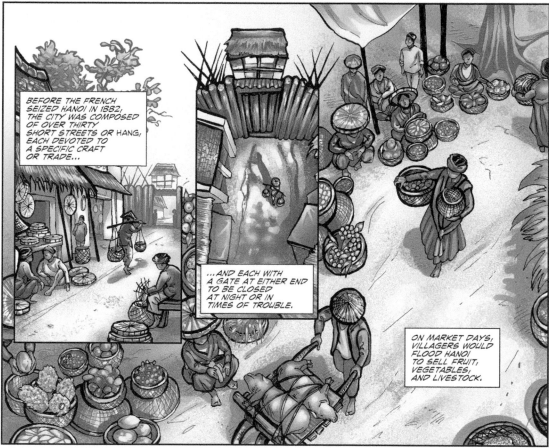

BEFORE THE FRENCH SEIZED HANOI IN 1882, THE CITY WAS COMPOSED OF OVER THIRTY SHORT STREETS OR HANG, EACH DEVOTED TO A SPECIFIC CRAFT OR TRADE...

...AND EACH WITH A GATE AT EITHER END TO BE CLOSED AT NIGHT OR IN TIMES OF TROUBLE.

ON MARKET DAYS, VILLAGERS WOULD FLOOD HANOI TO SELL FRUIT, VEGETABLES, AND LIVESTOCK.

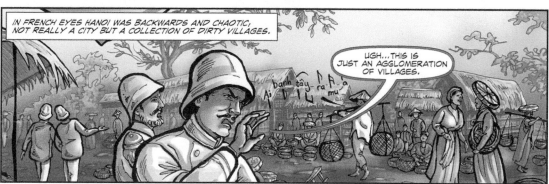

IN FRENCH EYES HANOI WAS BACKWARDS AND CHAOTIC, NOT REALLY A CITY BUT A COLLECTION OF DIRTY VILLAGES.

UGH...THIS IS JUST AN AGGLOMERATION OF VILLAGES.

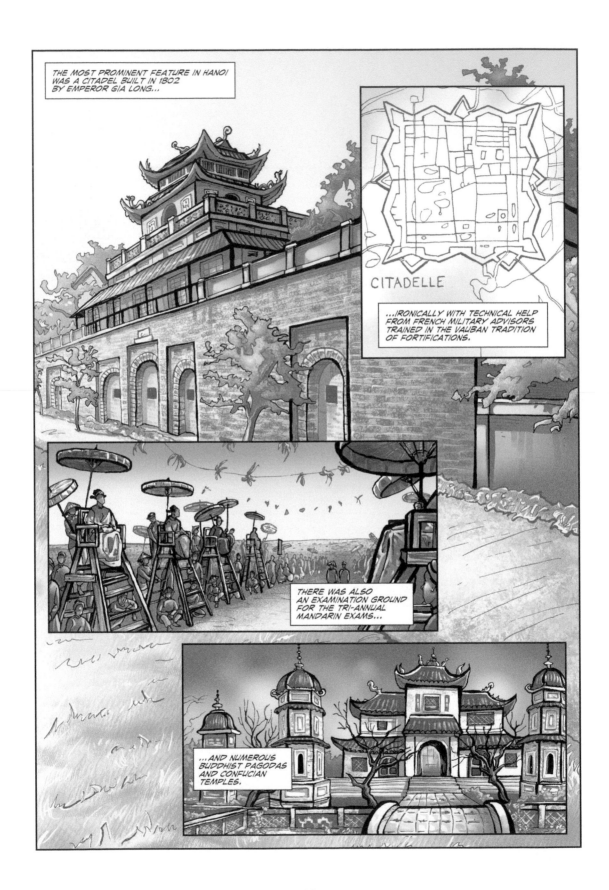

THE MOST PROMINENT FEATURE IN HANOI WAS A CITADEL BUILT IN 1802 BY EMPEROR GIA LONG...

CITADELLE

...IRONICALLY WITH TECHNICAL HELP FROM FRENCH MILITARY ADVISORS TRAINED IN THE VAUBAN TRADITION OF FORTIFICATIONS.

THERE WAS ALSO AN EXAMINATION GROUND FOR THE TRI-ANNUAL MANDARIN EXAMS...

...AND NUMEROUS BUDDHIST PAGODAS AND CONFUCIAN TEMPLES.

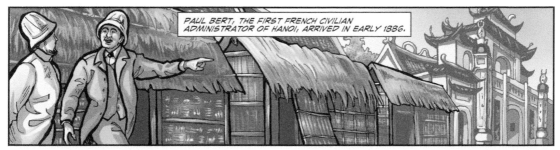

PAUL BERT, THE FIRST FRENCH CIVILIAN ADMINISTRATOR OF HANOI, ARRIVED IN EARLY 1886.

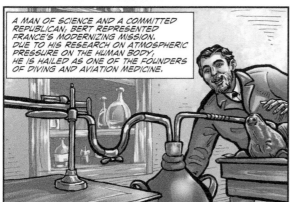

A MAN OF SCIENCE AND A COMMITTED REPUBLICAN, BERT REPRESENTED FRANCE'S MODERNIZING MISSION. DUE TO HIS RESEARCH ON ATMOSPHERIC PRESSURE ON THE HUMAN BODY, HE IS HAILED AS ONE OF THE FOUNDERS OF DIVING AND AVIATION MEDICINE.

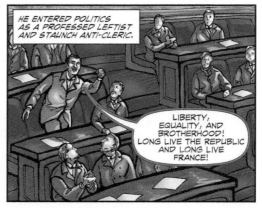

HE ENTERED POLITICS AS A PROFESSED LEFTIST AND STAUNCH ANTI-CLERIC.

LIBERTY, EQUALITY, AND BROTHERHOOD! LONG LIVE THE REPUBLIC AND LONG LIVE FRANCE!

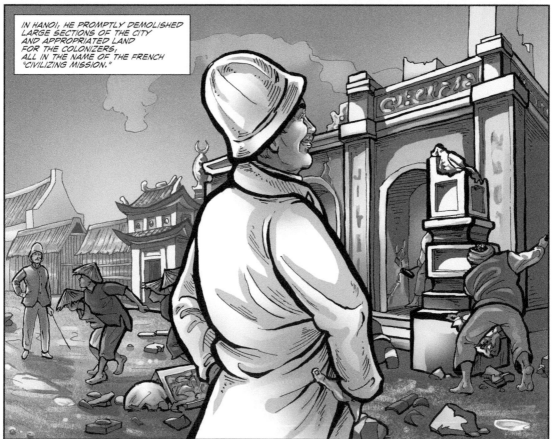

IN HANOI, HE PROMPTLY DEMOLISHED LARGE SECTIONS OF THE CITY AND APPROPRIATED LAND FOR THE COLONIZERS, ALL IN THE NAME OF THE FRENCH "CIVILIZING MISSION."

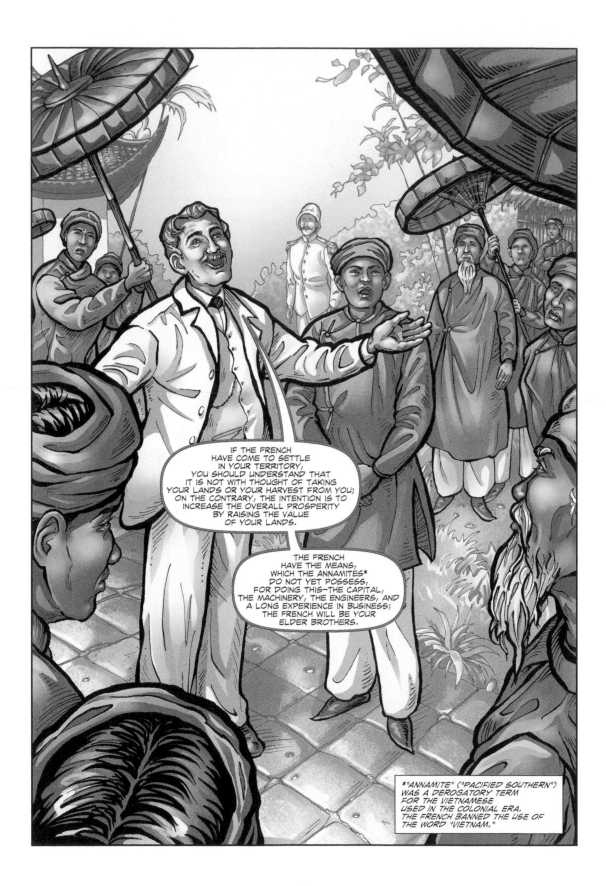

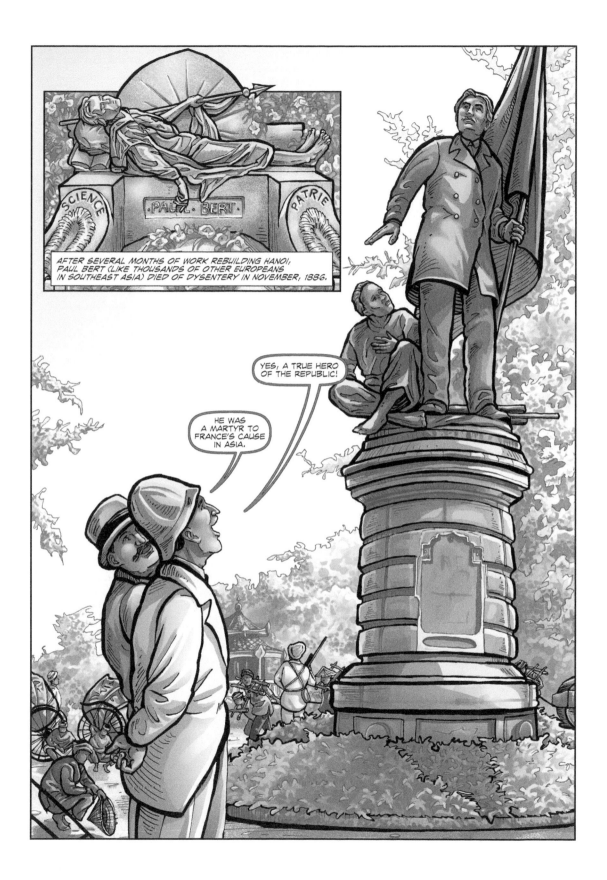

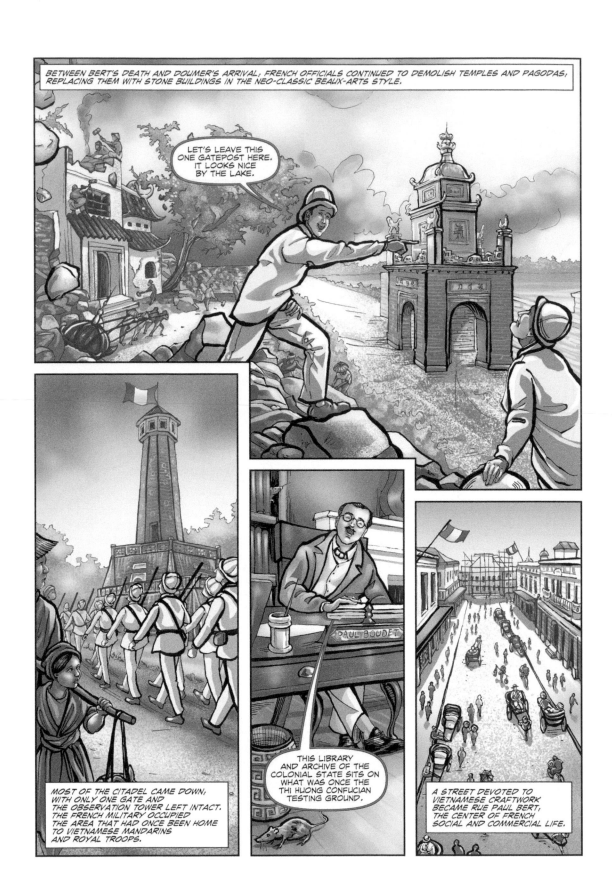

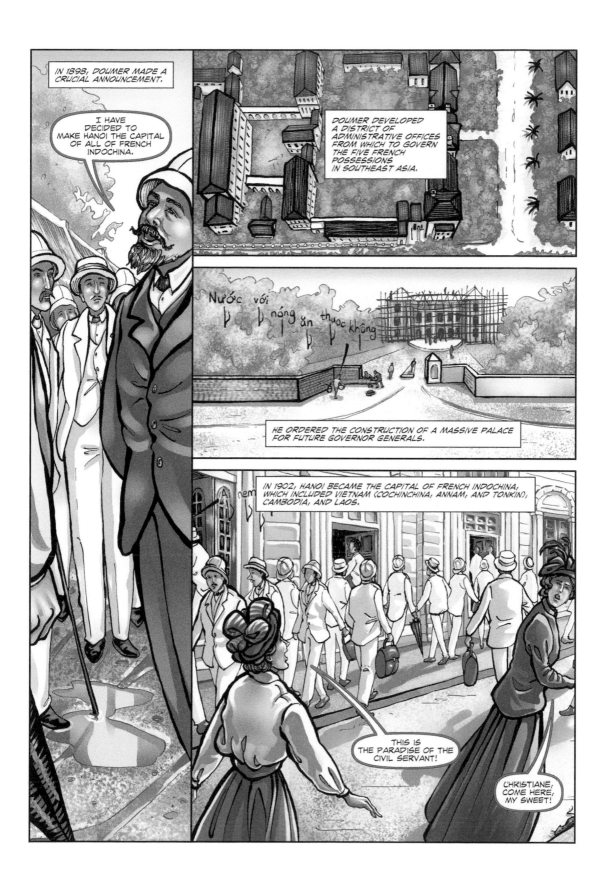

IN ADDITION TO THE IMPRESSIVE ARCHITECTURE, THE FRENCH DECORATED HANOI WITH A NUMBER OF STATUES AND MONUMENTS, CELEBRATING THEIR CONQUEST, CULTURE, AND VALUES.

AT THE CENTER OF THE CITY WAS HO HOAN KIEM, THE "LAKE OF THE RETURNED SWORD." ACCORDING TO LEGEND, A FISHERMAN DISCOVERED A MAGIC SWORD IN ITS WATERS WHICH INSPIRED HIM TO LIBERATE VIETNAM FROM THE CHINESE OCCUPATION AND BECOME THE KING LE LOI. AFTER HIS VICTORY, A MAGIC TURTLE TOOK THE SWORD FROM HIM AND DOVE BENEATH THE WATERS.

HOME TO SUCH A LEGEND, THE LAKE WAS A VERY SPECIAL PLACE IN THE VIETNAMESE NATIONALIST IMAGINATION. THE FRENCH, UNEASY WITH STORIES OF NATIONAL LIBERATION, CALL IT "LE PETIT LAC" (LITTLE LAKE).

THE DEATH OF CU RUA, A RARE HO HOAN KIEM TURTLE, IN 2016 WAS A NATIONAL EVENT.

IN THE 1890S, A FRENCH OFFICIAL WHO RECEIVED A SURPLUS COPY OF THE STATUE OF LIBERTY DECIDED TO PUT IT ON TOP OF THE TURTLE TOWER PAGODA IN THE LAKE.

SHE IS THE WIFE OF THAT OTHER STATUE, PAUL BERT, BUT SHE CHEATED ON HIM AND HE WAS ANGRY SO HE SENT HER HERE.

HOWEVER, WHEN THE WEIGHT OF THE STATUE CAUSED THE STRUCTURE TO LIST TO ONE SIDE, IT HAD TO BE MOVED TO A NEARBY PARK.

20

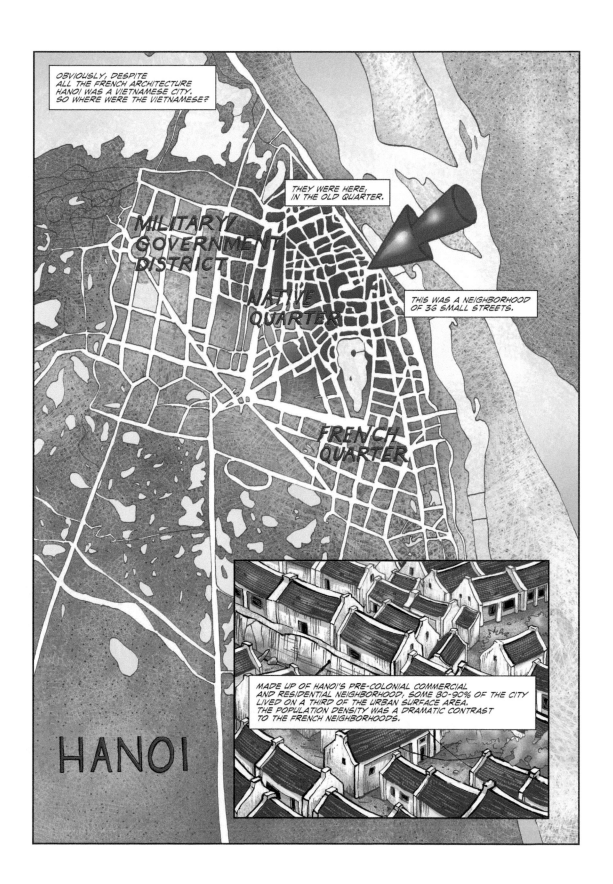

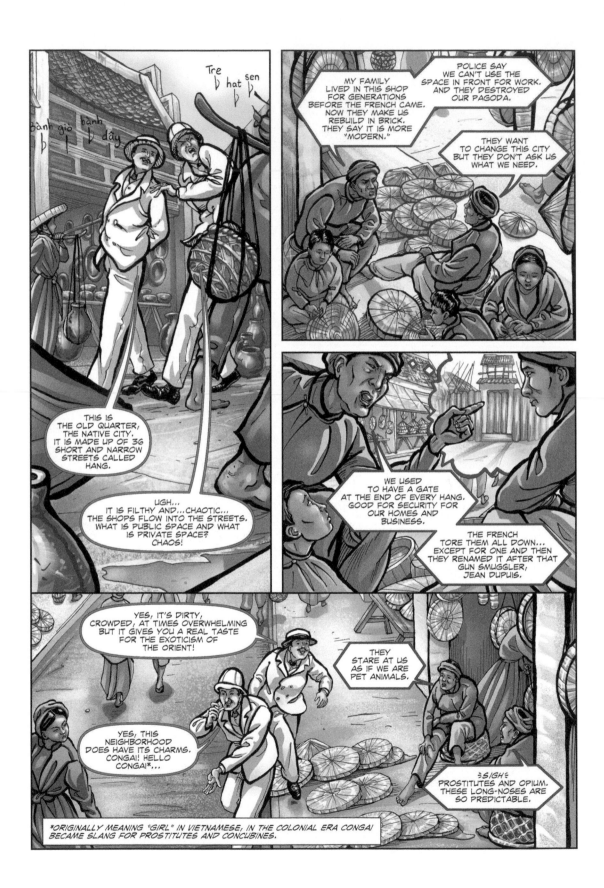

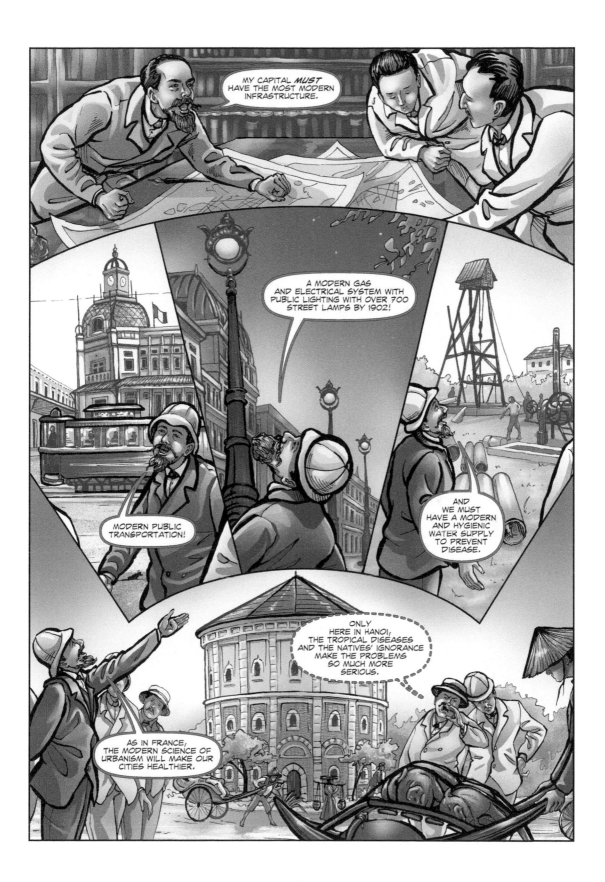

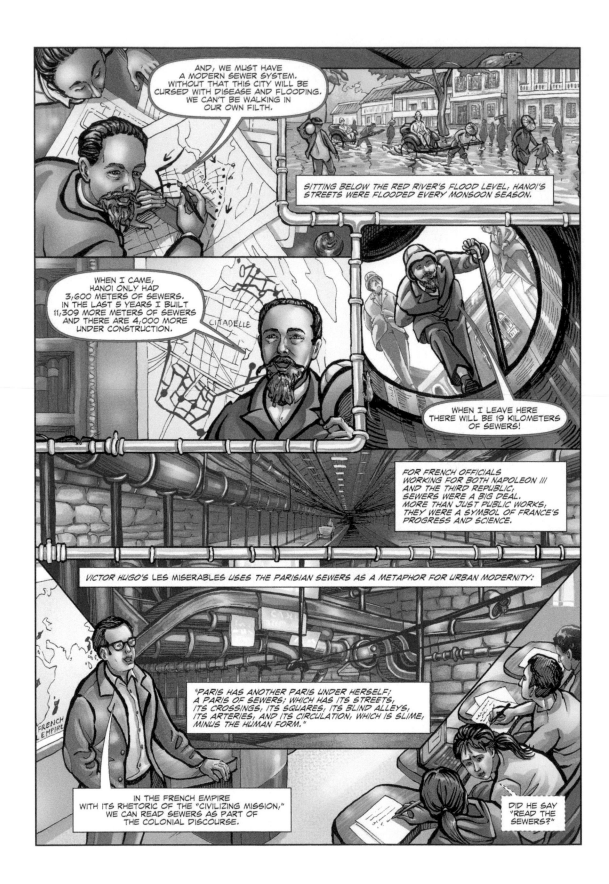

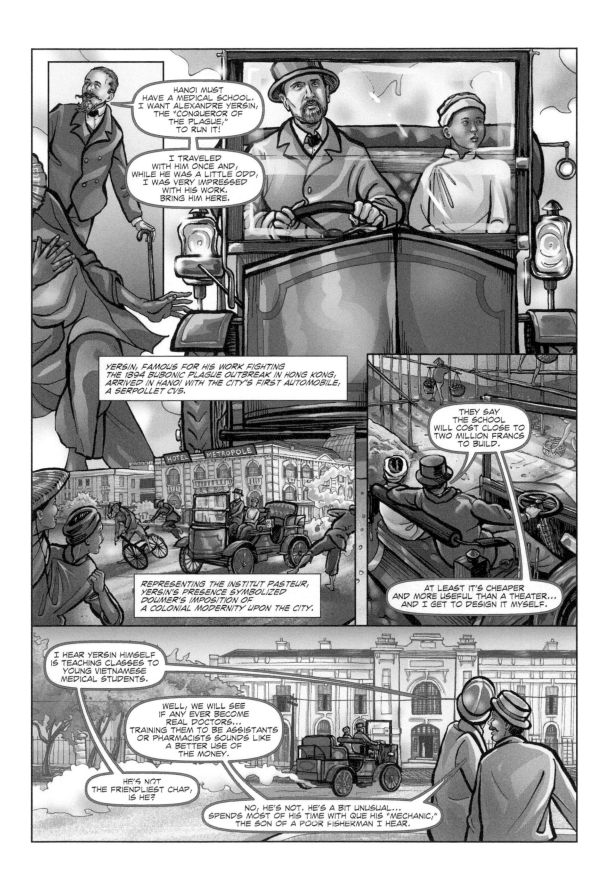

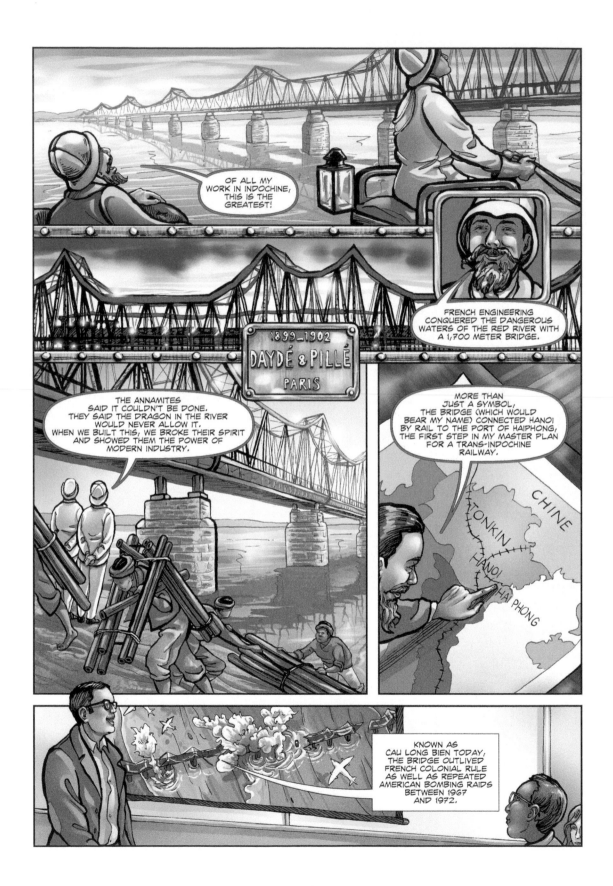

26

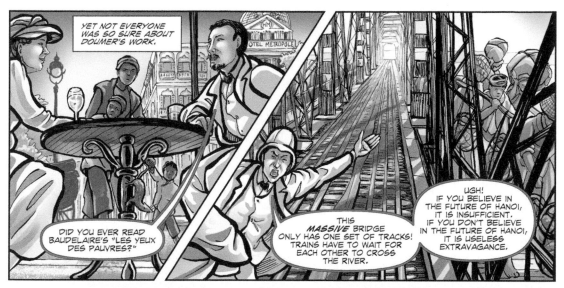

YET NOT EVERYONE WAS SO SURE ABOUT DOUMER'S WORK.

DID YOU EVER READ BAUDELAIRE'S "LES YEUX DES PAUVRES?"

THIS *MASSIVE* BRIDGE ONLY HAS ONE SET OF TRACKS! TRAINS HAVE TO WAIT FOR EACH OTHER TO CROSS THE RIVER.

UGH! IF YOU BELIEVE IN THE FUTURE OF HANOI, IT IS INSUFFICIENT. IF YOU DON'T BELIEVE IN THE FUTURE OF HANOI, IT IS USELESS EXTRAVAGANCE.

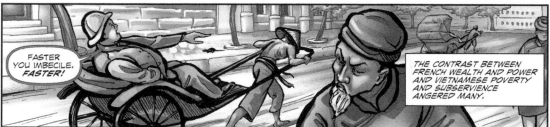

FASTER YOU IMBECILE, *FASTER!*

THE CONTRAST BETWEEN FRENCH WEALTH AND POWER AND VIETNAMESE POVERTY AND SUBSERVIENCE ANGERED MANY.

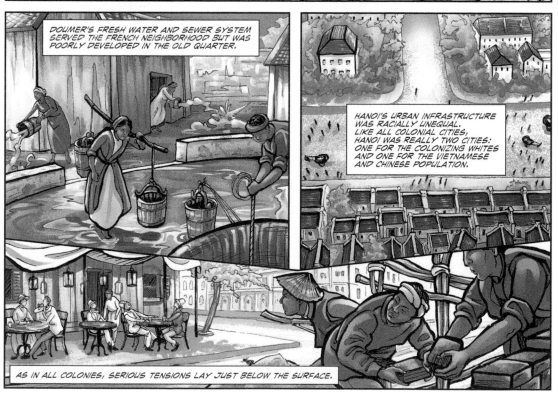

DOUMER'S FRESH WATER AND SEWER SYSTEM SERVED THE FRENCH NEIGHBORHOOD BUT WAS POORLY DEVELOPED IN THE OLD QUARTER.

HANOI'S URBAN INFRASTRUCTURE WAS RACIALLY UNEQUAL. LIKE ALL COLONIAL CITIES, HANOI WAS REALLY TWO CITIES: ONE FOR THE COLONIZING WHITES AND ONE FOR THE VIETNAMESE AND CHINESE POPULATION.

AS IN ALL COLONIES, SERIOUS TENSIONS LAY JUST BELOW THE SURFACE.

27

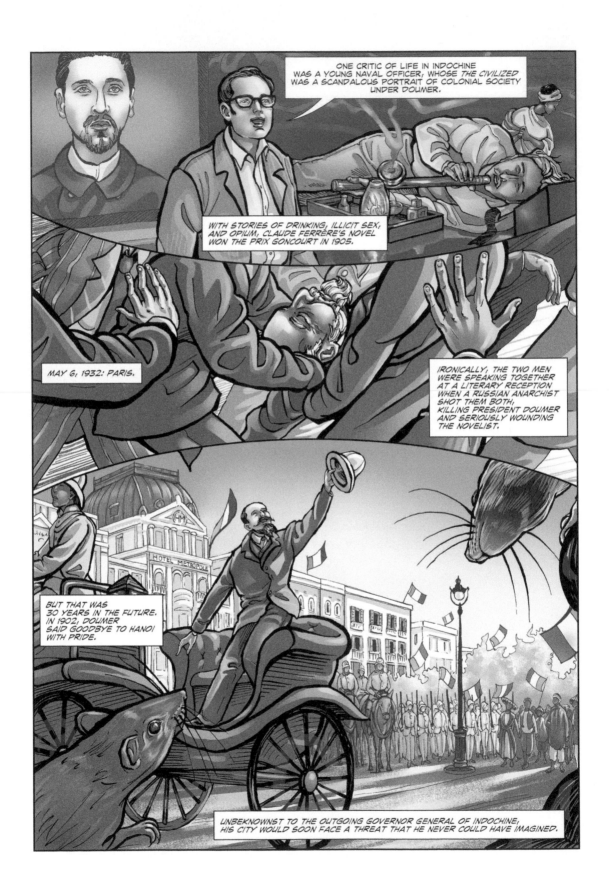

ONE CRITIC OF LIFE IN INDOCHINE WAS A YOUNG NAVAL OFFICER, WHOSE *THE CIVILIZED* WAS A SCANDALOUS PORTRAIT OF COLONIAL SOCIETY UNDER DOUMER.

WITH STORIES OF DRINKING, ILLICIT SEX, AND OPIUM, CLAUDE FERRÈRE'S NOVEL WON THE PRIX GONCOURT IN 1905.

MAY 6, 1932: PARIS.

IRONICALLY, THE TWO MEN WERE SPEAKING TOGETHER AT A LITERARY RECEPTION WHEN A RUSSIAN ANARCHIST SHOT THEM BOTH, KILLING PRESIDENT DOUMER AND SERIOUSLY WOUNDING THE NOVELIST.

BUT THAT WAS 30 YEARS IN THE FUTURE. IN 1902, DOUMER SAID GOODBYE TO HANOI WITH PRIDE.

UNBEKNOWNST TO THE OUTGOING GOVERNOR GENERAL OF INDOCHINE, HIS CITY WOULD SOON FACE A THREAT THAT HE NEVER COULD HAVE IMAGINED.

CHAPTER 2
WHY WAS HANOI FRENCH?

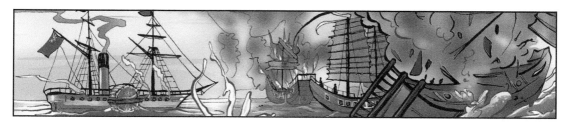

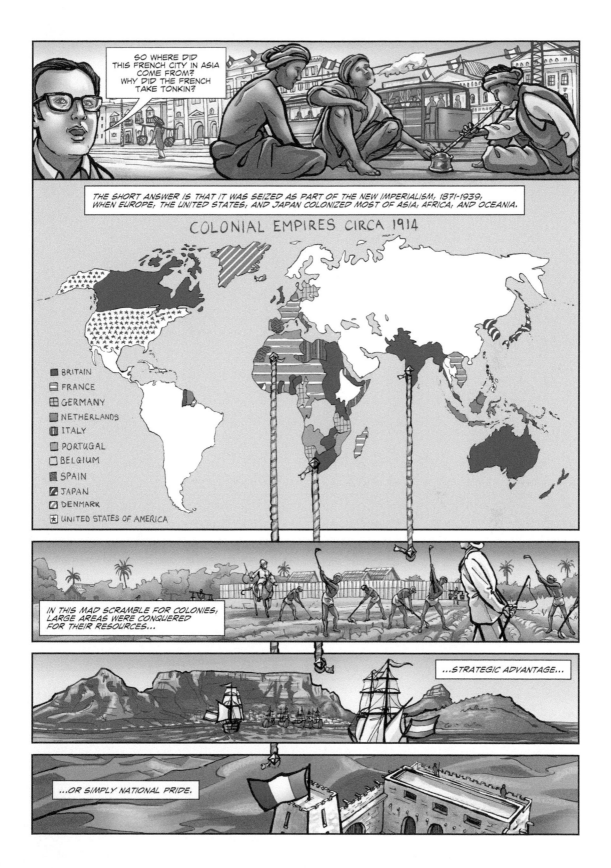

SO WHERE DID THIS FRENCH CITY IN ASIA COME FROM? WHY DID THE FRENCH TAKE TONKIN?

THE SHORT ANSWER IS THAT IT WAS SEIZED AS PART OF THE NEW IMPERIALISM, 1871-1939, WHEN EUROPE, THE UNITED STATES, AND JAPAN COLONIZED MOST OF ASIA, AFRICA, AND OCEANIA.

COLONIAL EMPIRES CIRCA 1914

BRITAIN
FRANCE
GERMANY
NETHERLANDS
ITALY
PORTUGAL
BELGIUM
SPAIN
JAPAN
DENMARK
UNITED STATES OF AMERICA

IN THIS MAD SCRAMBLE FOR COLONIES, LARGE AREAS WERE CONQUERED FOR THEIR RESOURCES...

...STRATEGIC ADVANTAGE...

...OR SIMPLY NATIONAL PRIDE.

31

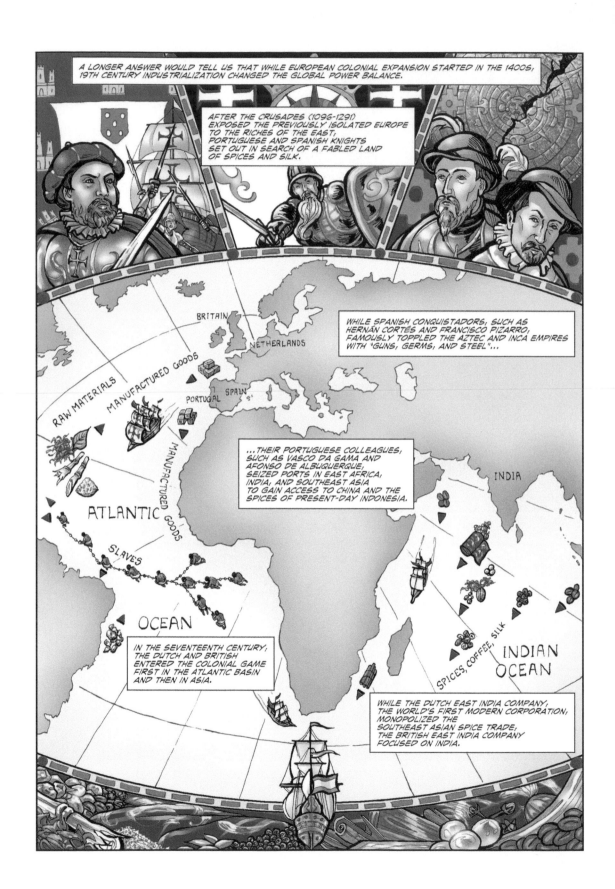

A LONGER ANSWER WOULD TELL US THAT WHILE EUROPEAN COLONIAL EXPANSION STARTED IN THE 1400S, 19TH CENTURY INDUSTRIALIZATION CHANGED THE GLOBAL POWER BALANCE.

AFTER THE CRUSADES (1096-1291) EXPOSED THE PREVIOUSLY ISOLATED EUROPE TO THE RICHES OF THE EAST, PORTUGUESE AND SPANISH KNIGHTS SET OUT IN SEARCH OF A FABLED LAND OF SPICES AND SILK.

WHILE SPANISH CONQUISTADORS, SUCH AS HERNÁN CORTÉS AND FRANCISCO PIZARRO, FAMOUSLY TOPPLED THE AZTEC AND INCA EMPIRES WITH "GUNS, GERMS, AND STEEL"...

...THEIR PORTUGUESE COLLEAGUES, SUCH AS VASCO DA GAMA AND AFONSO DE ALBUQUERQUE, SEIZED PORTS IN EAST AFRICA, INDIA, AND SOUTHEAST ASIA TO GAIN ACCESS TO CHINA AND THE SPICES OF PRESENT-DAY INDONESIA.

IN THE SEVENTEENTH CENTURY, THE DUTCH AND BRITISH ENTERED THE COLONIAL GAME FIRST IN THE ATLANTIC BASIN AND THEN IN ASIA.

WHILE THE DUTCH EAST INDIA COMPANY, THE WORLD'S FIRST MODERN CORPORATION, MONOPOLIZED THE SOUTHEAST ASIAN SPICE TRADE, THE BRITISH EAST INDIA COMPANY FOCUSED ON INDIA.

BRITAIN

NETHERLANDS

PORTUGAL   SPAIN

INDIA

RAW MATERIALS

MANUFACTURED GOODS

MANUFACTURED GOODS

ATLANTIC

SLAVES

OCEAN

SPICES, COFFEE, SILK

INDIAN OCEAN

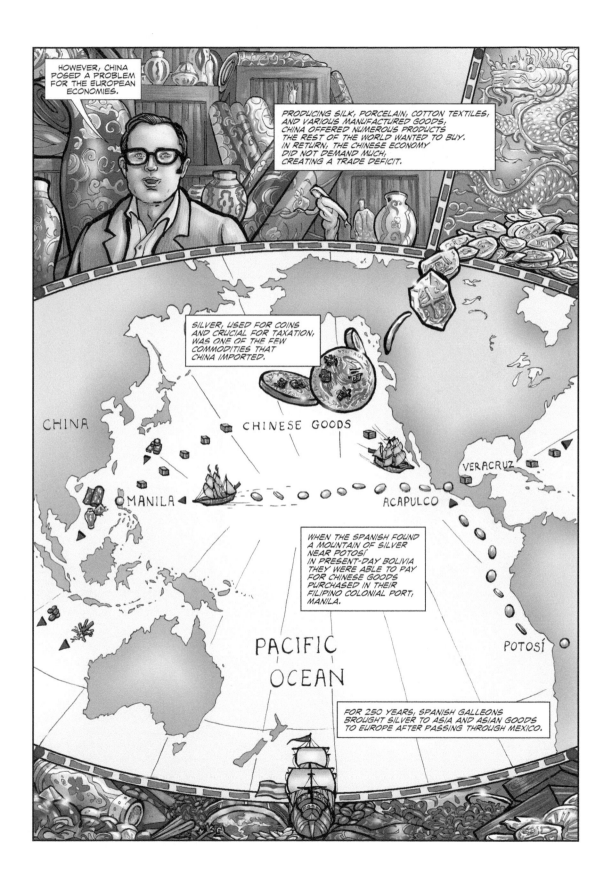

HOWEVER, CHINA POSED A PROBLEM FOR THE EUROPEAN ECONOMIES.

PRODUCING SILK, PORCELAIN, COTTON TEXTILES, AND VARIOUS MANUFACTURED GOODS, CHINA OFFERED NUMEROUS PRODUCTS THE REST OF THE WORLD WANTED TO BUY. IN RETURN, THE CHINESE ECONOMY DID NOT DEMAND MUCH, CREATING A TRADE DEFICIT.

SILVER, USED FOR COINS AND CRUCIAL FOR TAXATION, WAS ONE OF THE FEW COMMODITIES THAT CHINA IMPORTED.

CHINA

CHINESE GOODS

VERACRUZ

MANILA

ACAPULCO

WHEN THE SPANISH FOUND A MOUNTAIN OF SILVER NEAR POTOSÍ IN PRESENT-DAY BOLIVIA THEY WERE ABLE TO PAY FOR CHINESE GOODS PURCHASED IN THEIR FILIPINO COLONIAL PORT, MANILA.

PACIFIC OCEAN

POTOSÍ

FOR 250 YEARS, SPANISH GALLEONS BROUGHT SILVER TO ASIA AND ASIAN GOODS TO EUROPE AFTER PASSING THROUGH MEXICO.

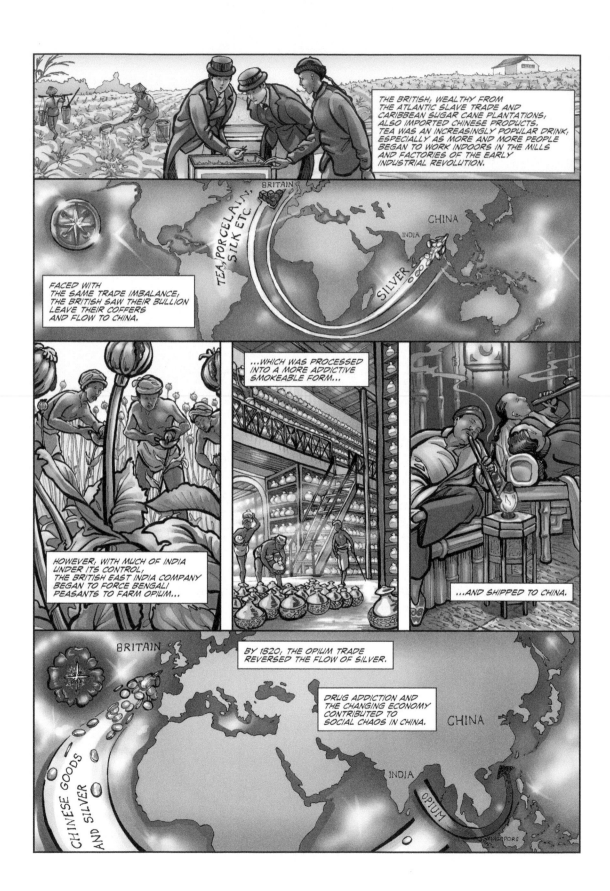

THE BRITISH, WEALTHY FROM THE ATLANTIC SLAVE TRADE AND CARIBBEAN SUGAR CANE PLANTATIONS, ALSO IMPORTED CHINESE PRODUCTS. TEA WAS AN INCREASINGLY POPULAR DRINK, ESPECIALLY AS MORE AND MORE PEOPLE BEGAN TO WORK INDOORS IN THE MILLS AND FACTORIES OF THE EARLY INDUSTRIAL REVOLUTION.

FACED WITH THE SAME TRADE IMBALANCE, THE BRITISH SAW THEIR BULLION LEAVE THEIR COFFERS AND FLOW TO CHINA.

...WHICH WAS PROCESSED INTO A MORE ADDICTIVE SMOKEABLE FORM...

HOWEVER, WITH MUCH OF INDIA UNDER ITS CONTROL, THE BRITISH EAST INDIA COMPANY BEGAN TO FORCE BENGALI PEASANTS TO FARM OPIUM...

...AND SHIPPED TO CHINA.

BY 1820, THE OPIUM TRADE REVERSED THE FLOW OF SILVER.

DRUG ADDICTION AND THE CHANGING ECONOMY CONTRIBUTED TO SOCIAL CHAOS IN CHINA.

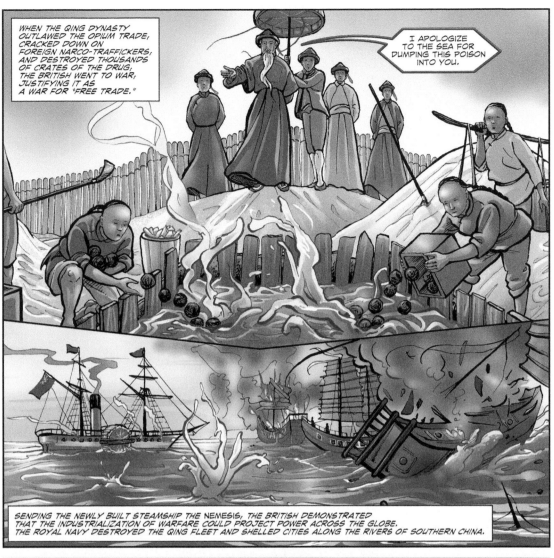

WHEN THE QING DYNASTY OUTLAWED THE OPIUM TRADE, CRACKED DOWN ON FOREIGN NARCO-TRAFFICKERS, AND DESTROYED THOUSANDS OF CRATES OF THE DRUG, THE BRITISH WENT TO WAR, JUSTIFYING IT AS A WAR FOR "FREE TRADE."

I APOLOGIZE TO THE SEA FOR DUMPING THIS POISON INTO YOU.

SENDING THE NEWLY BUILT STEAMSHIP THE NEMESIS, THE BRITISH DEMONSTRATED THAT THE INDUSTRIALIZATION OF WARFARE COULD PROJECT POWER ACROSS THE GLOBE. THE ROYAL NAVY DESTROYED THE QING FLEET AND SHELLED CITIES ALONG THE RIVERS OF SOUTHERN CHINA.

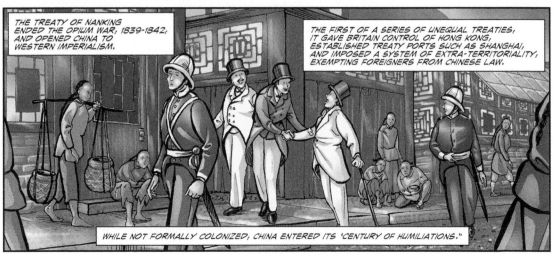

THE TREATY OF NANKING ENDED THE OPIUM WAR, 1839-1842, AND OPENED CHINA TO WESTERN IMPERIALISM.

THE FIRST OF A SERIES OF UNEQUAL TREATIES, IT GAVE BRITAIN CONTROL OF HONG KONG, ESTABLISHED TREATY PORTS SUCH AS SHANGHAI, AND IMPOSED A SYSTEM OF EXTRA-TERRITORIALITY, EXEMPTING FOREIGNERS FROM CHINESE LAW.

WHILE NOT FORMALLY COLONIZED, CHINA ENTERED ITS "CENTURY OF HUMILIATIONS."

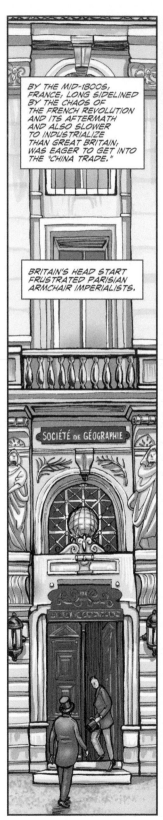

BY THE MID-1800S, FRANCE, LONG SIDELINED BY THE CHAOS OF THE FRENCH REVOLUTION AND ITS AFTERMATH AND ALSO SLOWER TO INDUSTRIALIZE THAN GREAT BRITAIN, WAS EAGER TO GET INTO THE "CHINA TRADE."

BRITAIN'S HEAD START FRUSTRATED PARISIAN ARMCHAIR IMPERIALISTS.

SOCIÉTÉ DE GÉOGRAPHIE

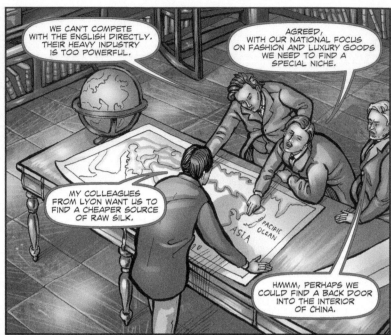

WE CAN'T COMPETE WITH THE ENGLISH DIRECTLY. THEIR HEAVY INDUSTRY IS TOO POWERFUL.

AGREED, WITH OUR NATIONAL FOCUS ON FASHION AND LUXURY GOODS WE NEED TO FIND A SPECIAL NICHE.

MY COLLEAGUES FROM LYON WANT US TO FIND A CHEAPER SOURCE OF RAW SILK.

HMMM, PERHAPS WE COULD FIND A BACK DOOR INTO THE INTERIOR OF CHINA.

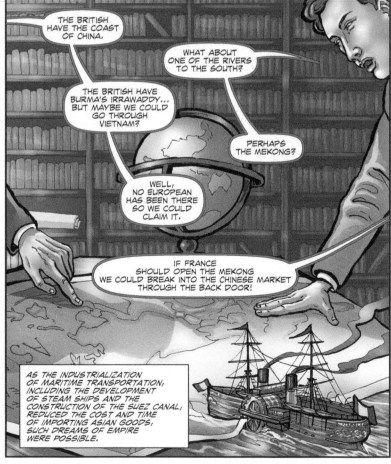

THE BRITISH HAVE THE COAST OF CHINA.

WHAT ABOUT ONE OF THE RIVERS TO THE SOUTH?

THE BRITISH HAVE BURMA'S IRRAWADDY... BUT MAYBE WE COULD GO THROUGH VIETNAM?

PERHAPS THE MEKONG?

WELL, NO EUROPEAN HAS BEEN THERE SO WE COULD CLAIM IT.

IF FRANCE SHOULD OPEN THE MEKONG WE COULD BREAK INTO THE CHINESE MARKET THROUGH THE BACK DOOR!

AS THE INDUSTRIALIZATION OF MARITIME TRANSPORTATION, INCLUDING THE DEVELOPMENT OF STEAM SHIPS AND THE CONSTRUCTION OF THE SUEZ CANAL, REDUCED THE COST AND TIME OF IMPORTING ASIAN GOODS, SUCH DREAMS OF EMPIRE WERE POSSIBLE.

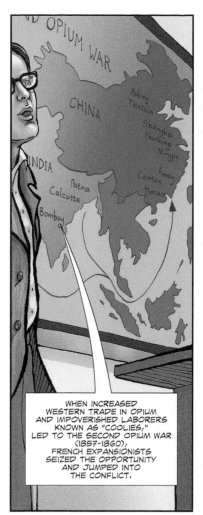

WHEN INCREASED
WESTERN TRADE IN OPIUM
AND IMPOVERISHED LABORERS
KNOWN AS "COOLIES,"
LED TO THE SECOND OPIUM WAR
(1857-1860),
FRENCH EXPANSIONISTS
SEIZED THE OPPORTUNITY
AND JUMPED INTO
THE CONFLICT.

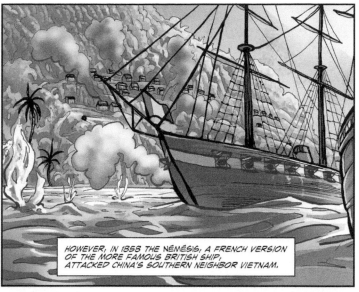

HOWEVER, IN 1858 THE NÉMÉSIS, A FRENCH VERSION
OF THE MORE FAMOUS BRITISH SHIP,
ATTACKED CHINA'S SOUTHERN NEIGHBOR VIETNAM.

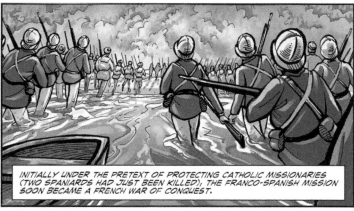

INITIALLY UNDER THE PRETEXT OF PROTECTING CATHOLIC MISSIONARIES
(TWO SPANIARDS HAD JUST BEEN KILLED), THE FRANCO-SPANISH MISSION
SOON BECAME A FRENCH WAR OF CONQUEST.

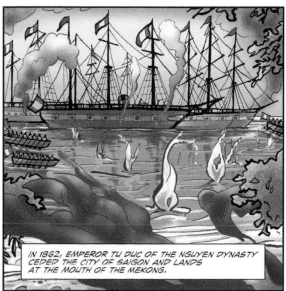

IN 1862, EMPEROR TU DUC OF THE NGUYEN DYNASTY
CEDED THE CITY OF SAIGON AND LANDS
AT THE MOUTH OF THE MEKONG.

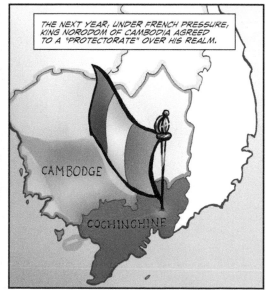

THE NEXT YEAR, UNDER FRENCH PRESSURE,
KING NORODOM OF CAMBODIA AGREED
TO A "PROTECTORATE" OVER HIS REALM.

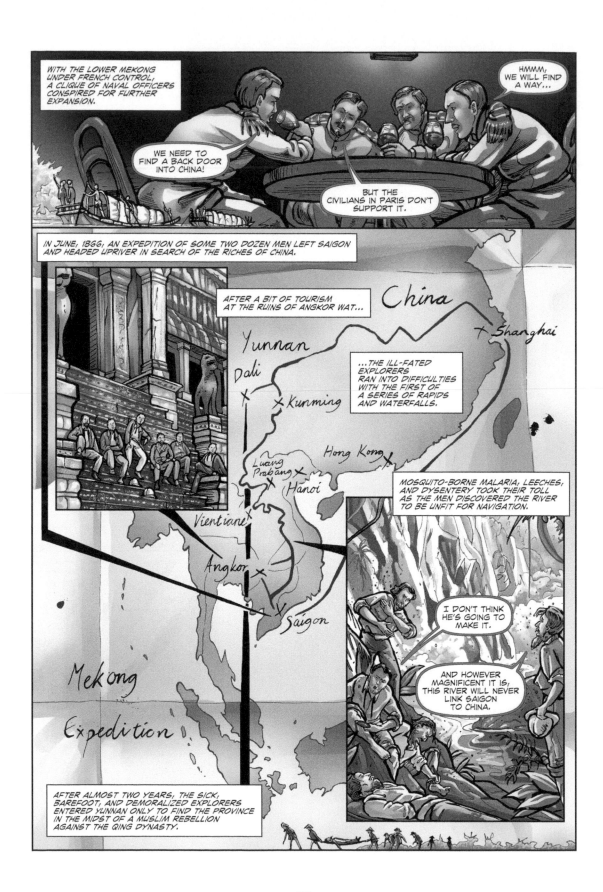

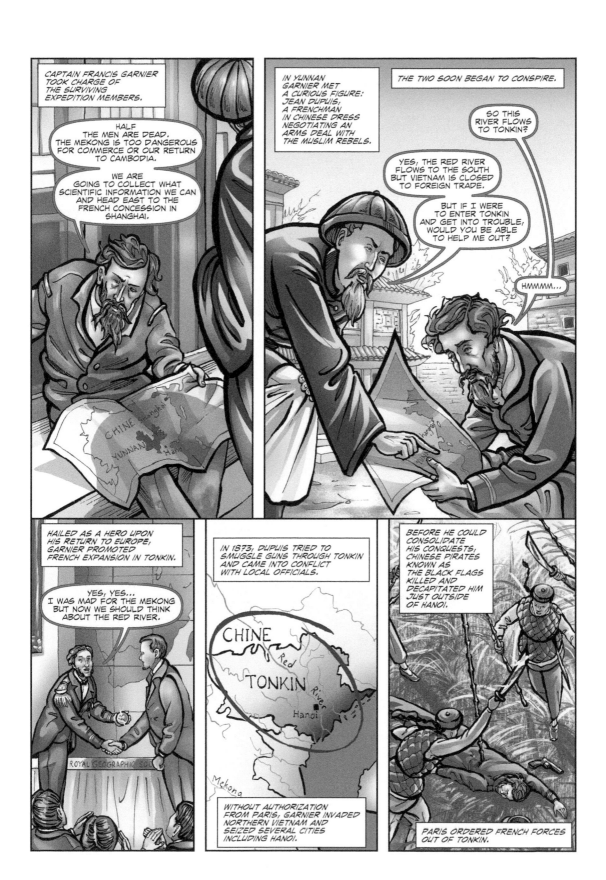

CAPTAIN FRANCIS GARNIER TOOK CHARGE OF THE SURVIVING EXPEDITION MEMBERS.

HALF THE MEN ARE DEAD. THE MEKONG IS TOO DANGEROUS FOR COMMERCE OR OUR RETURN TO CAMBODIA.

WE ARE GOING TO COLLECT WHAT SCIENTIFIC INFORMATION WE CAN AND HEAD EAST TO THE FRENCH CONCESSION IN SHANGHAI.

IN YUNNAN GARNIER MET A CURIOUS FIGURE: JEAN DUPUIS, A FRENCHMAN IN CHINESE DRESS NEGOTIATING AN ARMS DEAL WITH THE MUSLIM REBELS.

THE TWO SOON BEGAN TO CONSPIRE.

SO THIS RIVER FLOWS TO TONKIN?

YES, THE RED RIVER FLOWS TO THE SOUTH BUT VIETNAM IS CLOSED TO FOREIGN TRADE.

BUT IF I WERE TO ENTER TONKIN AND GET INTO TROUBLE, WOULD YOU BE ABLE TO HELP ME OUT?

HMMMM...

HAILED AS A HERO UPON HIS RETURN TO EUROPE, GARNIER PROMOTED FRENCH EXPANSION IN TONKIN.

YES, YES... I WAS MAD FOR THE MEKONG BUT NOW WE SHOULD THINK ABOUT THE RED RIVER.

ROYAL GEOGRAPHIC SOC.

IN 1873, DUPUIS TRIED TO SMUGGLE GUNS THROUGH TONKIN AND CAME INTO CONFLICT WITH LOCAL OFFICIALS.

CHINE

TONKIN

Red River

Hanoi

Mekong

WITHOUT AUTHORIZATION FROM PARIS, GARNIER INVADED NORTHERN VIETNAM AND SEIZED SEVERAL CITIES INCLUDING HANOI.

BEFORE HE COULD CONSOLIDATE HIS CONQUESTS, CHINESE PIRATES KNOWN AS THE BLACK FLAGS KILLED AND DECAPITATED HIM JUST OUTSIDE OF HANOI.

PARIS ORDERED FRENCH FORCES OUT OF TONKIN.

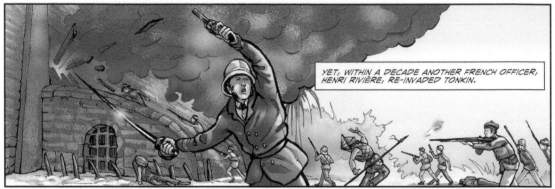

YET, WITHIN A DECADE ANOTHER FRENCH OFFICER, HENRI RIVIÈRE, RE-INVADED TONKIN.

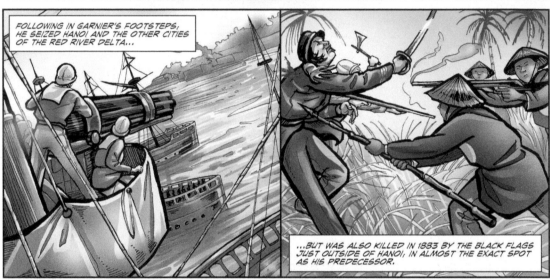

FOLLOWING IN GARNIER'S FOOTSTEPS, HE SEIZED HANOI AND THE OTHER CITIES OF THE RED RIVER DELTA...

...BUT WAS ALSO KILLED IN 1883 BY THE BLACK FLAGS JUST OUTSIDE OF HANOI, IN ALMOST THE EXACT SPOT AS HIS PREDECESSOR.

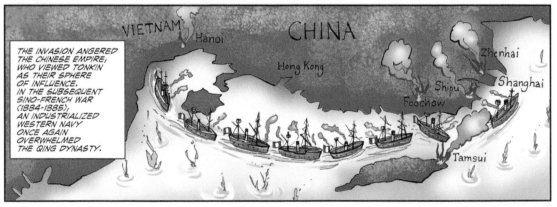

THE INVASION ANGERED THE CHINESE EMPIRE, WHO VIEWED TONKIN AS THEIR SPHERE OF INFLUENCE. IN THE SUBSEQUENT SINO-FRENCH WAR (1884-1885), AN INDUSTRIALIZED WESTERN NAVY ONCE AGAIN OVERWHELMED THE QING DYNASTY.

VIETNAM
Hanoi
CHINA
Hong Kong
Zhenhai
Shanghai
Shipu
Foochow
Tamsui

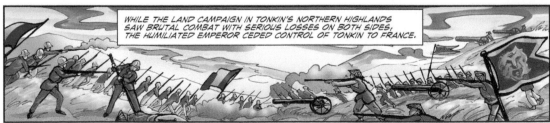

WHILE THE LAND CAMPAIGN IN TONKIN'S NORTHERN HIGHLANDS SAW BRUTAL COMBAT WITH SERIOUS LOSSES ON BOTH SIDES, THE HUMILIATED EMPEROR CEDED CONTROL OF TONKIN TO FRANCE.

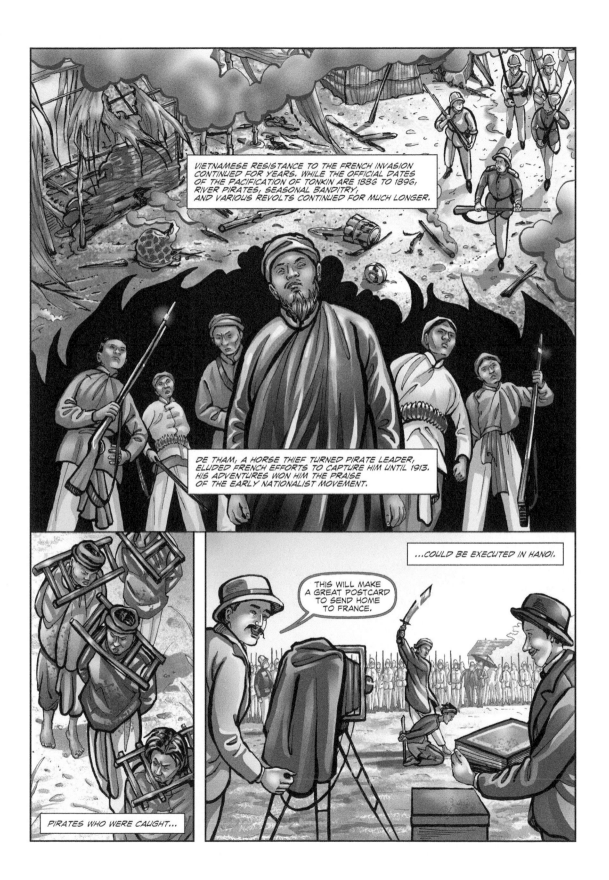

VIETNAMESE RESISTANCE TO THE FRENCH INVASION CONTINUED FOR YEARS. WHILE THE OFFICIAL DATES OF THE PACIFICATION OF TONKIN ARE 1886 TO 1896, RIVER PIRATES, SEASONAL BANDITRY, AND VARIOUS REVOLTS CONTINUED FOR MUCH LONGER.

DE THAM, A HORSE THIEF TURNED PIRATE LEADER, ELUDED FRENCH EFFORTS TO CAPTURE HIM UNTIL 1913. HIS ADVENTURES WON HIM THE PRAISE OF THE EARLY NATIONALIST MOVEMENT.

PIRATES WHO WERE CAUGHT...

...COULD BE EXECUTED IN HANOI.

THIS WILL MAKE A GREAT POSTCARD TO SEND HOME TO FRANCE.

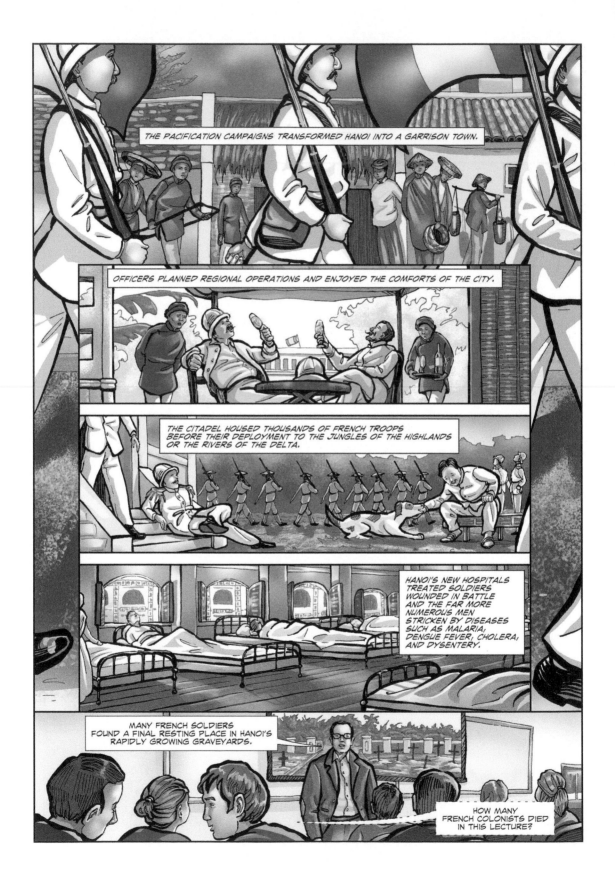

THE PACIFICATION CAMPAIGNS TRANSFORMED HANOI INTO A GARRISON TOWN.

OFFICERS PLANNED REGIONAL OPERATIONS AND ENJOYED THE COMFORTS OF THE CITY.

THE CITADEL HOUSED THOUSANDS OF FRENCH TROOPS BEFORE THEIR DEPLOYMENT TO THE JUNGLES OF THE HIGHLANDS OR THE RIVERS OF THE DELTA.

HANOI'S NEW HOSPITALS TREATED SOLDIERS WOUNDED IN BATTLE AND THE FAR MORE NUMEROUS MEN STRICKEN BY DISEASES SUCH AS MALARIA, DENGUE FEVER, CHOLERA, AND DYSENTERY.

MANY FRENCH SOLDIERS FOUND A FINAL RESTING PLACE IN HANOI'S RAPIDLY GROWING GRAVEYARDS.

HOW MANY FRENCH COLONISTS DIED IN THIS LECTURE?

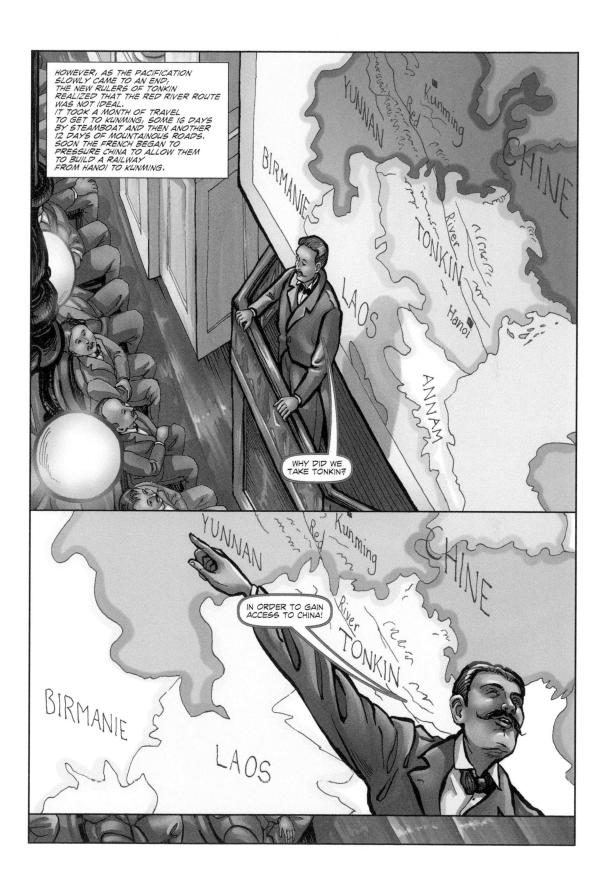

43

CHAPTER 3
WHO BUILT HANOI?

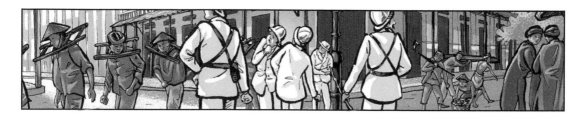

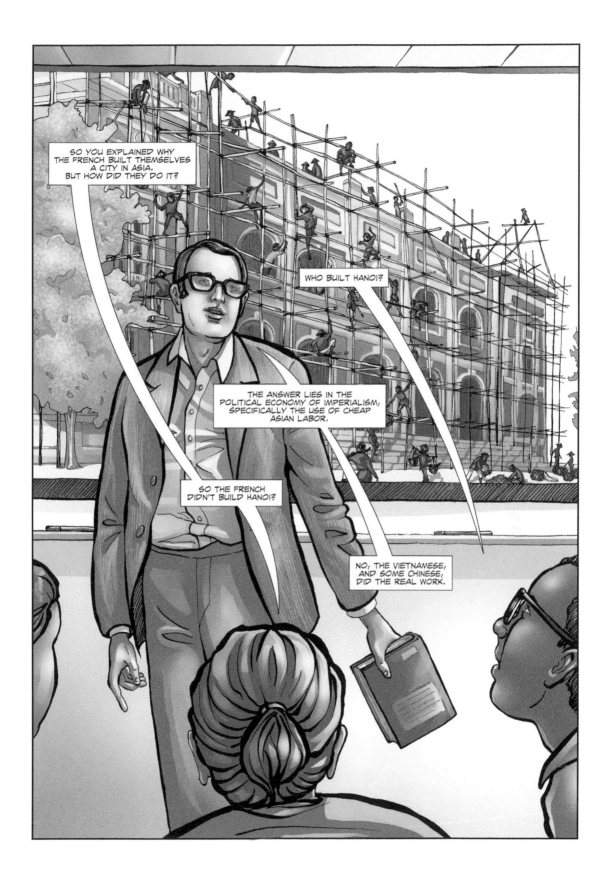

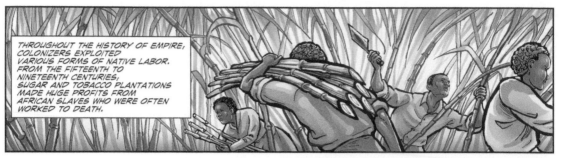

THROUGHOUT THE HISTORY OF EMPIRE, COLONIZERS EXPLOITED VARIOUS FORMS OF NATIVE LABOR. FROM THE FIFTEENTH TO NINETEENTH CENTURIES, SUGAR AND TOBACCO PLANTATIONS MADE HUGE PROFITS FROM AFRICAN SLAVES WHO WERE OFTEN WORKED TO DEATH.

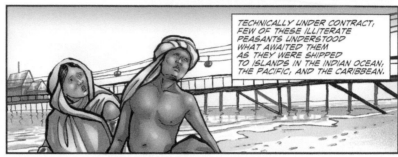

AFTER SLAVERY'S ABOLITION IN THE ATLANTIC, THE BRITISH AND THE FRENCH TURNED TO IMPOVERISHED INDIAN LABORERS KNOWN AS "COOLIES."

TECHNICALLY UNDER CONTRACT, FEW OF THESE ILLITERATE PEASANTS UNDERSTOOD WHAT AWAITED THEM AS THEY WERE SHIPPED TO ISLANDS IN THE INDIAN OCEAN, THE PACIFIC, AND THE CARIBBEAN.

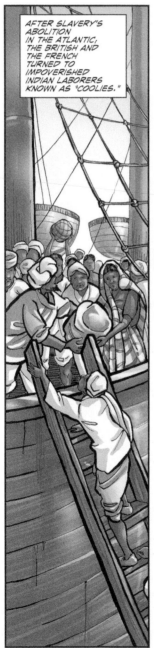

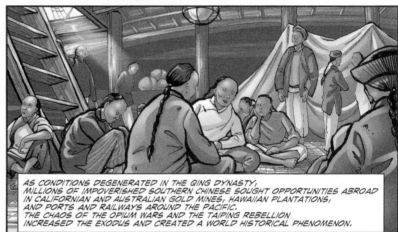

AS CONDITIONS DEGENERATED IN THE QING DYNASTY, MILLIONS OF IMPOVERISHED SOUTHERN CHINESE SOUGHT OPPORTUNITIES ABROAD IN CALIFORNIAN AND AUSTRALIAN GOLD MINES, HAWAIIAN PLANTATIONS, AND PORTS AND RAILWAYS AROUND THE PACIFIC. THE CHAOS OF THE OPIUM WARS AND THE TAIPING REBELLION INCREASED THE EXODUS AND CREATED A WORLD HISTORICAL PHENOMENON.

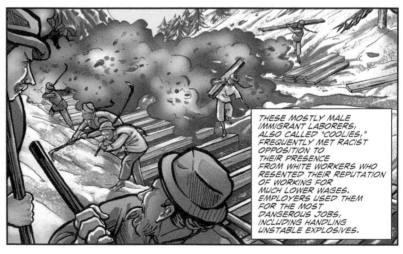

THESE MOSTLY MALE IMMIGRANT LABORERS, ALSO CALLED "COOLIES," FREQUENTLY MET RACIST OPPOSITION TO THEIR PRESENCE FROM WHITE WORKERS WHO RESENTED THEIR REPUTATION OF WORKING FOR MUCH LOWER WAGES. EMPLOYERS USED THEM FOR THE MOST DANGEROUS JOBS, INCLUDING HANDLING UNSTABLE EXPLOSIVES.

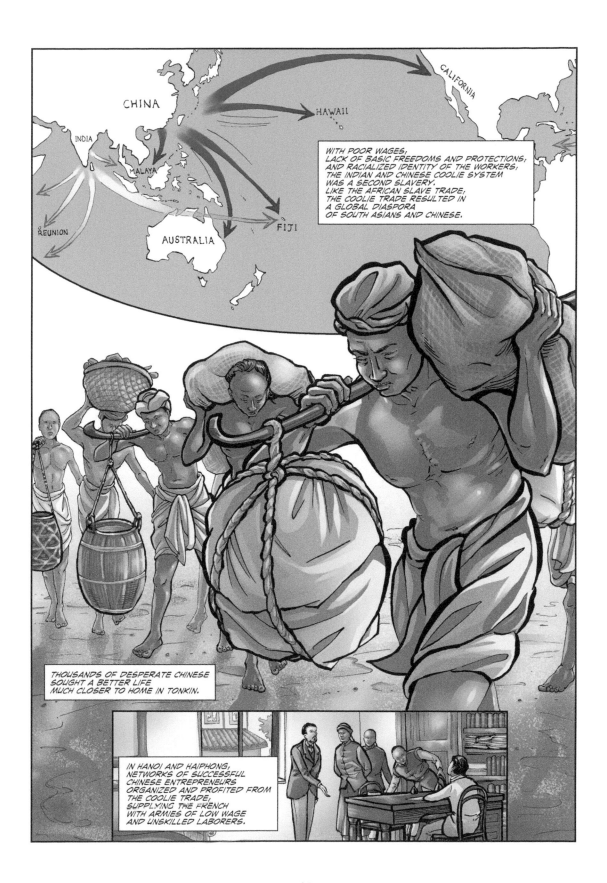

WITH POOR WAGES,
LACK OF BASIC FREEDOMS AND PROTECTIONS,
AND RACIALIZED IDENTITY OF THE WORKERS,
THE INDIAN AND CHINESE COOLIE SYSTEM
WAS A SECOND SLAVERY.
LIKE THE AFRICAN SLAVE TRADE,
THE COOLIE TRADE RESULTED IN
A GLOBAL DIASPORA
OF SOUTH ASIANS AND CHINESE.

THOUSANDS OF DESPERATE CHINESE
SOUGHT A BETTER LIFE
MUCH CLOSER TO HOME IN TONKIN.

IN HANOI AND HAIPHONG,
NETWORKS OF SUCCESSFUL
CHINESE ENTREPRENEURS
ORGANIZED AND PROFITED FROM
THE COOLIE TRADE,
SUPPLYING THE FRENCH
WITH ARMIES OF LOW WAGE
AND UNSKILLED LABORERS.

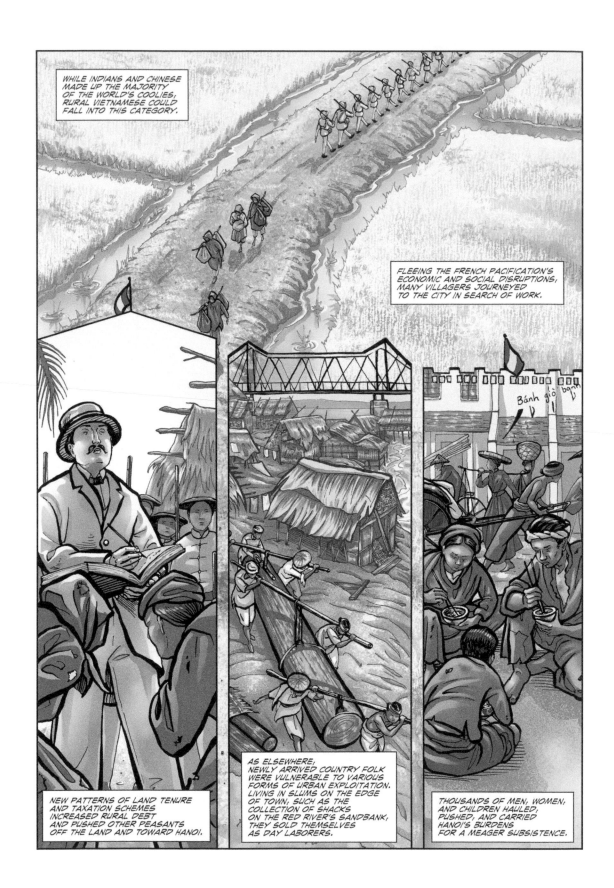

WHILE INDIANS AND CHINESE MADE UP THE MAJORITY OF THE WORLD'S COOLIES, RURAL VIETNAMESE COULD FALL INTO THIS CATEGORY.

FLEEING THE FRENCH PACIFICATION'S ECONOMIC AND SOCIAL DISRUPTIONS, MANY VILLAGERS JOURNEYED TO THE CITY IN SEARCH OF WORK.

Bánh giò banh

NEW PATTERNS OF LAND TENURE AND TAXATION SCHEMES INCREASED RURAL DEBT AND PUSHED OTHER PEASANTS OFF THE LAND AND TOWARD HANOI.

AS ELSEWHERE, NEWLY ARRIVED COUNTRY FOLK WERE VULNERABLE TO VARIOUS FORMS OF URBAN EXPLOITATION. LIVING IN SLUMS ON THE EDGE OF TOWN, SUCH AS THE COLLECTION OF SHACKS ON THE RED RIVER'S SANDBANK, THEY SOLD THEMSELVES AS DAY LABORERS.

THOUSANDS OF MEN, WOMEN, AND CHILDREN HAULED, PUSHED, AND CARRIED HANOI'S BURDENS FOR A MEAGER SUBSISTENCE.

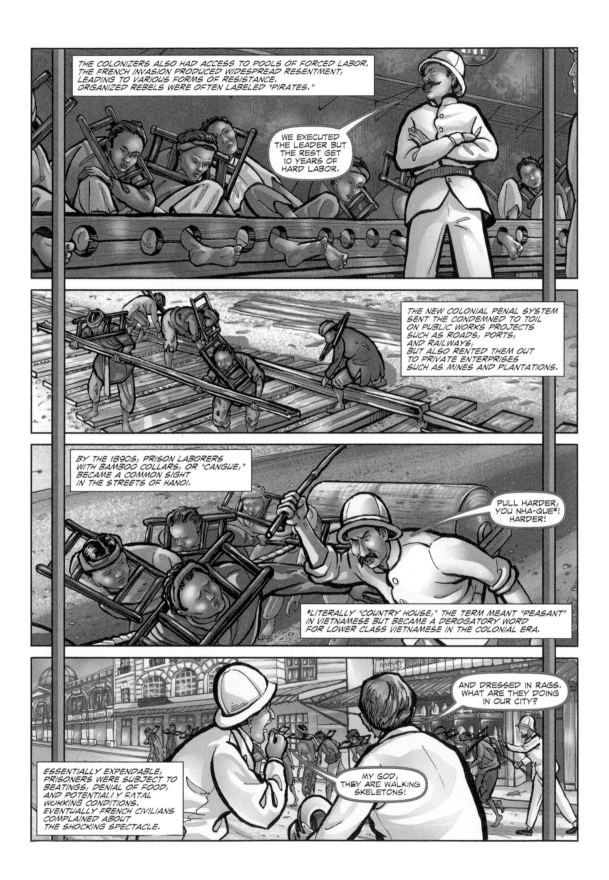

THE COLONIZERS ALSO HAD ACCESS TO POOLS OF FORCED LABOR. THE FRENCH INVASION PRODUCED WIDESPREAD RESENTMENT, LEADING TO VARIOUS FORMS OF RESISTANCE. ORGANIZED REBELS WERE OFTEN LABELED "PIRATES."

WE EXECUTED THE LEADER BUT THE REST GET 10 YEARS OF HARD LABOR.

THE NEW COLONIAL PENAL SYSTEM SENT THE CONDEMNED TO TOIL ON PUBLIC WORKS PROJECTS SUCH AS ROADS, PORTS, AND RAILWAYS, BUT ALSO RENTED THEM OUT TO PRIVATE ENTERPRISES SUCH AS MINES AND PLANTATIONS.

BY THE 1890S, PRISON LABORERS WITH BAMBOO COLLARS, OR "CANGUE," BECAME A COMMON SIGHT IN THE STREETS OF HANOI.

PULL HARDER, YOU NHA-QUE*! HARDER!

*LITERALLY "COUNTRY HOUSE," THE TERM MEANT "PEASANT" IN VIETNAMESE BUT BECAME A DEROGATORY WORD FOR LOWER CLASS VIETNAMESE IN THE COLONIAL ERA.

AND DRESSED IN RAGS, WHAT ARE THEY DOING IN OUR CITY?

ESSENTIALLY EXPENDABLE, PRISONERS WERE SUBJECT TO BEATINGS, DENIAL OF FOOD, AND POTENTIALLY FATAL WORKING CONDITIONS. EVENTUALLY FRENCH CIVILIANS COMPLAINED ABOUT THE SHOCKING SPECTACLE.

MY GOD, THEY ARE WALKING SKELETONS!

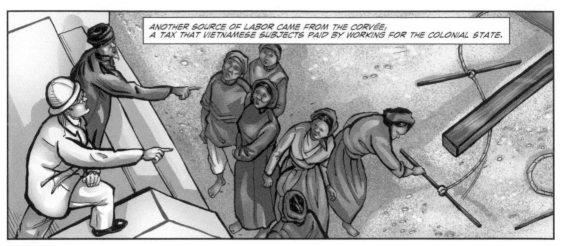

ANOTHER SOURCE OF LABOR CAME FROM THE CORVÉE;
A TAX THAT VIETNAMESE SUBJECTS PAID BY WORKING FOR THE COLONIAL STATE.

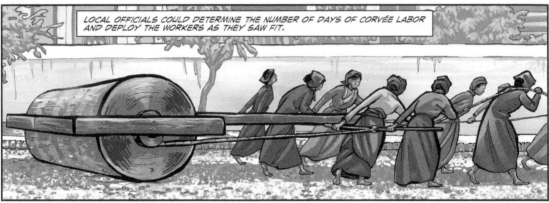

LOCAL OFFICIALS COULD DETERMINE THE NUMBER OF DAYS OF CORVÉE LABOR
AND DEPLOY THE WORKERS AS THEY SAW FIT.

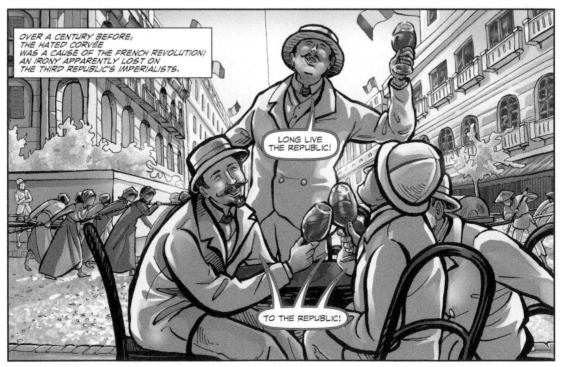

OVER A CENTURY BEFORE,
THE HATED CORVÉE
WAS A CAUSE OF THE FRENCH REVOLUTION;
AN IRONY APPARENTLY LOST ON
THE THIRD REPUBLIC'S IMPERIALISTS.

LONG LIVE
THE REPUBLIC!

TO THE REPUBLIC!

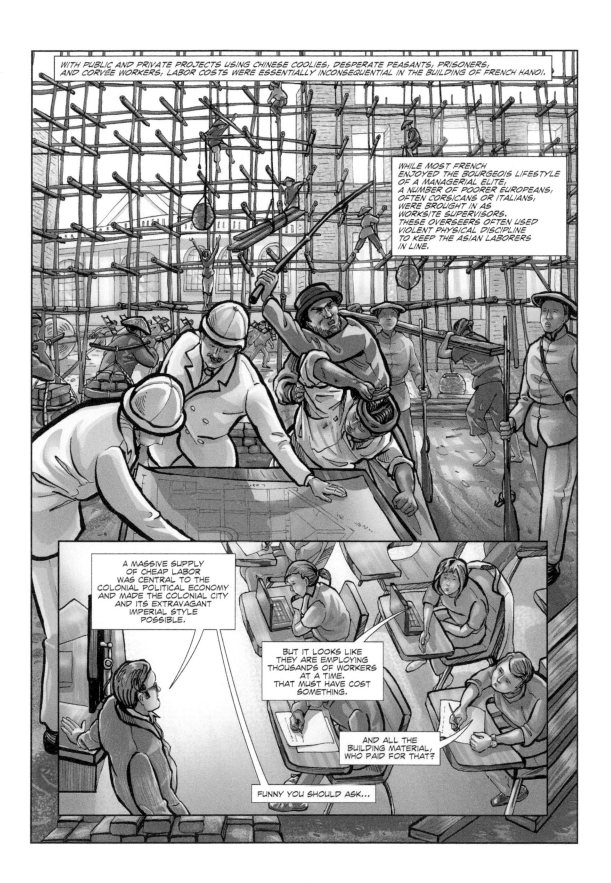

WITH PUBLIC AND PRIVATE PROJECTS USING CHINESE COOLIES, DESPERATE PEASANTS, PRISONERS, AND CORVÉE WORKERS, LABOR COSTS WERE ESSENTIALLY INCONSEQUENTIAL IN THE BUILDING OF FRENCH HANOI.

WHILE MOST FRENCH ENJOYED THE BOURGEOIS LIFESTYLE OF A MANAGERIAL ELITE, A NUMBER OF POORER EUROPEANS, OFTEN CORSICANS OR ITALIANS, WERE BROUGHT IN AS WORKSITE SUPERVISORS. THESE OVERSEERS OFTEN USED VIOLENT PHYSICAL DISCIPLINE TO KEEP THE ASIAN LABORERS IN LINE.

A MASSIVE SUPPLY OF CHEAP LABOR WAS CENTRAL TO THE COLONIAL POLITICAL ECONOMY AND MADE THE COLONIAL CITY AND ITS EXTRAVAGANT IMPERIAL STYLE POSSIBLE.

BUT IT LOOKS LIKE THEY ARE EMPLOYING THOUSANDS OF WORKERS AT A TIME. THAT MUST HAVE COST SOMETHING.

AND ALL THE BUILDING MATERIAL, WHO PAID FOR THAT?

FUNNY YOU SHOULD ASK...

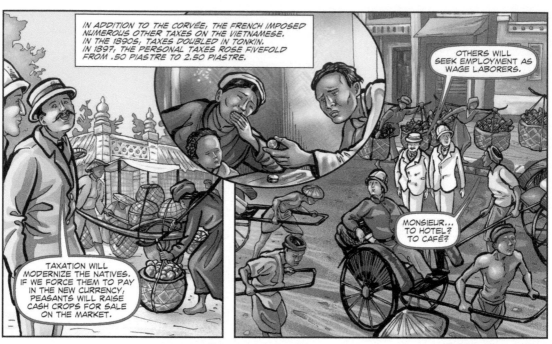

IN ADDITION TO THE CORVÉE, THE FRENCH IMPOSED NUMEROUS OTHER TAXES ON THE VIETNAMESE. IN THE 1890S, TAXES DOUBLED IN TONKIN. IN 1897, THE PERSONAL TAXES ROSE FIVEFOLD FROM .50 PIASTRE TO 2.50 PIASTRE.

OTHERS WILL SEEK EMPLOYMENT AS WAGE LABORERS.

MONSIEUR... TO HOTEL? TO CAFÉ?

TAXATION WILL MODERNIZE THE NATIVES. IF WE FORCE THEM TO PAY IN THE NEW CURRENCY, PEASANTS WILL RAISE CASH CROPS FOR SALE ON THE MARKET.

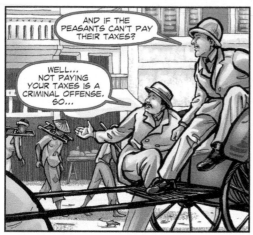

AND IF THE PEASANTS CAN'T PAY THEIR TAXES?

WELL... NOT PAYING YOUR TAXES IS A CRIMINAL OFFENSE. SO...

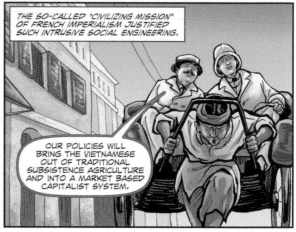

THE SO-CALLED "CIVILIZING MISSION" OF FRENCH IMPERIALISM JUSTIFIED SUCH INTRUSIVE SOCIAL ENGINEERING.

OUR POLICIES WILL BRING THE VIETNAMESE OUT OF TRADITIONAL SUBSISTENCE AGRICULTURE AND INTO A MARKET BASED CAPITALIST SYSTEM.

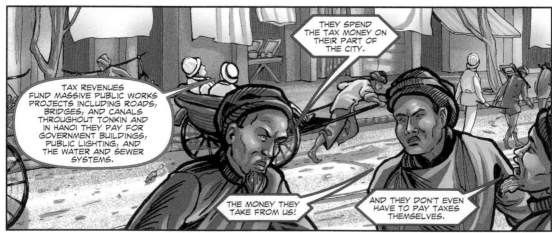

THEY SPEND THE TAX MONEY ON THEIR PART OF THE CITY.

TAX REVENUES FUND MASSIVE PUBLIC WORKS PROJECTS INCLUDING ROADS, BRIDGES, AND CANALS THROUGHOUT TONKIN AND IN HANOI THEY PAY FOR GOVERNMENT BUILDINGS, PUBLIC LIGHTING, AND THE WATER AND SEWER SYSTEMS.

THE MONEY THEY TAKE FROM US!

AND THEY DON'T EVEN HAVE TO PAY TAXES THEMSELVES.

WHEN PAUL DOUMER ARRIVED IN 1897, HE FOUND THE COLONY'S FISCAL SYSTEM TO BE ABSURDLY COMPLEX AND REDUNDANT, BUT ALSO INEFFICIENT.

WITHIN A FEW YEARS, HE HAD THE BOOKS OUT OF THE RED AND FIRMLY IN THE BLACK.

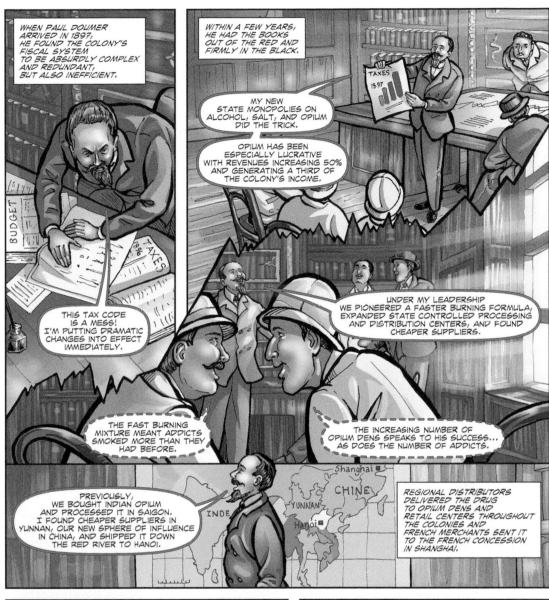

MY NEW STATE MONOPOLIES ON ALCOHOL, SALT, AND OPIUM DID THE TRICK.

OPIUM HAS BEEN ESPECIALLY LUCRATIVE WITH REVENUES INCREASING 50% AND GENERATING A THIRD OF THE COLONY'S INCOME.

THIS TAX CODE IS A MESS! I'M PUTTING DRAMATIC CHANGES INTO EFFECT IMMEDIATELY.

UNDER MY LEADERSHIP WE PIONEERED A FASTER BURNING FORMULA, EXPANDED STATE CONTROLLED PROCESSING AND DISTRIBUTION CENTERS, AND FOUND CHEAPER SUPPLIERS.

THE FAST BURNING MIXTURE MEANT ADDICTS SMOKED MORE THAN THEY HAD BEFORE.

THE INCREASING NUMBER OF OPIUM DENS SPEAKS TO HIS SUCCESS... AS DOES THE NUMBER OF ADDICTS.

PREVIOUSLY, WE BOUGHT INDIAN OPIUM AND PROCESSED IT IN SAIGON. I FOUND CHEAPER SUPPLIERS IN YUNNAN, OUR NEW SPHERE OF INFLUENCE IN CHINA, AND SHIPPED IT DOWN THE RED RIVER TO HANOI.

REGIONAL DISTRIBUTORS DELIVERED THE DRUG TO OPIUM DENS AND RETAIL CENTERS THROUGHOUT THE COLONIES AND FRENCH MERCHANTS SENT IT TO THE FRENCH CONCESSION IN SHANGHAI.

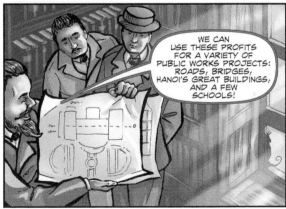

WE CAN USE THESE PROFITS FOR A VARIETY OF PUBLIC WORKS PROJECTS: ROADS, BRIDGES, HANOI'S GREAT BUILDINGS, AND A FEW SCHOOLS!

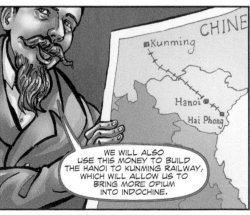

WE WILL ALSO USE THIS MONEY TO BUILD THE HANOI TO KUNMING RAILWAY, WHICH WILL ALLOW US TO BRING MORE OPIUM INTO INDOCHINE.

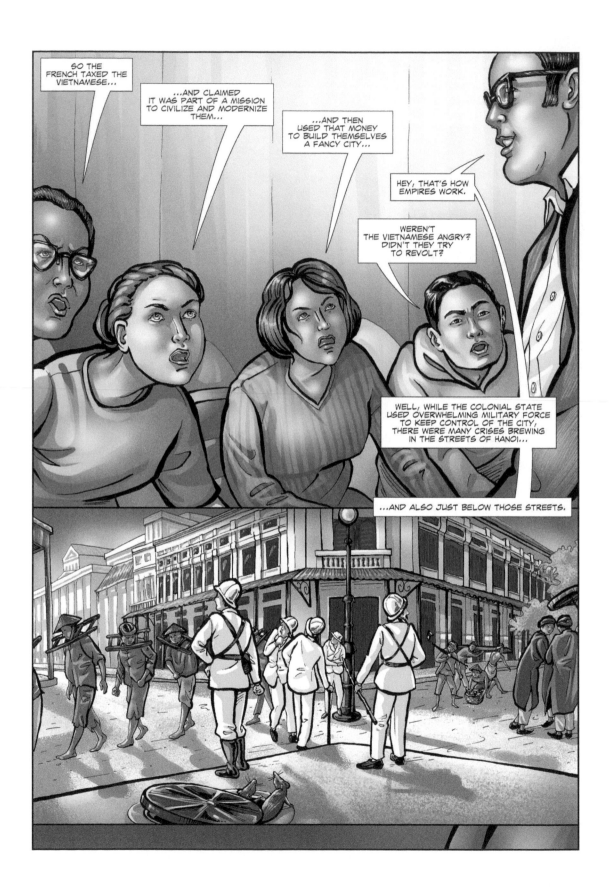

CHAPTER 4
THE ILLUSION OF CONTROL OR WHAT COULD POSSIBLY GO WRONG?

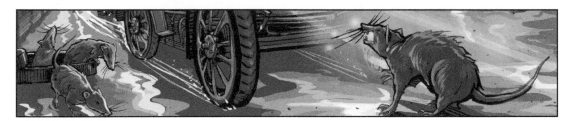

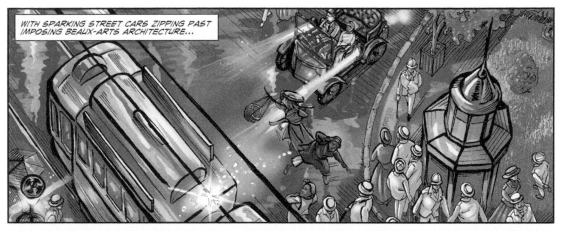

WITH SPARKING STREET CARS ZIPPING PAST IMPOSING BEAUX-ARTS ARCHITECTURE...

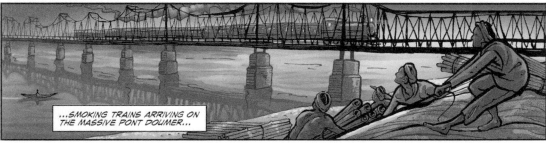

...SMOKING TRAINS ARRIVING ON THE MASSIVE PONT DOUMER...

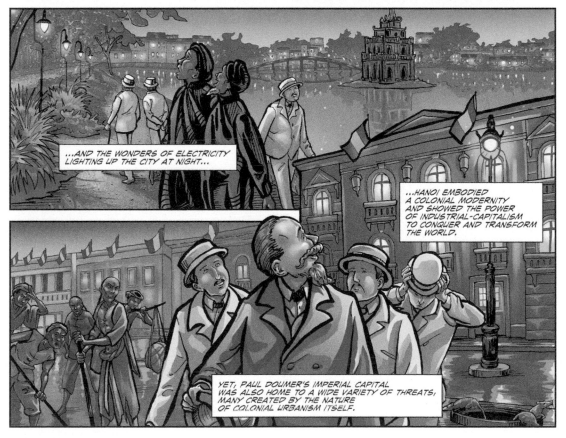

...AND THE WONDERS OF ELECTRICITY LIGHTING UP THE CITY AT NIGHT...

...HANOI EMBODIED A COLONIAL MODERNITY AND SHOWED THE POWER OF INDUSTRIAL-CAPITALISM TO CONQUER AND TRANSFORM THE WORLD.

YET, PAUL DOUMER'S IMPERIAL CAPITAL WAS ALSO HOME TO A WIDE VARIETY OF THREATS, MANY CREATED BY THE NATURE OF COLONIAL URBANISM ITSELF.

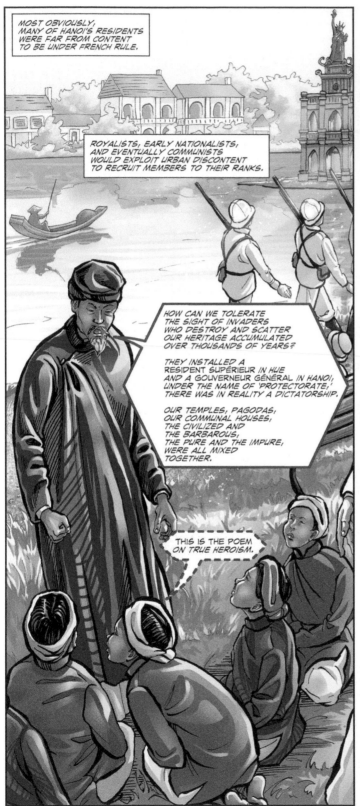

MOST OBVIOUSLY, MANY OF HANOI'S RESIDENTS WERE FAR FROM CONTENT TO BE UNDER FRENCH RULE.

ROYALISTS, EARLY NATIONALISTS, AND EVENTUALLY COMMUNISTS WOULD EXPLOIT URBAN DISCONTENT TO RECRUIT MEMBERS TO THEIR RANKS.

HOW CAN WE TOLERATE THE SIGHT OF INVADERS WHO DESTROY AND SCATTER OUR HERITAGE ACCUMULATED OVER THOUSANDS OF YEARS?

THEY INSTALLED A RESIDENT SUPÉRIEUR IN HUE AND A GOUVERNEUR GÉNÉRAL IN HANOI; UNDER THE NAME OF 'PROTECTORATE,' THERE WAS IN REALITY A DICTATORSHIP.

OUR TEMPLES, PAGODAS, OUR COMMUNAL HOUSES, THE CIVILIZED AND THE BARBAROUS, THE PURE AND THE IMPURE, WERE ALL MIXED TOGETHER.

THIS IS THE POEM ON TRUE HEROISM.

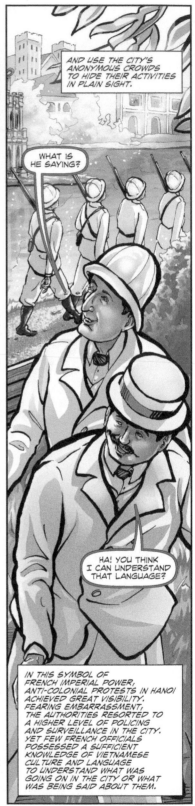

AND USE THE CITY'S ANONYMOUS CROWDS TO HIDE THEIR ACTIVITIES IN PLAIN SIGHT.

WHAT IS HE SAYING?

HA! YOU THINK I CAN UNDERSTAND THAT LANGUAGE?

IN THIS SYMBOL OF FRENCH IMPERIAL POWER, ANTI-COLONIAL PROTESTS IN HANOI ACHIEVED GREAT VISIBILITY. FEARING EMBARRASSMENT, THE AUTHORITIES RESORTED TO A HIGHER LEVEL OF POLICING AND SURVEILLANCE IN THE CITY. YET FEW FRENCH OFFICIALS POSSESSED A SUFFICIENT KNOWLEDGE OF VIETNAMESE CULTURE AND LANGUAGE TO UNDERSTAND WHAT WAS GOING ON IN THE CITY OR WHAT WAS BEING SAID ABOUT THEM.

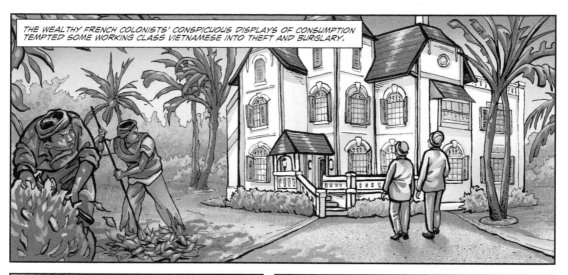

THE WEALTHY FRENCH COLONISTS' CONSPICUOUS DISPLAYS OF CONSUMPTION TEMPTED SOME WORKING CLASS VIETNAMESE INTO THEFT AND BURGLARY.

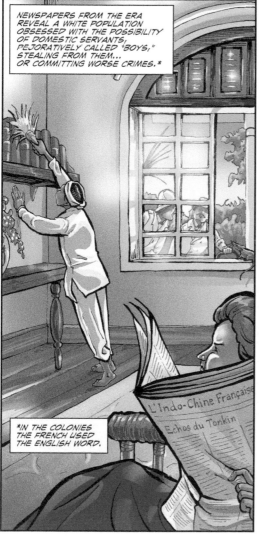

NEWSPAPERS FROM THE ERA REVEAL A WHITE POPULATION OBSESSED WITH THE POSSIBILITY OF DOMESTIC SERVANTS, PEJORATIVELY CALLED "BOYS," STEALING FROM THEM... OR COMMITTING WORSE CRIMES.*

L'Indo-Chine Française

Echos du Tonkin

*IN THE COLONIES THE FRENCH USED THE ENGLISH WORD.

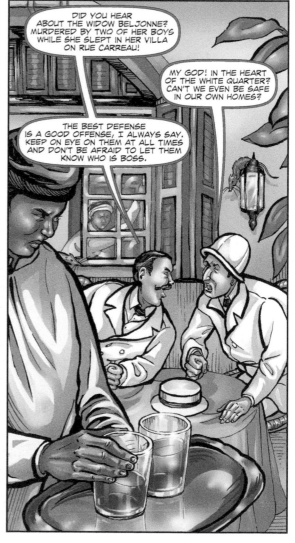

DID YOU HEAR ABOUT THE WIDOW BELJONNE? MURDERED BY TWO OF HER BOYS WHILE SHE SLEPT IN HER VILLA ON RUE CARREAU!

MY GOD! IN THE HEART OF THE WHITE QUARTER? CAN'T WE EVEN BE SAFE IN OUR OWN HOMES?

THE BEST DEFENSE IS A GOOD OFFENSE, I ALWAYS SAY. KEEP ON EYE ON THEM AT ALL TIMES AND DON'T BE AFRAID TO LET THEM KNOW WHO IS BOSS.

RÉPUBLIQUE F
LIBERTÉ — ÉGALITÉ — FRATERNITÉ

FACED WITH A RISE IN URBAN CRIME, FRENCH OFFICIALS BLAMED THE VIETNAMESE:

Report on the Political and Economic Situation in Indochine

The Résident Supérieur au Tonkin notes however, that these attacks against French denote a more and more troubling attitude in the native population immediately around the Europeans, either employees or domestic servants. It is thought that, faced with the audacity of these crimes, it is permitted to think that our French laws are not always of sufficient character to rapidly and severely repress criminality in the eyes of the natives. This attitude is most noticeable in the large cities or the centers inhabited by Europeans and natives more or less perverted by their time in the city. The majority of the population in the countryside remains honest, hard working, and respectful of authority.

RÉPUBLIQUE FRANÇAISE
LIBERTÉ — ÉGALITÉ — FRATERNITÉ

Political and Economic Situation in Tonkin.

At the same time that there have been audacious attempts at jail breaks, it should be noted that there is an augmentation of native criminality in the cities, that this all might be attributed to the ineffectiveness of our penal laws when applied to individuals of a mentality so different from our own.

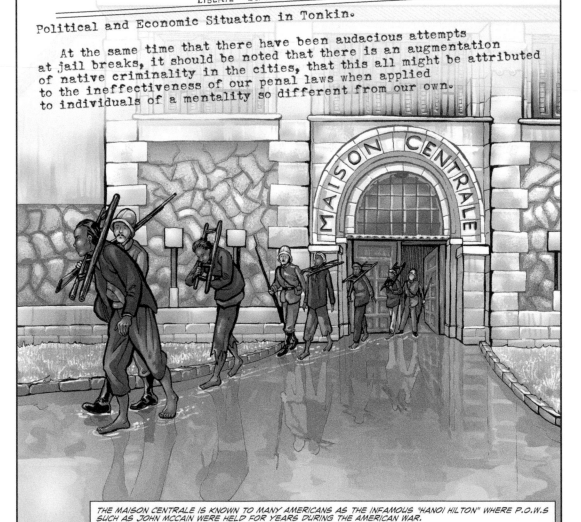

THE MAISON CENTRALE IS KNOWN TO MANY AMERICANS AS THE INFAMOUS "HANOI HILTON" WHERE P.O.W.S SUCH AS JOHN McCAIN WERE HELD FOR YEARS DURING THE AMERICAN WAR.

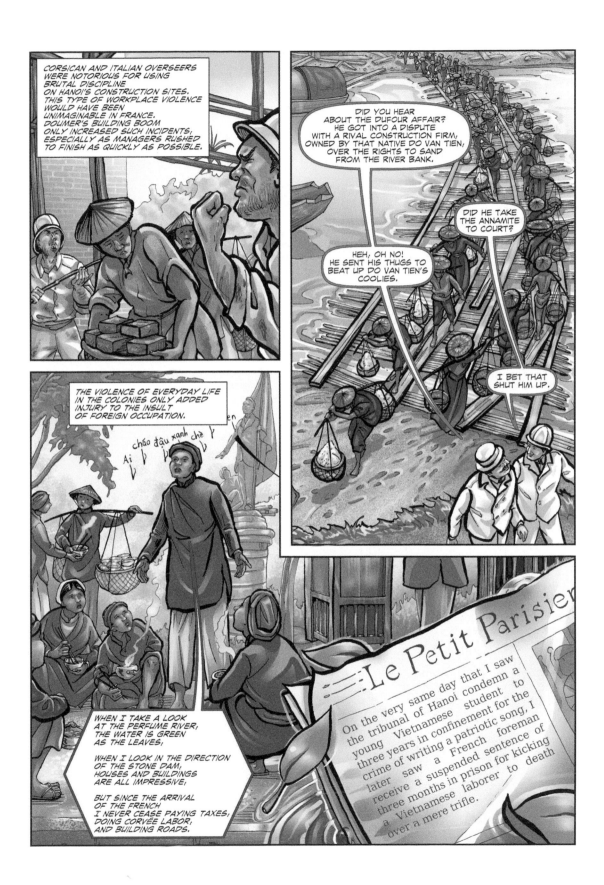

CORSICAN AND ITALIAN OVERSEERS WERE NOTORIOUS FOR USING BRUTAL DISCIPLINE ON HANOI'S CONSTRUCTION SITES. THIS TYPE OF WORKPLACE VIOLENCE WOULD HAVE BEEN UNIMAGINABLE IN FRANCE. DOUMER'S BUILDING BOOM ONLY INCREASED SUCH INCIDENTS, ESPECIALLY AS MANAGERS RUSHED TO FINISH AS QUICKLY AS POSSIBLE.

DID YOU HEAR ABOUT THE DUFOUR AFFAIR? HE GOT INTO A DISPUTE WITH A RIVAL CONSTRUCTION FIRM, OWNED BY THAT NATIVE DO VAN TIEN, OVER THE RIGHTS TO SAND FROM THE RIVER BANK.

DID HE TAKE THE ANNAMITE TO COURT?

HEH, OH NO! HE SENT HIS THUGS TO BEAT UP DO VAN TIEN'S COOLIES.

I BET THAT SHUT HIM UP.

THE VIOLENCE OF EVERYDAY LIFE IN THE COLONIES ONLY ADDED INJURY TO THE INSULT OF FOREIGN OCCUPATION.

WHEN I TAKE A LOOK AT THE PERFUME RIVER, THE WATER IS GREEN AS THE LEAVES;

WHEN I LOOK IN THE DIRECTION OF THE STONE DAM, HOUSES AND BUILDINGS ARE ALL IMPRESSIVE;

BUT SINCE THE ARRIVAL OF THE FRENCH I NEVER CEASE PAYING TAXES, DOING CORVÉE LABOR, AND BUILDING ROADS.

Le Petit Parisien

On the very same day that I saw the tribunal of Hanoi condemn a young Vietnamese student to three years in confinement for the crime of writing a patriotic song, I later saw a French foreman receive a suspended sentence of three months in prison for kicking a Vietnamese laborer to death over a mere trifle.

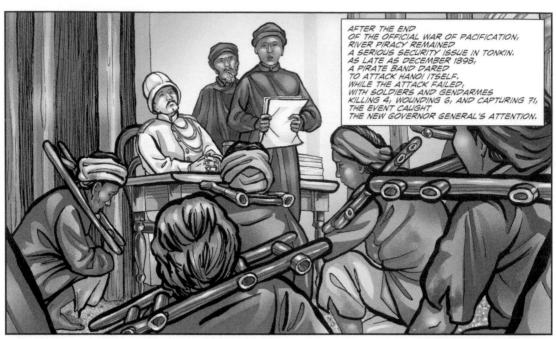

AFTER THE END
OF THE OFFICIAL WAR OF PACIFICATION,
RIVER PIRACY REMAINED
A SERIOUS SECURITY ISSUE IN TONKIN.
AS LATE AS DECEMBER 1898,
A PIRATE BAND DARED
TO ATTACK HANOI ITSELF.
WHILE THE ATTACK FAILED,
WITH SOLDIERS AND GENDARMES
KILLING 4, WOUNDING 6, AND CAPTURING 71,
THE EVENT CAUGHT
THE NEW GOVERNOR GENERAL'S ATTENTION.

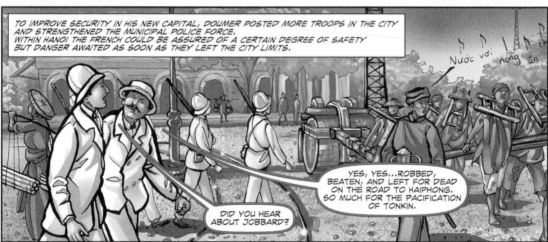

TO IMPROVE SECURITY IN HIS NEW CAPITAL, DOUMER POSTED MORE TROOPS IN THE CITY
AND STRENGTHENED THE MUNICIPAL POLICE FORCE.
WITHIN HANOI THE FRENCH COULD BE ASSURED OF A CERTAIN DEGREE OF SAFETY
BUT DANGER AWAITED AS SOON AS THEY LEFT THE CITY LIMITS.

Nước với nông ăn

DID YOU HEAR
ABOUT JOBBARD?

YES, YES...ROBBED,
BEATEN, AND LEFT FOR DEAD
ON THE ROAD TO HAIPHONG.
SO MUCH FOR THE PACIFICATION
OF TONKIN.

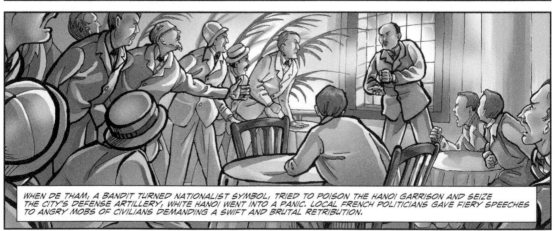

WHEN DE THAM, A BANDIT TURNED NATIONALIST SYMBOL, TRIED TO POISON THE HANOI GARRISON AND SEIZE
THE CITY'S DEFENSE ARTILLERY, WHITE HANOI WENT INTO A PANIC. LOCAL FRENCH POLITICIANS GAVE FIERY SPEECHES
TO ANGRY MOBS OF CIVILIANS DEMANDING A SWIFT AND BRUTAL RETRIBUTION.

HANOI'S CHINESE INHABITANTS ALSO MADE THE FRENCH UNEASY. COMPOSED OF BOTH IMPOVERISHED LABORERS AND SUCCESSFUL ENTREPRENEURS, THE CHINESE COMMUNITY ORGANIZED REGIONAL SOCIETIES KNOWN AS HUI FOR COLLECTIVE WELFARE AND COMMERCIAL COOPERATION.

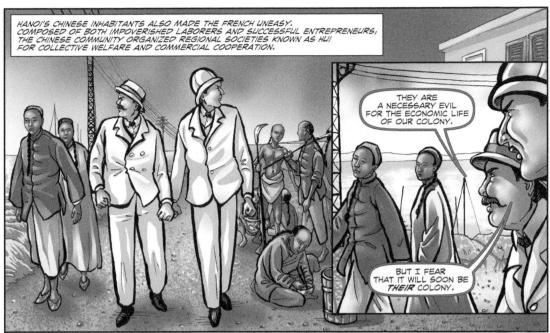

THEY ARE A NECESSARY EVIL FOR THE ECONOMIC LIFE OF OUR COLONY.

BUT I FEAR THAT IT WILL SOON BE *THEIR* COLONY.

THE POROUS BORDER TO THE NORTH BELIED THE FACT THAT IT WAS A RECENT CREATION, AN ARTIFICIAL BARRIER DISRUPTING 2,000 YEARS OF TRADE NETWORKS.

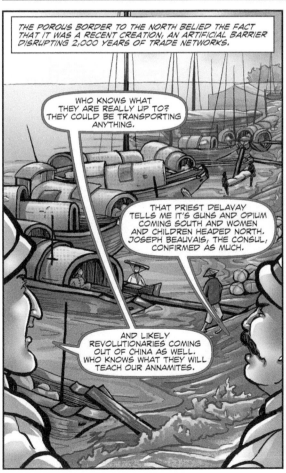

WHO KNOWS WHAT THEY ARE REALLY UP TO? THEY COULD BE TRANSPORTING ANYTHING.

THAT PRIEST DELAVAY TELLS ME IT'S GUNS AND OPIUM COMING SOUTH AND WOMEN AND CHILDREN HEADED NORTH. JOSEPH BEAUVAIS, THE CONSUL, CONFIRMED AS MUCH.

AND LIKELY REVOLUTIONARIES COMING OUT OF CHINA AS WELL. WHO KNOWS WHAT THEY WILL TEACH OUR ANNAMITES.

INDEED, SUN YAT-SEN WAS IN HANOI TO ESTABLISH A LOCAL CHAPTER OF HSING CHUNG HUI (REVIVE CHINA SOCIETY) FOR MOST OF 1902 AND INTO 1903. THIS HUI WOULD BECOME THE KUOMINTANG (CHINESE NATIONALIST PARTY).

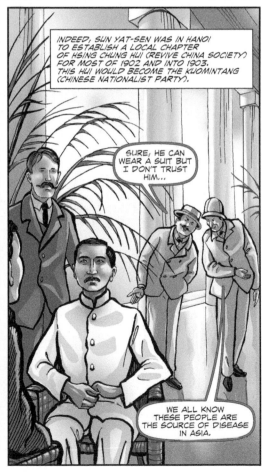

SURE, HE CAN WEAR A SUIT BUT I DON'T TRUST HIM...

WE ALL KNOW THESE PEOPLE ARE THE SOURCE OF DISEASE IN ASIA.

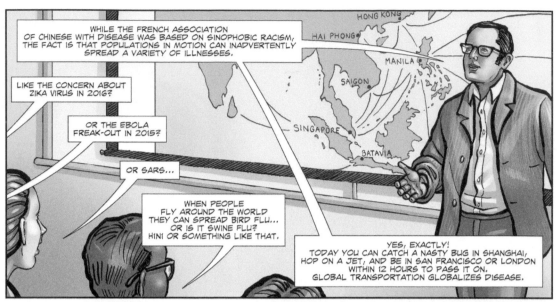

WHILE THE FRENCH ASSOCIATION OF CHINESE WITH DISEASE WAS BASED ON SINOPHOBIC RACISM, THE FACT IS THAT POPULATIONS IN MOTION CAN INADVERTENTLY SPREAD A VARIETY OF ILLNESSES.

LIKE THE CONCERN ABOUT ZIKA VIRUS IN 2016?

OR THE EBOLA FREAK-OUT IN 2015?

OR SARS...

WHEN PEOPLE FLY AROUND THE WORLD THEY CAN SPREAD BIRD FLU... OR IS IT SWINE FLU? H1N1 OR SOMETHING LIKE THAT.

YES, EXACTLY! TODAY YOU CAN CATCH A NASTY BUG IN SHANGHAI, HOP ON A JET, AND BE IN SAN FRANCISCO OR LONDON WITHIN 12 HOURS TO PASS IT ON. GLOBAL TRANSPORTATION GLOBALIZES DISEASE.

HONG KONG
HAI PHONG
MANILA
SAIGON
SINGAPORE
BATAVIA

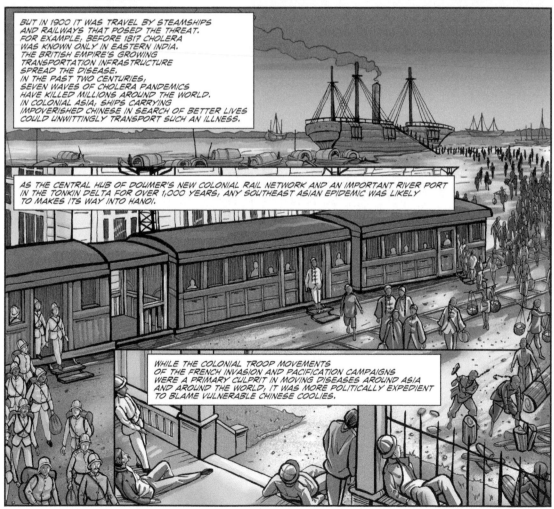

BUT IN 1900 IT WAS TRAVEL BY STEAMSHIPS AND RAILWAYS THAT POSED THE THREAT. FOR EXAMPLE, BEFORE 1817 CHOLERA WAS KNOWN ONLY IN EASTERN INDIA. THE BRITISH EMPIRE'S GROWING TRANSPORTATION INFRASTRUCTURE SPREAD THE DISEASE. IN THE PAST TWO CENTURIES, SEVEN WAVES OF CHOLERA PANDEMICS HAVE KILLED MILLIONS AROUND THE WORLD. IN COLONIAL ASIA, SHIPS CARRYING IMPOVERISHED CHINESE IN SEARCH OF BETTER LIVES COULD UNWITTINGLY TRANSPORT SUCH AN ILLNESS.

AS THE CENTRAL HUB OF DOUMER'S NEW COLONIAL RAIL NETWORK AND AN IMPORTANT RIVER PORT IN THE TONKIN DELTA FOR OVER 1,000 YEARS, ANY SOUTHEAST ASIAN EPIDEMIC WAS LIKELY TO MAKES ITS WAY INTO HANOI.

WHILE THE COLONIAL TROOP MOVEMENTS OF THE FRENCH INVASION AND PACIFICATION CAMPAIGNS WERE A PRIMARY CULPRIT IN MOVING DISEASES AROUND ASIA AND AROUND THE WORLD, IT WAS MORE POLITICALLY EXPEDIENT TO BLAME VULNERABLE CHINESE COOLIES.

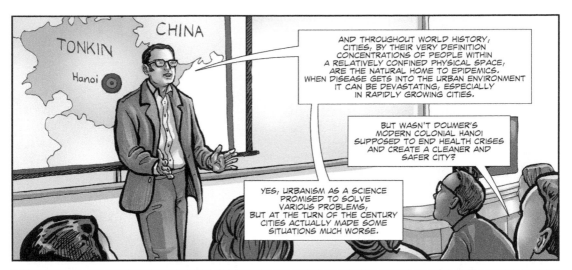

AND THROUGHOUT WORLD HISTORY, CITIES, BY THEIR VERY DEFINITION CONCENTRATIONS OF PEOPLE WITHIN A RELATIVELY CONFINED PHYSICAL SPACE, ARE THE NATURAL HOME TO EPIDEMICS. WHEN DISEASE GETS INTO THE URBAN ENVIRONMENT IT CAN BE DEVASTATING, ESPECIALLY IN RAPIDLY GROWING CITIES.

BUT WASN'T DOUMER'S MODERN COLONIAL HANOI SUPPOSED TO END HEALTH CRISES AND CREATE A CLEANER AND SAFER CITY?

YES, URBANISM AS A SCIENCE PROMISED TO SOLVE VARIOUS PROBLEMS, BUT AT THE TURN OF THE CENTURY CITIES ACTUALLY MADE SOME SITUATIONS MUCH WORSE.

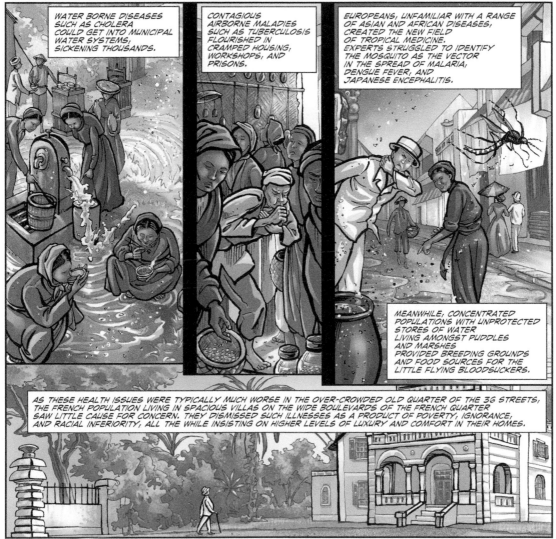

WATER BORNE DISEASES SUCH AS CHOLERA COULD GET INTO MUNICIPAL WATER SYSTEMS, SICKENING THOUSANDS.

CONTAGIOUS AIRBORNE MALADIES SUCH AS TUBERCULOSIS FLOURISHED IN CRAMPED HOUSING, WORKSHOPS, AND PRISONS.

EUROPEANS, UNFAMILIAR WITH A RANGE OF ASIAN AND AFRICAN DISEASES, CREATED THE NEW FIELD OF TROPICAL MEDICINE. EXPERTS STRUGGLED TO IDENTIFY THE MOSQUITO AS THE VECTOR IN THE SPREAD OF MALARIA, DENGUE FEVER, AND JAPANESE ENCEPHALITIS.

MEANWHILE, CONCENTRATED POPULATIONS WITH UNPROTECTED STORES OF WATER LIVING AMONGST PUDDLES AND MARSHES PROVIDED BREEDING GROUNDS AND FOOD SOURCES FOR THE LITTLE FLYING BLOODSUCKERS.

AS THESE HEALTH ISSUES WERE TYPICALLY MUCH WORSE IN THE OVER-CROWDED OLD QUARTER OF THE 36 STREETS, THE FRENCH POPULATION LIVING IN SPACIOUS VILLAS ON THE WIDE BOULEVARDS OF THE FRENCH QUARTER SAW LITTLE CAUSE FOR CONCERN. THEY DISMISSED SUCH ILLNESSES AS A PRODUCT OF POVERTY, IGNORANCE, AND RACIAL INFERIORITY; ALL THE WHILE INSISTING ON HIGHER LEVELS OF LUXURY AND COMFORT IN THEIR HOMES.

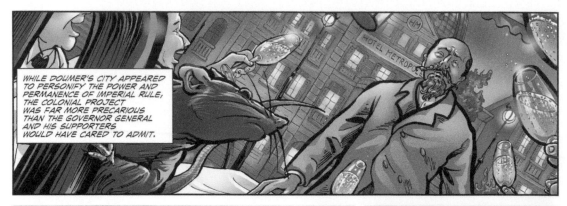

WHILE DOUMER'S CITY APPEARED TO PERSONIFY THE POWER AND PERMANENCE OF IMPERIAL RULE, THE COLONIAL PROJECT WAS FAR MORE PRECARIOUS THAN THE GOVERNOR GENERAL AND HIS SUPPORTERS WOULD HAVE CARED TO ADMIT.

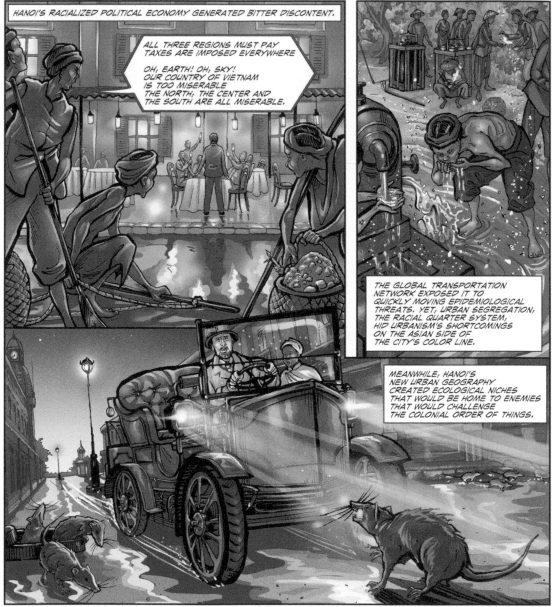

HANOI'S RACIALIZED POLITICAL ECONOMY GENERATED BITTER DISCONTENT.

ALL THREE REGIONS MUST PAY TAXES ARE IMPOSED EVERYWHERE

OH, EARTH! OH, SKY! OUR COUNTRY OF VIETNAM IS TOO MISERABLE THE NORTH, THE CENTER AND THE SOUTH ARE ALL MISERABLE.

THE GLOBAL TRANSPORTATION NETWORK EXPOSED IT TO QUICKLY MOVING EPIDEMIOLOGICAL THREATS. YET, URBAN SEGREGATION, THE RACIAL QUARTER SYSTEM, HID URBANISM'S SHORTCOMINGS ON THE ASIAN SIDE OF THE CITY'S COLOR LINE.

MEANWHILE, HANOI'S NEW URBAN GEOGRAPHY CREATED ECOLOGICAL NICHES THAT WOULD BE HOME TO ENEMIES THAT WOULD CHALLENGE THE COLONIAL ORDER OF THINGS.

CHAPTER 5
BLACK DEATH IN THE WHITE CITY!

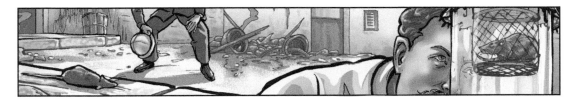

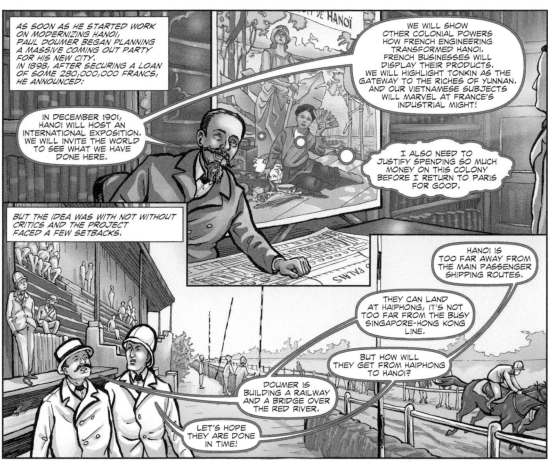

AS SOON AS HE STARTED WORK ON MODERNIZING HANOI, PAUL DOUMER BEGAN PLANNING A MASSIVE COMING OUT PARTY FOR HIS NEW CITY. IN 1898, AFTER SECURING A LOAN OF SOME 280,000,000 FRANCS, HE ANNOUNCED:

IN DECEMBER 1901, HANOI WILL HOST AN INTERNATIONAL EXPOSITION. WE WILL INVITE THE WORLD TO SEE WHAT WE HAVE DONE HERE.

WE WILL SHOW OTHER COLONIAL POWERS HOW FRENCH ENGINEERING TRANSFORMED HANOI. FRENCH BUSINESSES WILL DISPLAY THEIR PRODUCTS. WE WILL HIGHLIGHT TONKIN AS THE GATEWAY TO THE RICHES OF YUNNAN. AND OUR VIETNAMESE SUBJECTS WILL MARVEL AT FRANCE'S INDUSTRIAL MIGHT!

I ALSO NEED TO JUSTIFY SPENDING SO MUCH MONEY ON THIS COLONY BEFORE I RETURN TO PARIS FOR GOOD.

BUT THE IDEA WAS WITH NOT WITHOUT CRITICS AND THE PROJECT FACED A FEW SETBACKS.

HANOI IS TOO FAR AWAY FROM THE MAIN PASSENGER SHIPPING ROUTES.

THEY CAN LAND AT HAIPHONG, IT'S NOT TOO FAR FROM THE BUSY SINGAPORE-HONG KONG LINE.

BUT HOW WILL THEY GET FROM HAIPHONG TO HANOI?

DOUMER IS BUILDING A RAILWAY AND A BRIDGE OVER THE RED RIVER.

LET'S HOPE THEY ARE DONE IN TIME!

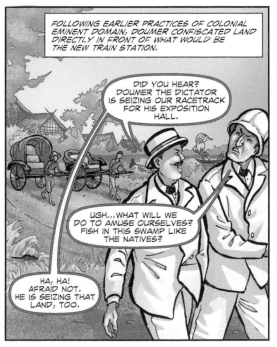

FOLLOWING EARLIER PRACTICES OF COLONIAL EMINENT DOMAIN, DOUMER CONFISCATED LAND DIRECTLY IN FRONT OF WHAT WOULD BE THE NEW TRAIN STATION.

DID YOU HEAR? DOUMER THE DICTATOR IS SEIZING OUR RACETRACK FOR HIS EXPOSITION HALL.

UGH...WHAT WILL WE DO TO AMUSE OURSELVES? FISH IN THIS SWAMP LIKE THE NATIVES?

HA, HA! AFRAID NOT. HE IS SEIZING THAT LAND, TOO.

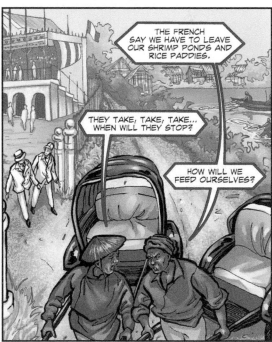

THE FRENCH SAY WE HAVE TO LEAVE OUR SHRIMP PONDS AND RICE PADDIES.

THEY TAKE, TAKE, TAKE... WHEN WILL THEY STOP?

HOW WILL WE FEED OURSELVES?

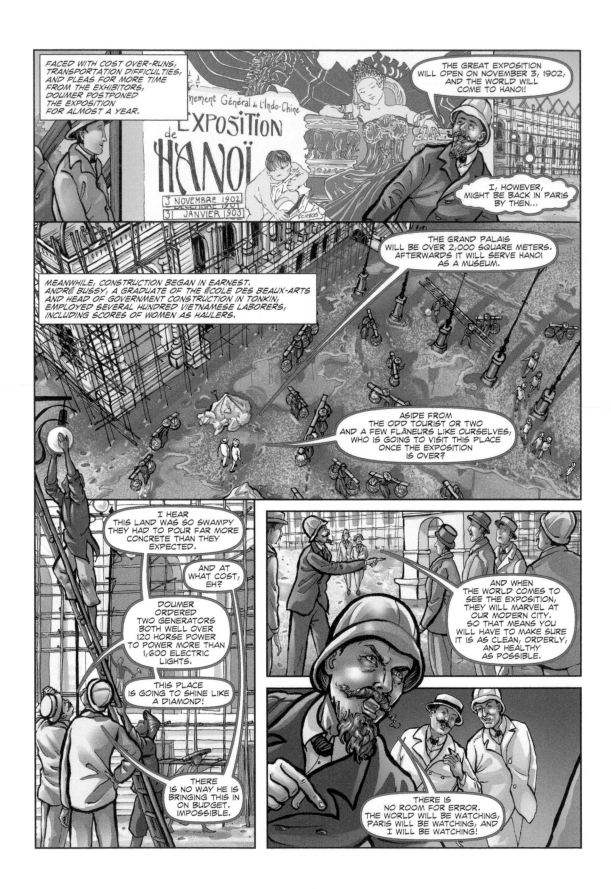

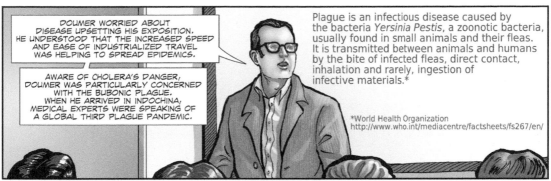

DOUMER WORRIED ABOUT DISEASE UPSETTING HIS EXPOSITION. HE UNDERSTOOD THAT THE INCREASED SPEED AND EASE OF INDUSTRIALIZED TRAVEL WAS HELPING TO SPREAD EPIDEMICS.

AWARE OF CHOLERA'S DANGER, DOUMER WAS PARTICULARLY CONCERNED WITH THE BUBONIC PLAGUE. WHEN HE ARRIVED IN INDOCHINA, MEDICAL EXPERTS WERE SPEAKING OF A GLOBAL THIRD PLAGUE PANDEMIC.

Plague is an infectious disease caused by the bacteria *Yersinia Pestis*, a zoonotic bacteria, usually found in small animals and their fleas. It is transmitted between animals and humans by the bite of infected fleas, direct contact, inhalation and rarely, ingestion of infective materials.*

*World Health Organization
http://www.who.int/mediacentre/factsheets/fs267/en/

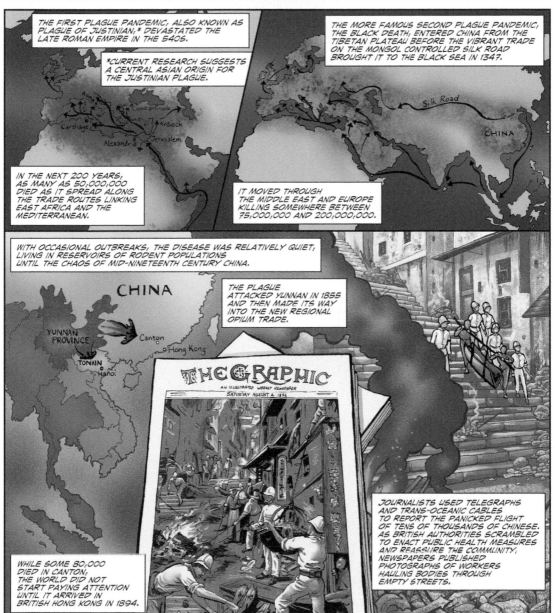

THE FIRST PLAGUE PANDEMIC, ALSO KNOWN AS PLAGUE OF JUSTINIAN,* DEVASTATED THE LATE ROMAN EMPIRE IN THE 540S.

*CURRENT RESEARCH SUGGESTS A CENTRAL ASIAN ORIGIN FOR THE JUSTINIAN PLAGUE.

IN THE NEXT 200 YEARS, AS MANY AS 50,000,000 DIED AS IT SPREAD ALONG THE TRADE ROUTES LINKING EAST AFRICA AND THE MEDITERRANEAN.

THE MORE FAMOUS SECOND PLAGUE PANDEMIC, THE BLACK DEATH, ENTERED CHINA FROM THE TIBETAN PLATEAU BEFORE THE VIBRANT TRADE ON THE MONGOL CONTROLLED SILK ROAD BROUGHT IT TO THE BLACK SEA IN 1347.

IT MOVED THROUGH THE MIDDLE EAST AND EUROPE KILLING SOMEWHERE BETWEEN 75,000,000 AND 200,000,000.

WITH OCCASIONAL OUTBREAKS, THE DISEASE WAS RELATIVELY QUIET, LIVING IN RESERVOIRS OF RODENT POPULATIONS UNTIL THE CHAOS OF MID-NINETEENTH CENTURY CHINA.

THE PLAGUE ATTACKED YUNNAN IN 1855 AND THEN MADE ITS WAY INTO THE NEW REGIONAL OPIUM TRADE.

WHILE SOME 80,000 DIED IN CANTON, THE WORLD DID NOT START PAYING ATTENTION UNTIL IT ARRIVED IN BRITISH HONG KONG IN 1894.

JOURNALISTS USED TELEGRAPHS AND TRANS-OCEANIC CABLES TO REPORT THE PANICKED FLIGHT OF TENS OF THOUSANDS OF CHINESE. AS BRITISH AUTHORITIES SCRAMBLED TO ENACT PUBLIC HEALTH MEASURES AND REASSURE THE COMMUNITY, NEWSPAPERS PUBLISHED PHOTOGRAPHS OF WORKERS HAULING BODIES THROUGH EMPTY STREETS.

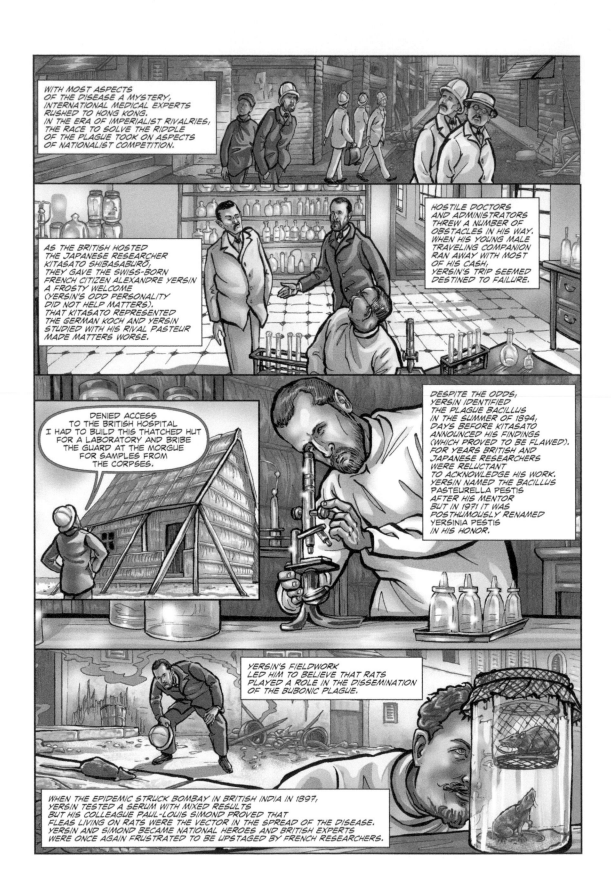

WITH MOST ASPECTS OF THE DISEASE A MYSTERY, INTERNATIONAL MEDICAL EXPERTS RUSHED TO HONG KONG. IN THE ERA OF IMPERIALIST RIVALRIES, THE RACE TO SOLVE THE RIDDLE OF THE PLAGUE TOOK ON ASPECTS OF NATIONALIST COMPETITION.

AS THE BRITISH HOSTED THE JAPANESE RESEARCHER KITASATO SHIBASABURO, THEY GAVE THE SWISS-BORN FRENCH CITIZEN ALEXANDRE YERSIN A FROSTY WELCOME (YERSIN'S ODD PERSONALITY DID NOT HELP MATTERS). THAT KITASATO REPRESENTED THE GERMAN KOCH AND YERSIN STUDIED WITH HIS RIVAL PASTEUR MADE MATTERS WORSE.

HOSTILE DOCTORS AND ADMINISTRATORS THREW A NUMBER OF OBSTACLES IN HIS WAY. WHEN HIS YOUNG MALE TRAVELING COMPANION RAN AWAY WITH MOST OF HIS CASH, YERSIN'S TRIP SEEMED DESTINED TO FAILURE.

DENIED ACCESS TO THE BRITISH HOSPITAL I HAD TO BUILD THIS THATCHED HUT FOR A LABORATORY AND BRIBE THE GUARD AT THE MORGUE FOR SAMPLES FROM THE CORPSES.

DESPITE THE ODDS, YERSIN IDENTIFIED THE PLAGUE BACILLUS IN THE SUMMER OF 1894, DAYS BEFORE KITASATO ANNOUNCED HIS FINDINGS (WHICH PROVED TO BE FLAWED). FOR YEARS BRITISH AND JAPANESE RESEARCHERS WERE RELUCTANT TO ACKNOWLEDGE HIS WORK. YERSIN NAMED THE BACILLUS PASTEURELLA PESTIS AFTER HIS MENTOR BUT IN 1971 IT WAS POSTHUMOUSLY RENAMED YERSINIA PESTIS IN HIS HONOR.

YERSIN'S FIELDWORK LED HIM TO BELIEVE THAT RATS PLAYED A ROLE IN THE DISSEMINATION OF THE BUBONIC PLAGUE.

WHEN THE EPIDEMIC STRUCK BOMBAY IN BRITISH INDIA IN 1897, YERSIN TESTED A SERUM WITH MIXED RESULTS BUT HIS COLLEAGUE PAUL-LOUIS SIMOND PROVED THAT FLEAS LIVING ON RATS WERE THE VECTOR IN THE SPREAD OF THE DISEASE. YERSIN AND SIMOND BECAME NATIONAL HEROES AND BRITISH EXPERTS WERE ONCE AGAIN FRUSTRATED TO BE UPSTAGED BY FRENCH RESEARCHERS.

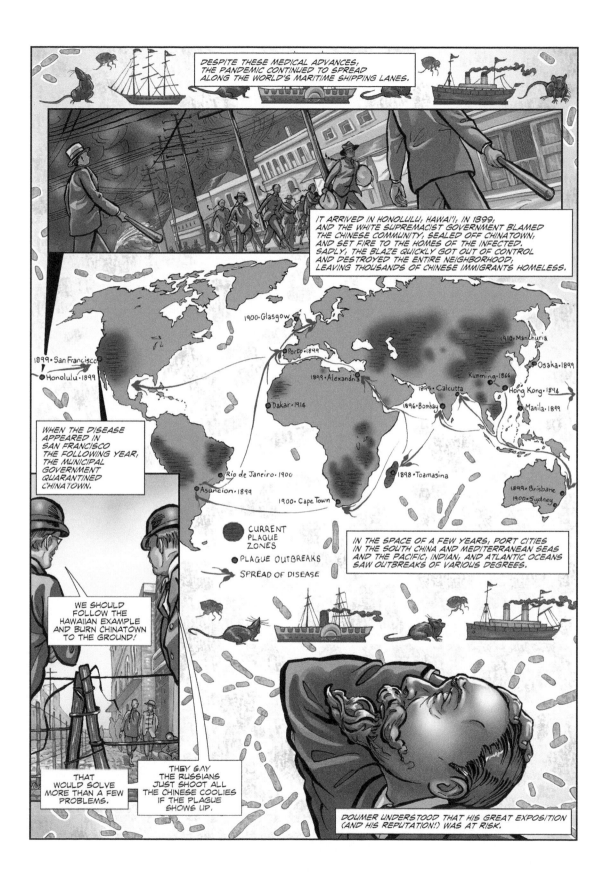

DESPITE THESE MEDICAL ADVANCES, THE PANDEMIC CONTINUED TO SPREAD ALONG THE WORLD'S MARITIME SHIPPING LANES.

IT ARRIVED IN HONOLULU, HAWAI'I, IN 1899, AND THE WHITE SUPREMACIST GOVERNMENT BLAMED THE CHINESE COMMUNITY, SEALED OFF CHINATOWN, AND SET FIRE TO THE HOMES OF THE INFECTED. SADLY, THE BLAZE QUICKLY GOT OUT OF CONTROL AND DESTROYED THE ENTIRE NEIGHBORHOOD, LEAVING THOUSANDS OF CHINESE IMMIGRANTS HOMELESS.

WHEN THE DISEASE APPEARED IN SAN FRANCISCO THE FOLLOWING YEAR, THE MUNICIPAL GOVERNMENT QUARANTINED CHINATOWN.

1900·Glasgow
1899·San Francisco
Honolulu·1899
Porto·1899
1899·Alexandria
Dakar·1914
1910·Manchuria
Osaka·1899
Kunming·1866
1895·Calcutta
Hong Kong·1894
1896·Bombay
Manila·1899
Rio de Janeiro·1900
Asuncion·1899
1900·Cape Town
1898·Toamasina
1899·Brisbane
1900·Sydney

CURRENT PLAGUE ZONES
PLAGUE OUTBREAKS
SPREAD OF DISEASE

IN THE SPACE OF A FEW YEARS, PORT CITIES IN THE SOUTH CHINA AND MEDITERRANEAN SEAS AND THE PACIFIC, INDIAN, AND ATLANTIC OCEANS SAW OUTBREAKS OF VARIOUS DEGREES.

WE SHOULD FOLLOW THE HAWAIIAN EXAMPLE AND BURN CHINATOWN TO THE GROUND!

THAT WOULD SOLVE MORE THAN A FEW PROBLEMS.

THEY GAY THE RUSSIANS JUST SHOOT ALL THE CHINESE COOLIES IF THE PLAGUE SHOWS UP.

DOUMER UNDERSTOOD THAT HIS GREAT EXPOSITION (AND HIS REPUTATION!) WAS AT RISK.

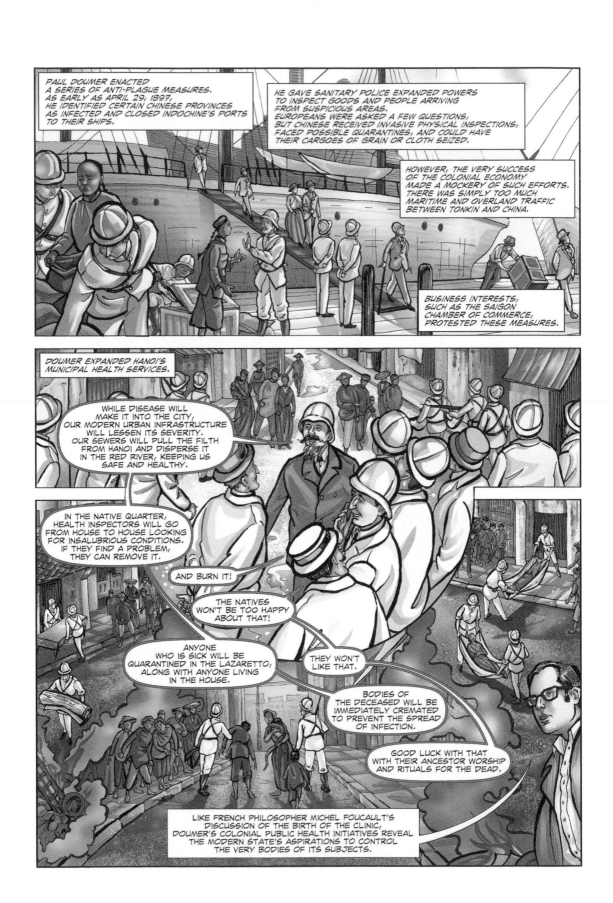

PAUL DOUMER ENACTED A SERIES OF ANTI-PLAGUE MEASURES. AS EARLY AS APRIL 29, 1897, HE IDENTIFIED CERTAIN CHINESE PROVINCES AS INFECTED AND CLOSED INDOCHINE'S PORTS TO THEIR SHIPS.

HE GAVE SANITARY POLICE EXPANDED POWERS TO INSPECT GOODS AND PEOPLE ARRIVING FROM SUSPICIOUS AREAS. EUROPEANS WERE ASKED A FEW QUESTIONS, BUT CHINESE RECEIVED INVASIVE PHYSICAL INSPECTIONS, FACED POSSIBLE QUARANTINES, AND COULD HAVE THEIR CARGOES OF GRAIN OR CLOTH SEIZED.

HOWEVER, THE VERY SUCCESS OF THE COLONIAL ECONOMY MADE A MOCKERY OF SUCH EFFORTS. THERE WAS SIMPLY TOO MUCH MARITIME AND OVERLAND TRAFFIC BETWEEN TONKIN AND CHINA.

BUSINESS INTERESTS, SUCH AS THE SAIGON CHAMBER OF COMMERCE, PROTESTED THESE MEASURES.

DOUMER EXPANDED HANOI'S MUNICIPAL HEALTH SERVICES.

WHILE DISEASE WILL MAKE IT INTO THE CITY, OUR MODERN URBAN INFRASTRUCTURE WILL LESSEN ITS SEVERITY. OUR SEWERS WILL PULL THE FILTH FROM HANOI AND DISPERSE IT IN THE RED RIVER, KEEPING US SAFE AND HEALTHY.

IN THE NATIVE QUARTER, HEALTH INSPECTORS WILL GO FROM HOUSE TO HOUSE LOOKING FOR INSALUBRIOUS CONDITIONS. IF THEY FIND A PROBLEM, THEY CAN REMOVE IT.

AND BURN IT!

THE NATIVES WON'T BE TOO HAPPY ABOUT THAT!

ANYONE WHO IS SICK WILL BE QUARANTINED IN THE LAZARETTO, ALONG WITH ANYONE LIVING IN THE HOUSE.

THEY WON'T LIKE THAT.

BODIES OF THE DECEASED WILL BE IMMEDIATELY CREMATED TO PREVENT THE SPREAD OF INFECTION.

GOOD LUCK WITH THAT WITH THEIR ANCESTOR WORSHIP AND RITUALS FOR THE DEAD.

LIKE FRENCH PHILOSOPHER MICHEL FOUCAULT'S DISCUSSION OF THE BIRTH OF THE CLINIC, DOUMER'S COLONIAL PUBLIC HEALTH INITIATIVES REVEAL THE MODERN STATE'S ASPIRATIONS TO CONTROL THE VERY BODIES OF ITS SUBJECTS.

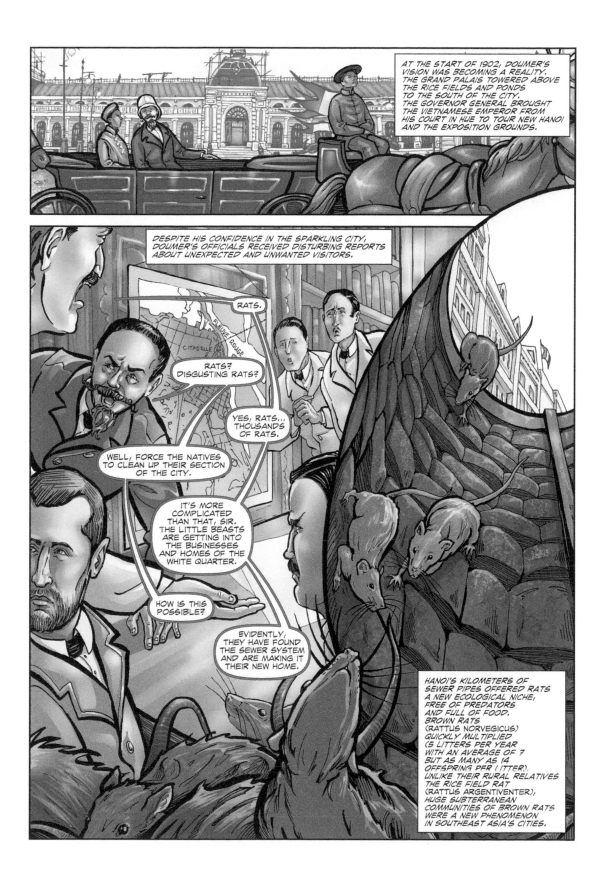

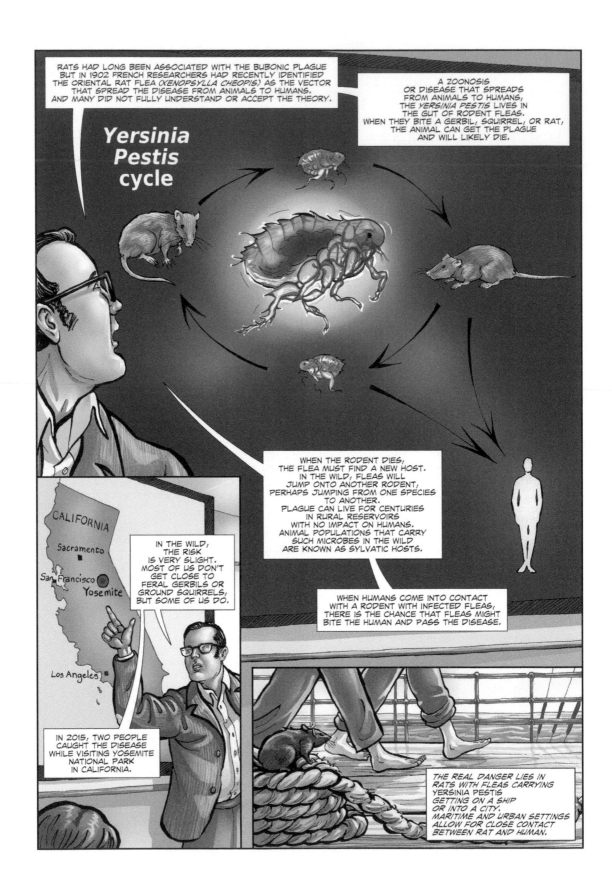

RATS HAD LONG BEEN ASSOCIATED WITH THE BUBONIC PLAGUE BUT IN 1902 FRENCH RESEARCHERS HAD RECENTLY IDENTIFIED THE ORIENTAL RAT FLEA (*XENOPSYLLA CHEOPIS*) AS THE VECTOR THAT SPREAD THE DISEASE FROM ANIMALS TO HUMANS, AND MANY DID NOT FULLY UNDERSTAND OR ACCEPT THE THEORY.

A ZOONOSIS OR DISEASE THAT SPREADS FROM ANIMALS TO HUMANS, THE *YERSINIA PESTIS* LIVES IN THE GUT OF RODENT FLEAS. WHEN THEY BITE A GERBIL, SQUIRREL, OR RAT, THE ANIMAL CAN GET THE PLAGUE AND WILL LIKELY DIE.

Yersinia Pestis cycle

WHEN THE RODENT DIES, THE FLEA MUST FIND A NEW HOST. IN THE WILD, FLEAS WILL JUMP ONTO ANOTHER RODENT, PERHAPS JUMPING FROM ONE SPECIES TO ANOTHER. PLAGUE CAN LIVE FOR CENTURIES IN RURAL RESERVOIRS WITH NO IMPACT ON HUMANS. ANIMAL POPULATIONS THAT CARRY SUCH MICROBES IN THE WILD ARE KNOWN AS SYLVATIC HOSTS.

IN THE WILD, THE RISK IS VERY SLIGHT. MOST OF US DON'T GET CLOSE TO FERAL GERBILS OR GROUND SQUIRRELS, BUT SOME OF US DO.

WHEN HUMANS COME INTO CONTACT WITH A RODENT WITH INFECTED FLEAS, THERE IS THE CHANCE THAT FLEAS MIGHT BITE THE HUMAN AND PASS THE DISEASE.

CALIFORNIA
Sacramento
San Francisco
Yosemite
Los Angeles

IN 2015, TWO PEOPLE CAUGHT THE DISEASE WHILE VISITING YOSEMITE NATIONAL PARK IN CALIFORNIA.

THE REAL DANGER LIES IN RATS WITH FLEAS CARRYING YERSINIA PESTIS GETTING ON A SHIP OR INTO A CITY. MARITIME AND URBAN SETTINGS ALLOW FOR CLOSE CONTACT BETWEEN RAT AND HUMAN.

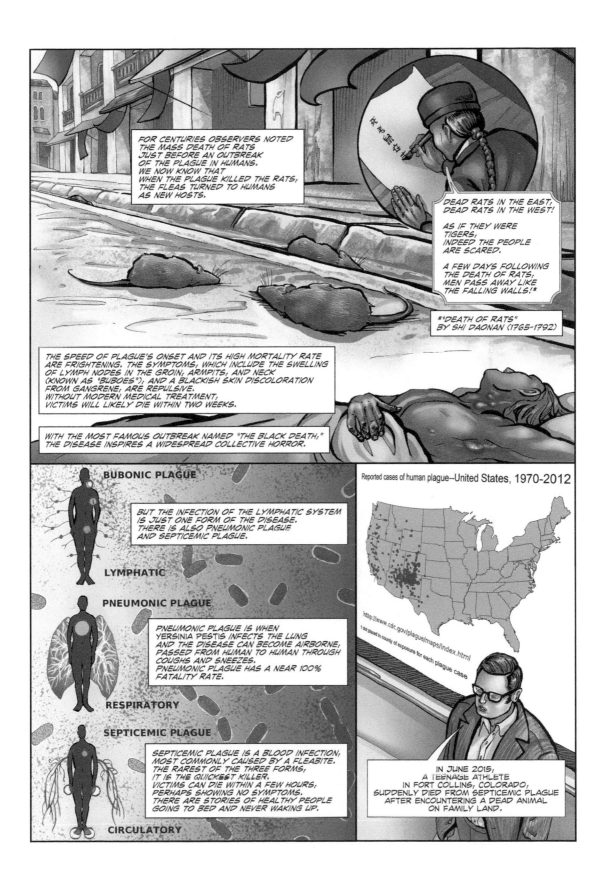

FOR CENTURIES OBSERVERS NOTED THE MASS DEATH OF RATS JUST BEFORE AN OUTBREAK OF THE PLAGUE IN HUMANS. WE NOW KNOW THAT WHEN THE PLAGUE KILLED THE RATS, THE FLEAS TURNED TO HUMANS AS NEW HOSTS.

DEAD RATS IN THE EAST, DEAD RATS IN THE WEST!

AS IF THEY WERE TIGERS, INDEED THE PEOPLE ARE SCARED.

A FEW DAYS FOLLOWING THE DEATH OF RATS, MEN PASS AWAY LIKE THE FALLING WALLS!*

*"DEATH OF RATS" BY SHI DAONAN (1765-1792)

THE SPEED OF PLAGUE'S ONSET AND ITS HIGH MORTALITY RATE ARE FRIGHTENING. THE SYMPTOMS, WHICH INCLUDE THE SWELLING OF LYMPH NODES IN THE GROIN, ARMPITS, AND NECK (KNOWN AS "BUBOES"), AND A BLACKISH SKIN DISCOLORATION FROM GANGRENE, ARE REPULSIVE. WITHOUT MODERN MEDICAL TREATMENT, VICTIMS WILL LIKELY DIE WITHIN TWO WEEKS.

WITH THE MOST FAMOUS OUTBREAK NAMED "THE BLACK DEATH," THE DISEASE INSPIRES A WIDESPREAD COLLECTIVE HORROR.

BUBONIC PLAGUE

BUT THE INFECTION OF THE LYMPHATIC SYSTEM IS JUST ONE FORM OF THE DISEASE. THERE IS ALSO PNEUMONIC PLAGUE AND SEPTICEMIC PLAGUE.

LYMPHATIC

PNEUMONIC PLAGUE

PNEUMONIC PLAGUE IS WHEN YERSINIA PESTIS INFECTS THE LUNG AND THE DISEASE CAN BECOME AIRBORNE, PASSED FROM HUMAN TO HUMAN THROUGH COUGHS AND SNEEZES. PNEUMONIC PLAGUE HAS A NEAR 100% FATALITY RATE.

RESPIRATORY

SEPTICEMIC PLAGUE

SEPTICEMIC PLAGUE IS A BLOOD INFECTION, MOST COMMONLY CAUSED BY A FLEABITE. THE RAREST OF THE THREE FORMS, IT IS THE QUICKEST KILLER. VICTIMS CAN DIE WITHIN A FEW HOURS, PERHAPS SHOWING NO SYMPTOMS. THERE ARE STORIES OF HEALTHY PEOPLE GOING TO BED AND NEVER WAKING UP.

CIRCULATORY

Reported cases of human plague--United States, 1970-2012

http://www.cdc.gov/plague/maps/index.html

1 dot placed in county of exposure for each plague case

IN JUNE 2015, A TEENAGE ATHLETE IN FORT COLLINS, COLORADO, SUDDENLY DIED FROM SEPTICEMIC PLAGUE AFTER ENCOUNTERING A DEAD ANIMAL ON FAMILY LAND.

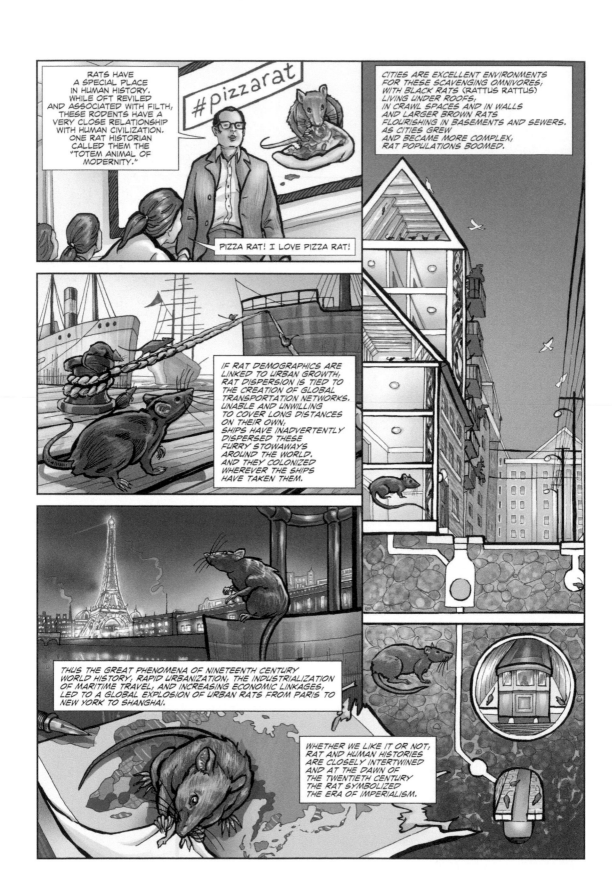

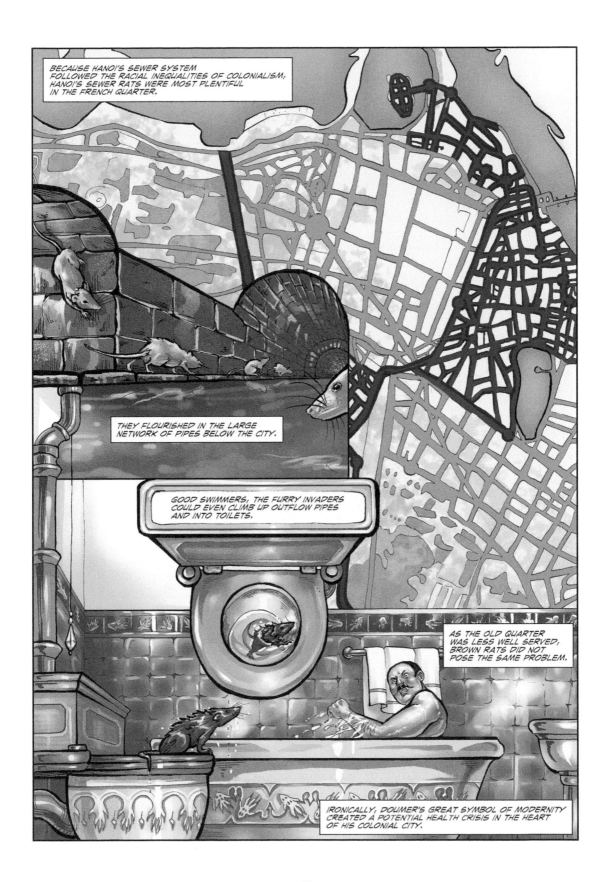

BECAUSE HANOI'S SEWER SYSTEM FOLLOWED THE RACIAL INEQUALITIES OF COLONIALISM, HANOI'S SEWER RATS WERE MOST PLENTIFUL IN THE FRENCH QUARTER.

THEY FLOURISHED IN THE LARGE NETWORK OF PIPES BELOW THE CITY.

GOOD SWIMMERS, THE FURRY INVADERS COULD EVEN CLIMB UP OUTFLOW PIPES AND INTO TOILETS.

AS THE OLD QUARTER WAS LESS WELL SERVED, BROWN RATS DID NOT POSE THE SAME PROBLEM.

IRONICALLY, DOUMER'S GREAT SYMBOL OF MODERNITY CREATED A POTENTIAL HEALTH CRISIS IN THE HEART OF HIS COLONIAL CITY.

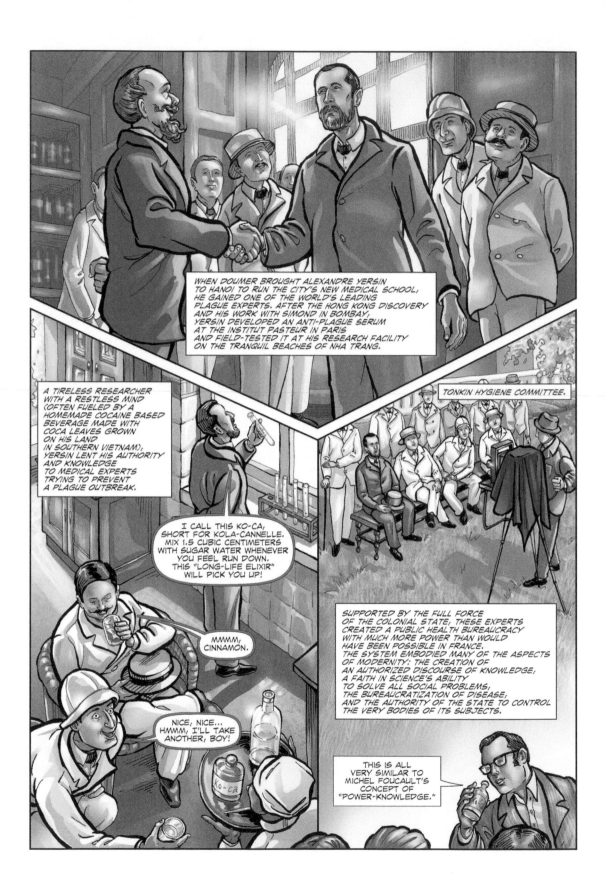

WHEN DOUMER BROUGHT ALEXANDRE YERSIN TO HANOI TO RUN THE CITY'S NEW MEDICAL SCHOOL, HE GAINED ONE OF THE WORLD'S LEADING PLAGUE EXPERTS. AFTER THE HONG KONG DISCOVERY AND HIS WORK WITH SIMOND IN BOMBAY, YERSIN DEVELOPED AN ANTI-PLAGUE SERUM AT THE INSTITUT PASTEUR IN PARIS AND FIELD-TESTED IT AT HIS RESEARCH FACILITY ON THE TRANQUIL BEACHES OF NHA TRANG.

A TIRELESS RESEARCHER WITH A RESTLESS MIND (OFTEN FUELED BY A HOMEMADE COCAINE BASED BEVERAGE MADE WITH COCA LEAVES GROWN ON HIS LAND IN SOUTHERN VIETNAM), YERSIN LENT HIS AUTHORITY AND KNOWLEDGE TO MEDICAL EXPERTS TRYING TO PREVENT A PLAGUE OUTBREAK.

I CALL THIS KO-CA, SHORT FOR KOLA-CANNELLE. MIX 1.5 CUBIC CENTIMETERS WITH SUGAR WATER WHENEVER YOU FEEL RUN DOWN. THIS "LONG-LIFE ELIXIR" WILL PICK YOU UP!

MMMM, CINNAMON.

NICE, NICE... HMMM, I'LL TAKE ANOTHER, BOY!

TONKIN HYGIENE COMMITTEE.

SUPPORTED BY THE FULL FORCE OF THE COLONIAL STATE, THESE EXPERTS CREATED A PUBLIC HEALTH BUREAUCRACY WITH MUCH MORE POWER THAN WOULD HAVE BEEN POSSIBLE IN FRANCE. THE SYSTEM EMBODIED MANY OF THE ASPECTS OF MODERNITY: THE CREATION OF AN AUTHORIZED DISCOURSE OF KNOWLEDGE; A FAITH IN SCIENCE'S ABILITY TO SOLVE ALL SOCIAL PROBLEMS; THE BUREAUCRATIZATION OF DISEASE; AND THE AUTHORITY OF THE STATE TO CONTROL THE VERY BODIES OF ITS SUBJECTS.

THIS IS ALL VERY SIMILAR TO MICHEL FOUCAULT'S CONCEPT OF "POWER-KNOWLEDGE."

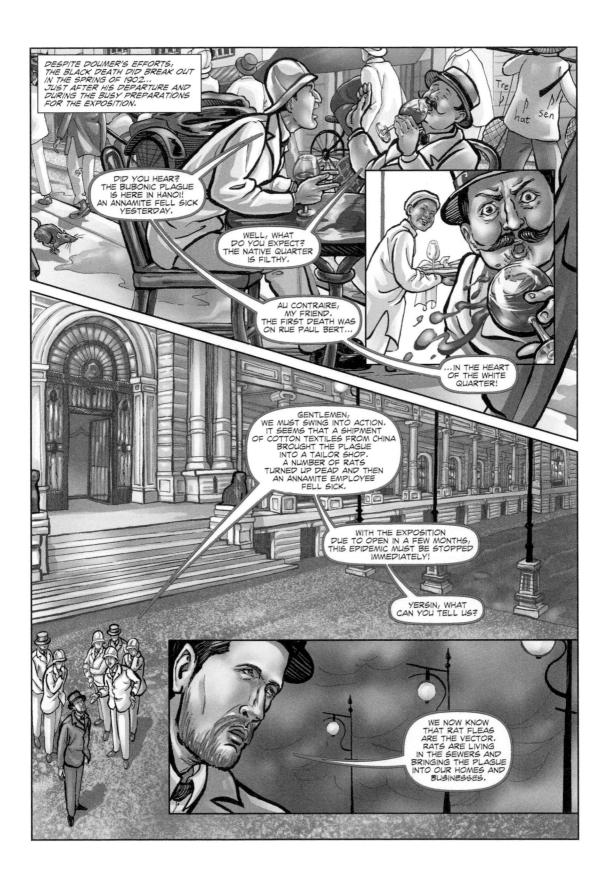

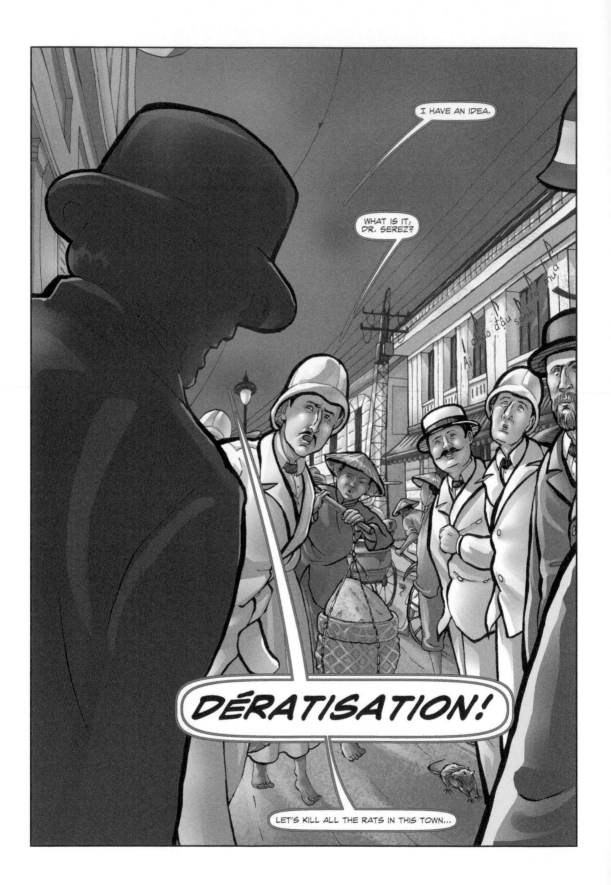

CHAPTER 6
THE GREAT RAT HUNT

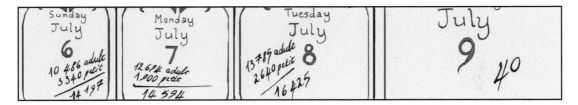

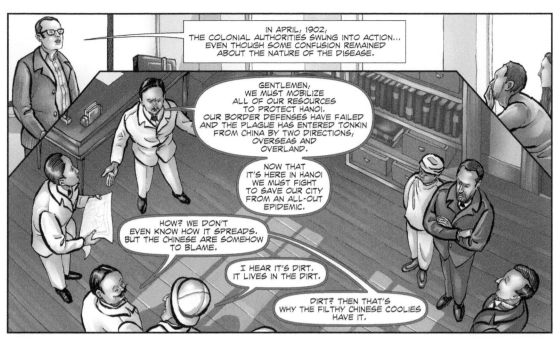

IN APRIL, 1902, THE COLONIAL AUTHORITIES SWUNG INTO ACTION... EVEN THOUGH SOME CONFUSION REMAINED ABOUT THE NATURE OF THE DISEASE.

GENTLEMEN, WE MUST MOBILIZE ALL OF OUR RESOURCES TO PROTECT HANOI. OUR BORDER DEFENSES HAVE FAILED AND THE PLAGUE HAS ENTERED TONKIN FROM CHINA BY TWO DIRECTIONS, OVERSEAS AND OVERLAND.

NOW THAT IT'S HERE IN HANOI WE MUST FIGHT TO SAVE OUR CITY FROM AN ALL-OUT EPIDEMIC.

HOW? WE DON'T EVEN KNOW HOW IT SPREADS. BUT THE CHINESE ARE SOMEHOW TO BLAME.

I HEAR IT'S DIRT. IT LIVES IN THE DIRT.

DIRT? THEN THAT'S WHY THE FILTHY CHINESE COOLIES HAVE IT.

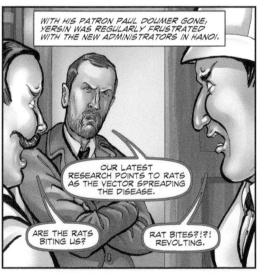

WITH HIS PATRON PAUL DOUMER GONE, YERSIN WAS REGULARLY FRUSTRATED WITH THE NEW ADMINISTRATORS IN HANOI.

OUR LATEST RESEARCH POINTS TO RATS AS THE VECTOR SPREADING THE DISEASE.

ARE THE RATS BITING US?

RAT BITES?!?! REVOLTING.

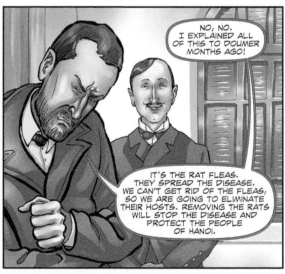

NO, NO. I EXPLAINED ALL OF THIS TO DOUMER MONTHS AGO!

IT'S THE RAT FLEAS. THEY SPREAD THE DISEASE. WE CAN'T GET RID OF THE FLEAS, SO WE ARE GOING TO ELIMINATE THEIR HOSTS. REMOVING THE RATS WILL STOP THE DISEASE AND PROTECT THE PEOPLE OF HANOI.

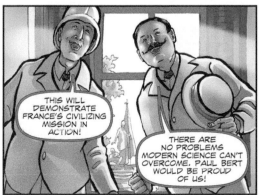

THIS WILL DEMONSTRATE FRANCE'S CIVILIZING MISSION IN ACTION!

THERE ARE NO PROBLEMS MODERN SCIENCE CAN'T OVERCOME. PAUL BERT WOULD BE PROUD OF US!

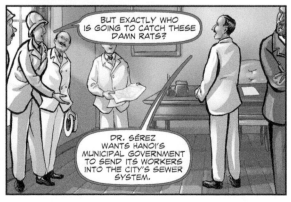

BUT EXACTLY WHO IS GOING TO CATCH THESE DAMN RATS?

DR. SÉREZ WANTS HANOI'S MUNICIPAL GOVERNMENT TO SEND ITS WORKERS INTO THE CITY'S SEWER SYSTEM.

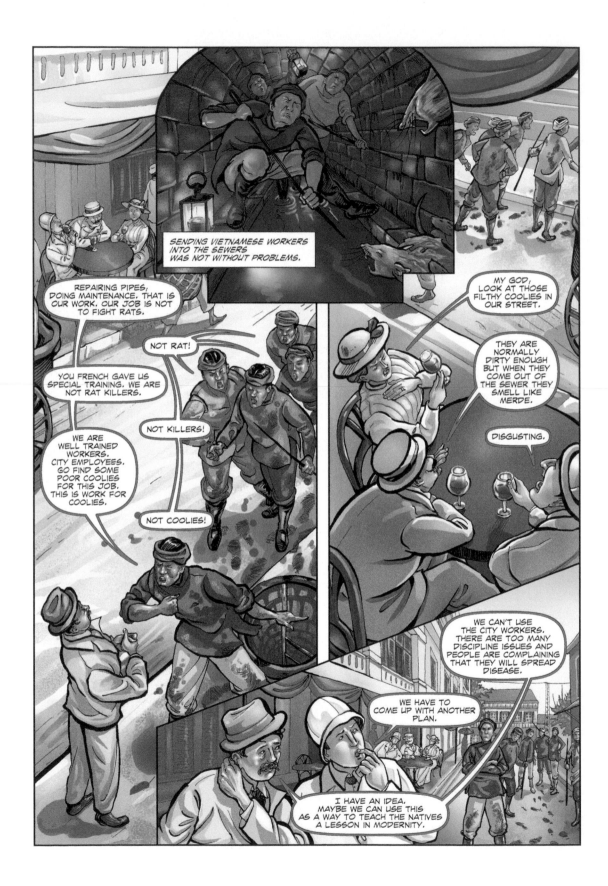

88

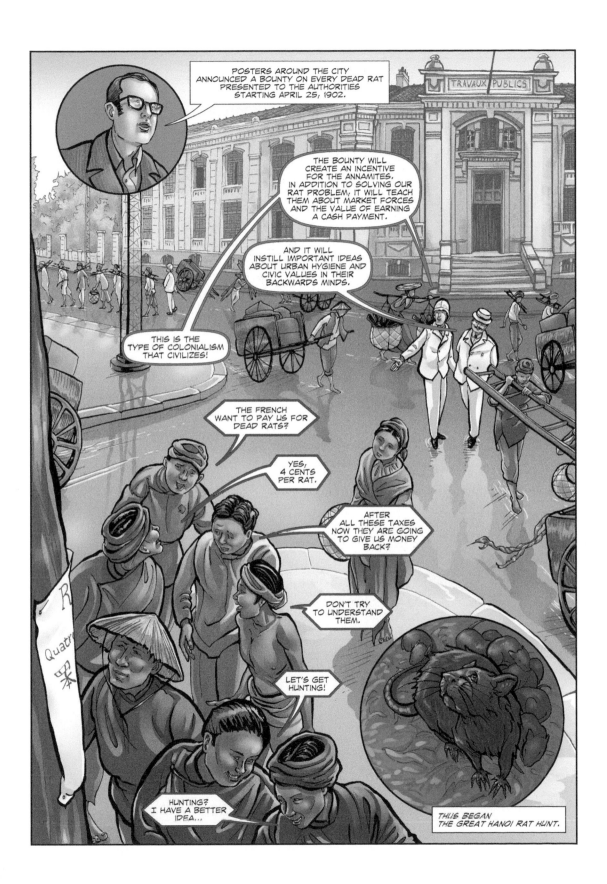

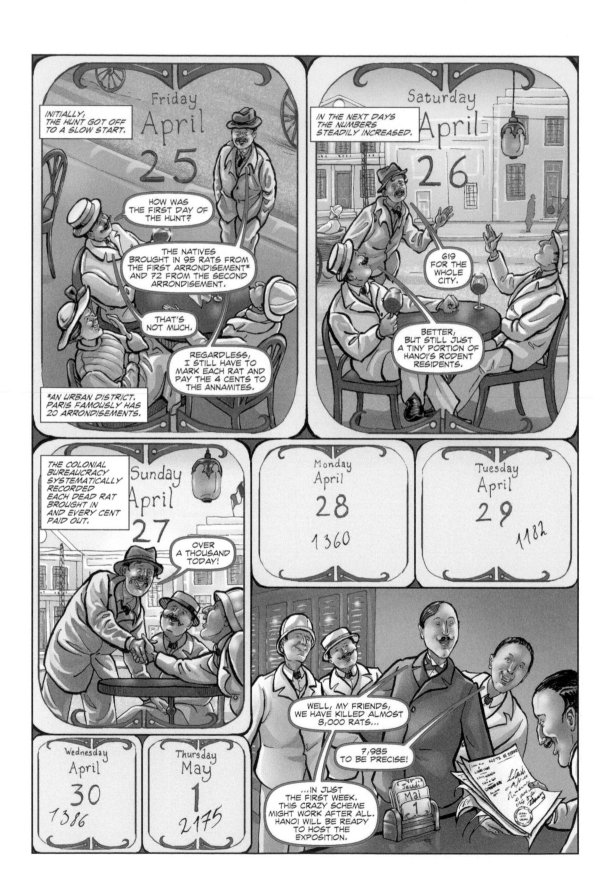

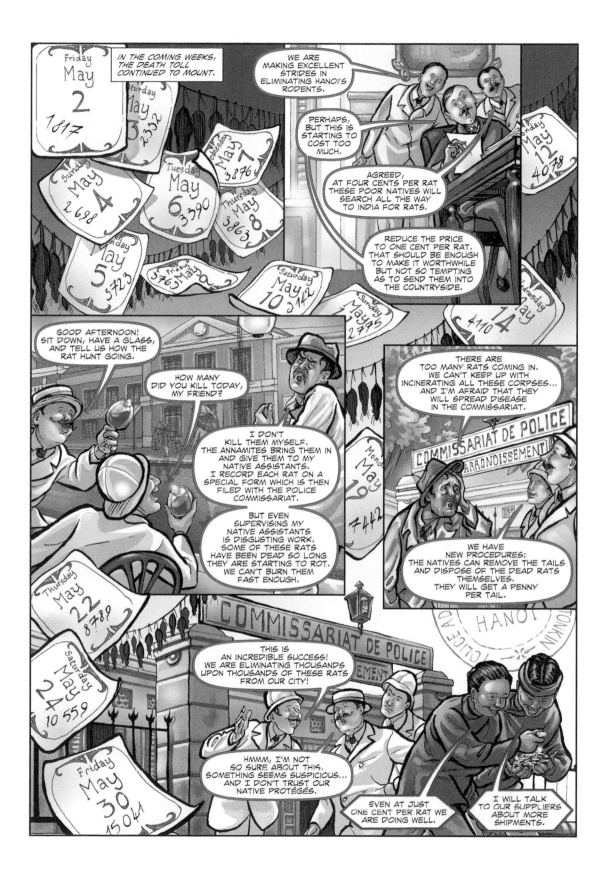

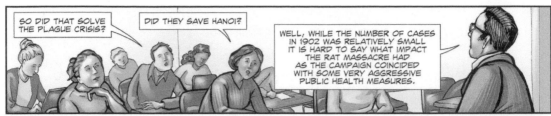

SO DID THAT SOLVE THE PLAGUE CRISIS?

DID THEY SAVE HANOI?

WELL, WHILE THE NUMBER OF CASES IN 1902 WAS RELATIVELY SMALL IT IS HARD TO SAY WHAT IMPACT THE RAT MASSACRE HAD AS THE CAMPAIGN COINCIDED WITH SOME VERY AGGRESSIVE PUBLIC HEALTH MEASURES.

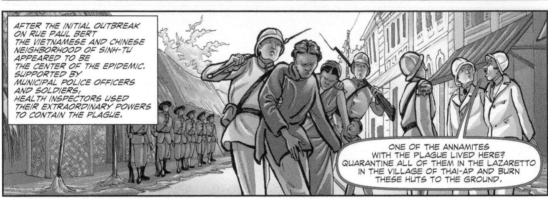

AFTER THE INITIAL OUTBREAK ON RUE PAUL BERT THE VIETNAMESE AND CHINESE NEIGHBORHOOD OF SINH-TU APPEARED TO BE THE CENTER OF THE EPIDEMIC. SUPPORTED BY MUNICIPAL POLICE OFFICERS AND SOLDIERS, HEALTH INSPECTORS USED THEIR EXTRAORDINARY POWERS TO CONTAIN THE PLAGUE.

ONE OF THE ANNAMITES WITH THE PLAGUE LIVED HERE? QUARANTINE ALL OF THEM IN THE LAZARETTO IN THE VILLAGE OF THAI-AP AND BURN THESE HUTS TO THE GROUND.

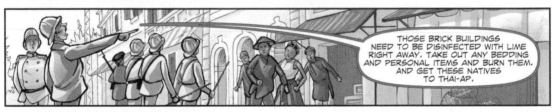

THOSE BRICK BUILDINGS NEED TO BE DISINFECTED WITH LIME RIGHT AWAY. TAKE OUT ANY BEDDING AND PERSONAL ITEMS AND BURN THEM. AND GET THESE NATIVES TO THAI-AP.

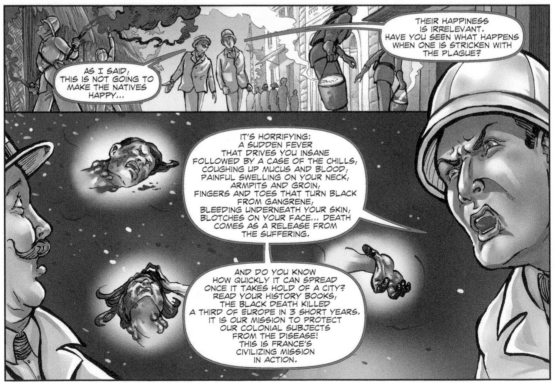

THEIR HAPPINESS IS IRRELEVANT. HAVE YOU SEEN WHAT HAPPENS WHEN ONE IS STRICKEN WITH THE PLAGUE?

AS I SAID, THIS IS NOT GOING TO MAKE THE NATIVES HAPPY...

IT'S HORRIFYING: A SUDDEN FEVER THAT DRIVES YOU INSANE FOLLOWED BY A CASE OF THE CHILLS, COUGHING UP MUCUS AND BLOOD, PAINFUL SWELLING ON YOUR NECK, ARMPITS AND GROIN, FINGERS AND TOES THAT TURN BLACK FROM GANGRENE, BLEEDING UNDERNEATH YOUR SKIN; BLOTCHES ON YOUR FACE... DEATH COMES AS A RELEASE FROM THE SUFFERING.

AND DO YOU KNOW HOW QUICKLY IT CAN SPREAD ONCE IT TAKES HOLD OF A CITY? READ YOUR HISTORY BOOKS, THE BLACK DEATH KILLED A THIRD OF EUROPE IN 3 SHORT YEARS. IT IS OUR MISSION TO PROTECT OUR COLONIAL SUBJECTS FROM THE DISEASE! THIS IS FRANCE'S CIVILIZING MISSION IN ACTION.

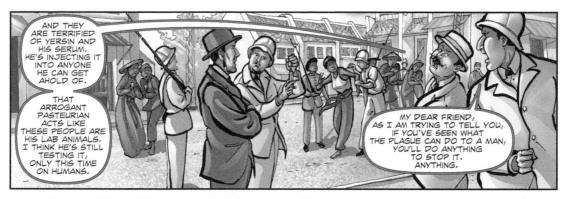

AND THEY ARE TERRIFIED OF YERSIN AND HIS SERUM. HE'S INJECTING IT INTO ANYONE HE CAN GET AHOLD OF.

THAT ARROGANT PASTEURIAN ACTS LIKE THESE PEOPLE ARE HIS LAB ANIMALS. I THINK HE'S STILL TESTING IT, ONLY THIS TIME ON HUMANS.

MY DEAR FRIEND, AS I AM TRYING TO TELL YOU, IF YOU'VE SEEN WHAT THE PLAGUE CAN DO TO A MAN, YOU'LL DO ANYTHING TO STOP IT. ANYTHING.

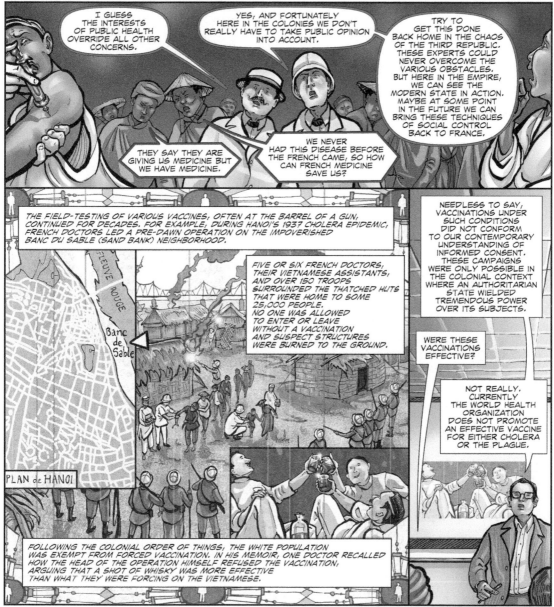

I GUESS THE INTERESTS OF PUBLIC HEALTH OVERRIDE ALL OTHER CONCERNS.

YES, AND FORTUNATELY HERE IN THE COLONIES WE DON'T REALLY HAVE TO TAKE PUBLIC OPINION INTO ACCOUNT.

TRY TO GET THIS DONE BACK HOME IN THE CHAOS OF THE THIRD REPUBLIC. THESE EXPERTS COULD NEVER OVERCOME THE VARIOUS OBSTACLES. BUT HERE IN THE EMPIRE, WE CAN SEE THE MODERN STATE IN ACTION. MAYBE AT SOME POINT IN THE FUTURE WE CAN BRING THESE TECHNIQUES OF SOCIAL CONTROL BACK TO FRANCE.

THEY SAY THEY ARE GIVING US MEDICINE BUT WE HAVE MEDICINE.

WE NEVER HAD THIS DISEASE BEFORE THE FRENCH CAME, SO HOW CAN FRENCH MEDICINE SAVE US?

THE FIELD-TESTING OF VARIOUS VACCINES, OFTEN AT THE BARREL OF A GUN, CONTINUED FOR DECADES. FOR EXAMPLE, DURING HANOI'S 1937 CHOLERA EPIDEMIC, FRENCH DOCTORS LED A PRE-DAWN OPERATION ON THE IMPOVERISHED BANC DU SABLE (SAND BANK) NEIGHBORHOOD.

NEEDLESS TO SAY, VACCINATIONS UNDER SUCH CONDITIONS DID NOT CONFORM TO OUR CONTEMPORARY UNDERSTANDING OF INFORMED CONSENT. THESE CAMPAIGNS WERE ONLY POSSIBLE IN THE COLONIAL CONTEXT WHERE AN AUTHORITARIAN STATE WIELDED TREMENDOUS POWER OVER ITS SUBJECTS.

FIVE OR SIX FRENCH DOCTORS, THEIR VIETNAMESE ASSISTANTS, AND OVER 150 TROOPS SURROUNDED THE THATCHED HUTS THAT WERE HOME TO SOME 25,000 PEOPLE. NO ONE WAS ALLOWED TO ENTER OR LEAVE WITHOUT A VACCINATION AND SUSPECT STRUCTURES WERE BURNED TO THE GROUND.

WERE THESE VACCINATIONS EFFECTIVE?

NOT REALLY. CURRENTLY THE WORLD HEALTH ORGANIZATION DOES NOT PROMOTE AN EFFECTIVE VACCINE FOR EITHER CHOLERA OR THE PLAGUE.

FLEUVE ROUGE

Banc de Sable

PLAN de HANOI

FOLLOWING THE COLONIAL ORDER OF THINGS, THE WHITE POPULATION WAS EXEMPT FROM FORCED VACCINATION. IN HIS MEMOIR, ONE DOCTOR RECALLED HOW THE HEAD OF THE OPERATION HIMSELF REFUSED THE VACCINATION, ARGUING THAT A SHOT OF WHISKY WAS MORE EFFECTIVE THAN WHAT THEY WERE FORCING ON THE VIETNAMESE.

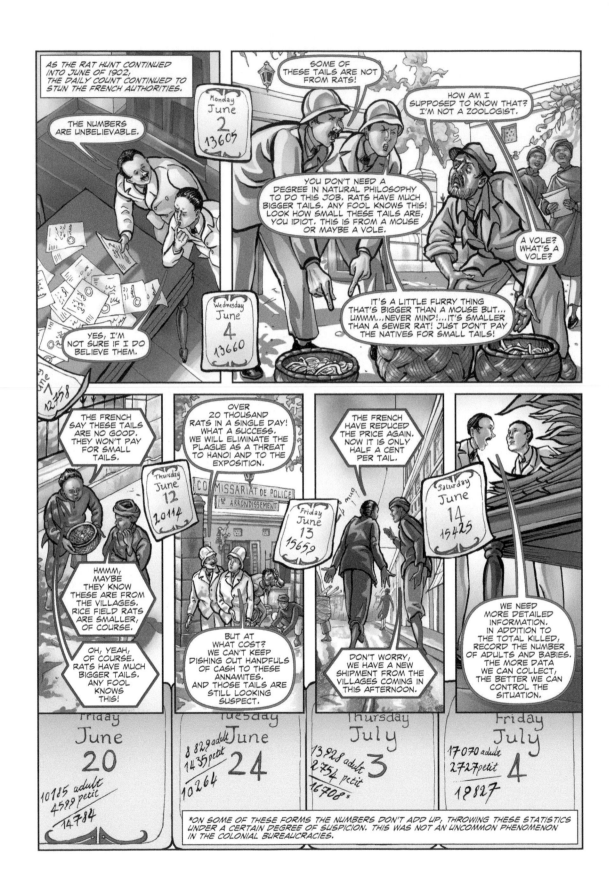

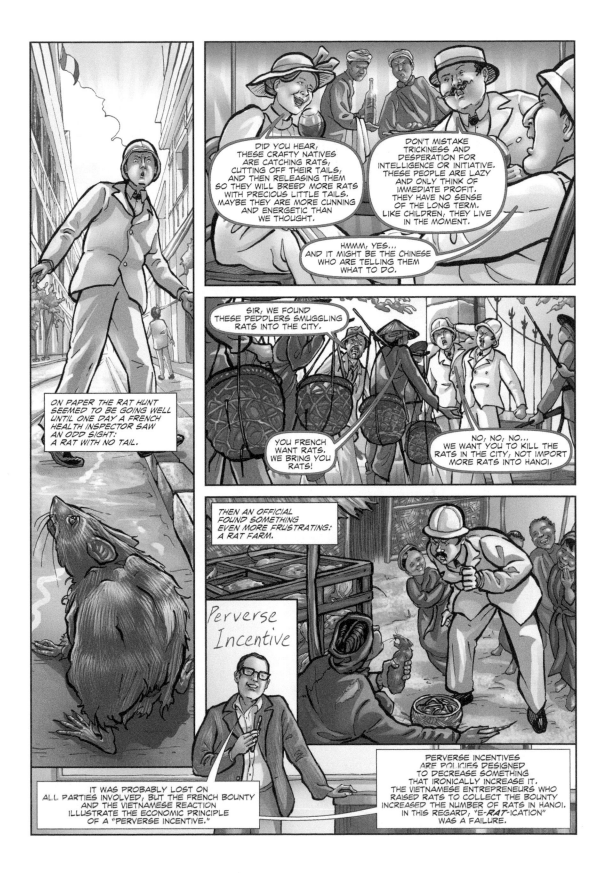

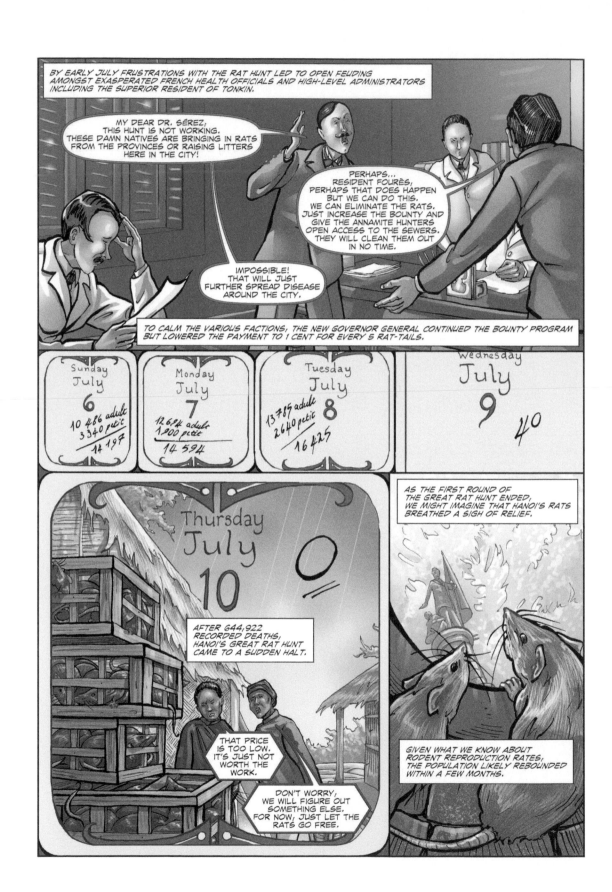

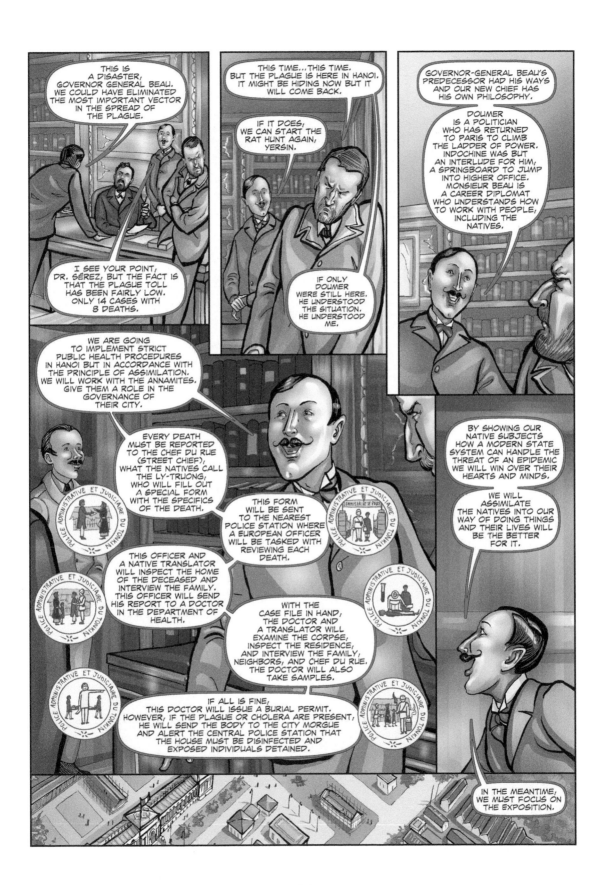

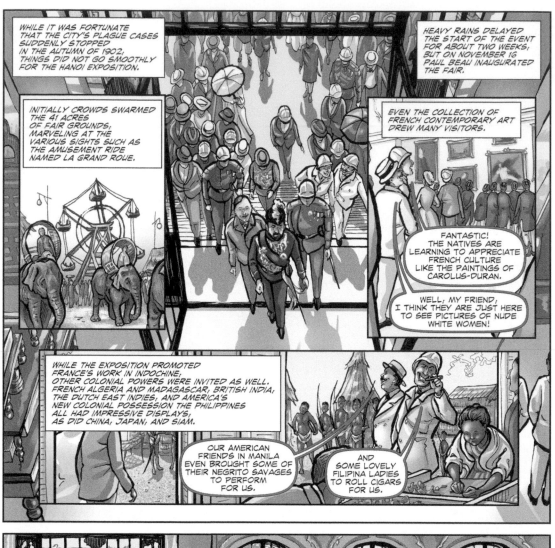

WHILE IT WAS FORTUNATE THAT THE CITY'S PLAGUE CASES SUDDENLY STOPPED IN THE AUTUMN OF 1902, THINGS DID NOT GO SMOOTHLY FOR THE HANOI EXPOSITION.

HEAVY RAINS DELAYED THE START OF THE EVENT FOR ABOUT TWO WEEKS, BUT ON NOVEMBER 16 PAUL BEAU INAUGURATED THE FAIR.

INITIALLY CROWDS SWARMED THE 41 ACRES OF FAIR GROUNDS, MARVELING AT THE VARIOUS SIGHTS SUCH AS THE AMUSEMENT RIDE NAMED LA GRAND ROUE.

EVEN THE COLLECTION OF FRENCH CONTEMPORARY ART DREW MANY VISITORS.

FANTASTIC! THE NATIVES ARE LEARNING TO APPRECIATE FRENCH CULTURE LIKE THE PAINTINGS OF CAROLUS-DURAN.

WELL, MY FRIEND, I THINK THEY ARE JUST HERE TO SEE PICTURES OF NUDE WHITE WOMEN!

WHILE THE EXPOSITION PROMOTED FRANCE'S WORK IN INDOCHINE, OTHER COLONIAL POWERS WERE INVITED AS WELL. FRENCH ALGERIA AND MADAGASCAR, BRITISH INDIA, THE DUTCH EAST INDIES, AND AMERICA'S NEW COLONIAL POSSESSION THE PHILIPPINES ALL HAD IMPRESSIVE DISPLAYS, AS DID CHINA, JAPAN, AND SIAM.

OUR AMERICAN FRIENDS IN MANILA EVEN BROUGHT SOME OF THEIR NEGRITO SAVAGES TO PERFORM FOR US.

AND SOME LOVELY FILIPINA LADIES TO ROLL CIGARS FOR US.

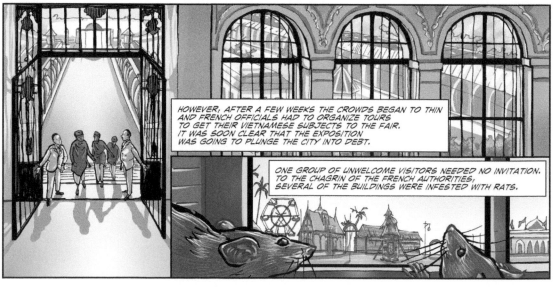

HOWEVER, AFTER A FEW WEEKS THE CROWDS BEGAN TO THIN AND FRENCH OFFICIALS HAD TO ORGANIZE TOURS TO GET THEIR VIETNAMESE SUBJECTS TO THE FAIR. IT WAS SOON CLEAR THAT THE EXPOSITION WAS GOING TO PLUNGE THE CITY INTO DEBT.

ONE GROUP OF UNWELCOME VISITORS NEEDED NO INVITATION. TO THE CHAGRIN OF THE FRENCH AUTHORITIES, SEVERAL OF THE BUILDINGS WERE INFESTED WITH RATS.

CHAPTER 7
THE BEST LAID SCHEMES OF RATS AND MEN

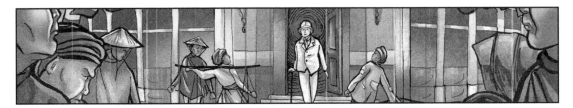

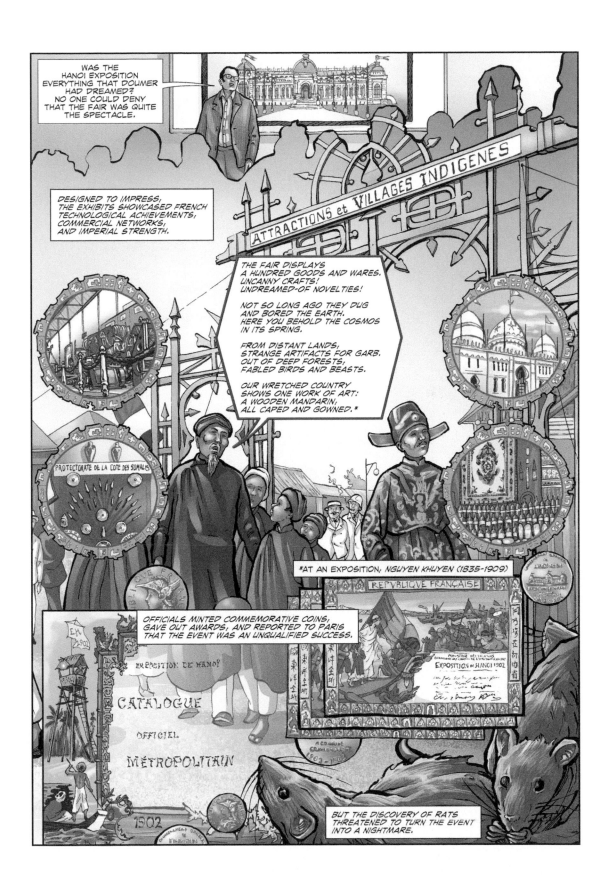

WAS THE HANOI EXPOSITION EVERYTHING THAT DOUMER HAD DREAMED? NO ONE COULD DENY THAT THE FAIR WAS QUITE THE SPECTACLE.

DESIGNED TO IMPRESS, THE EXHIBITS SHOWCASED FRENCH TECHNOLOGICAL ACHIEVEMENTS, COMMERCIAL NETWORKS, AND IMPERIAL STRENGTH.

ATTRACTIONS et VILLAGES INDIGENES

THE FAIR DISPLAYS
A HUNDRED GOODS AND WARES.
UNCANNY CRAFTS!
UNDREAMED-OF NOVELTIES!

NOT SO LONG AGO THEY DUG
AND BORED THE EARTH.
HERE YOU BEHOLD THE COSMOS
IN ITS SPRING.

FROM DISTANT LANDS,
STRANGE ARTIFACTS FOR GARB.
OUT OF DEEP FORESTS,
FABLED BIRDS AND BEASTS.

OUR WRETCHED COUNTRY
SHOWS ONE WORK OF ART:
A WOODEN MANDARIN,
ALL CAPED AND GOWNED. *

PROTECTORATE DE LA COTE DES SOMALIS

*AT AN EXPOSITION, NGUYEN KHUYEN (1835-1909)

OFFICIALS MINTED COMMEMORATIVE COINS, GAVE OUT AWARDS, AND REPORTED TO PARIS THAT THE EVENT WAS AN UNQUALIFIED SUCCESS.

REPVBLIQVE FRANÇAISE

EXPOSITION DE HANOI

CATALOGUE

OFFICIEL

MÉTROPOLITAIN

1902

BUT THE DISCOVERY OF RATS THREATENED TO TURN THE EVENT INTO A NIGHTMARE.

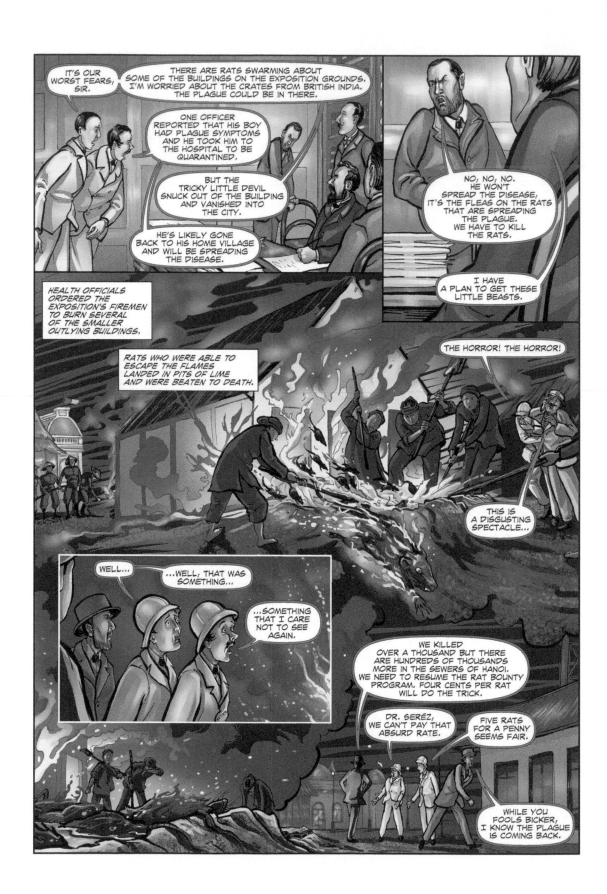

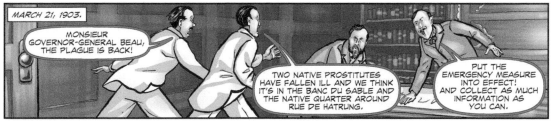

MARCH 21, 1903.

MONSIEUR GOVERNOR-GENERAL BEAU, THE PLAGUE IS BACK!

TWO NATIVE PROSTITUTES HAVE FALLEN ILL AND WE THINK IT'S IN THE BANC DU SABLE AND THE NATIVE QUARTER AROUND RUE DE HATRUNG.

PUT THE EMERGENCY MEASURE INTO EFFECT! AND COLLECT AS MUCH INFORMATION AS YOU CAN.

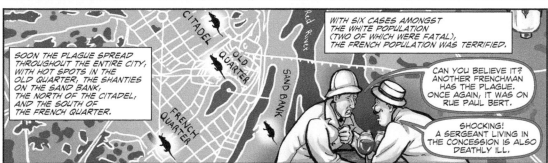

SOON THE PLAGUE SPREAD THROUGHOUT THE ENTIRE CITY, WITH HOT SPOTS IN THE OLD QUARTER, THE SHANTIES ON THE SAND BANK, THE NORTH OF THE CITADEL, AND THE SOUTH OF THE FRENCH QUARTER.

CITADEL

OLD QUARTER

FRENCH QUARTER

SAND BANK

WITH SIX CASES AMONGST THE WHITE POPULATION (TWO OF WHICH WERE FATAL), THE FRENCH POPULATION WAS TERRIFIED.

CAN YOU BELIEVE IT? ANOTHER FRENCHMAN HAS THE PLAGUE. ONCE AGAIN, IT WAS ON RUE PAUL BERT.

SHOCKING! A SERGEANT LIVING IN THE CONCESSION IS ALSO DEATHLY ILL.

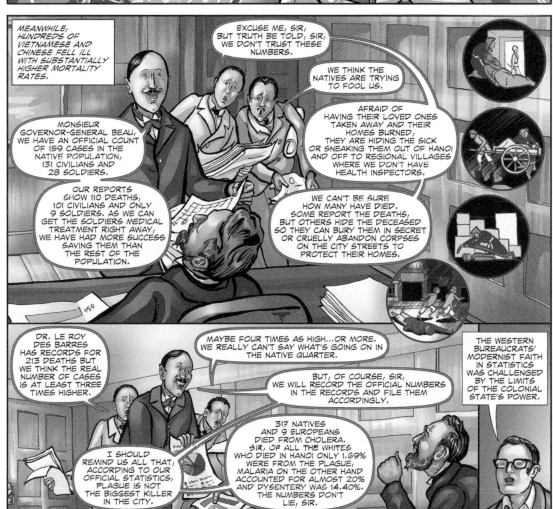

MEANWHILE, HUNDREDS OF VIETNAMESE AND CHINESE FELL ILL WITH SUBSTANTIALLY HIGHER MORTALITY RATES.

EXCUSE ME, SIR, BUT TRUTH BE TOLD, SIR, WE DON'T TRUST THESE NUMBERS.

WE THINK THE NATIVES ARE TRYING TO FOOL US.

AFRAID OF HAVING THEIR LOVED ONES TAKEN AWAY AND THEIR HOMES BURNED, THEY ARE HIDING THE SICK OR SNEAKING THEM OUT OF HANOI AND OFF TO REGIONAL VILLAGES WHERE WE DON'T HAVE HEALTH INSPECTORS.

MONSIEUR GOVERNOR-GENERAL BEAU, WE HAVE AN OFFICIAL COUNT OF 159 CASES IN THE NATIVE POPULATION, 131 CIVILIANS AND 28 SOLDIERS.

OUR REPORTS SHOW 110 DEATHS, 101 CIVILIANS AND ONLY 9 SOLDIERS. AS WE CAN GET THE SOLDIERS MEDICAL TREATMENT RIGHT AWAY, WE HAVE HAD MORE SUCCESS SAVING THEM THAN THE REST OF THE POPULATION.

WE CAN'T BE SURE HOW MANY HAVE DIED. SOME REPORT THE DEATHS, BUT OTHERS HIDE THE DECEASED SO THEY CAN BURY THEM IN SECRET OR CRUELLY ABANDON CORPSES ON THE CITY STREETS TO PROTECT THEIR HOMES.

DR. LE ROY DES BARRES HAS RECORDS FOR 213 DEATHS BUT WE THINK THE REAL NUMBER OF CASES IS AT LEAST THREE TIMES HIGHER.

MAYBE FOUR TIMES AS HIGH...OR MORE. WE REALLY CAN'T SAY WHAT'S GOING ON IN THE NATIVE QUARTER.

BUT, OF COURSE, SIR, WE WILL RECORD THE OFFICIAL NUMBERS IN THE RECORDS AND FILE THEM ACCORDINGLY.

THE WESTERN BUREAUCRATS' MODERNIST FAITH IN STATISTICS WAS CHALLENGED BY THE LIMITS OF THE COLONIAL STATE'S POWER.

I SHOULD REMIND US ALL THAT, ACCORDING TO OUR OFFICIAL STATISTICS, PLAGUE IS NOT THE BIGGEST KILLER IN THE CITY.

317 NATIVES AND 9 EUROPEANS DIED FROM CHOLERA. SIR, OF ALL THE WHITES WHO DIED IN HANOI ONLY 1.69% WERE FROM THE PLAGUE; MALARIA ON THE OTHER HAND ACCOUNTED FOR ALMOST 20% AND DYSENTERY WAS 14.40%. THE NUMBERS DON'T LIE, SIR.

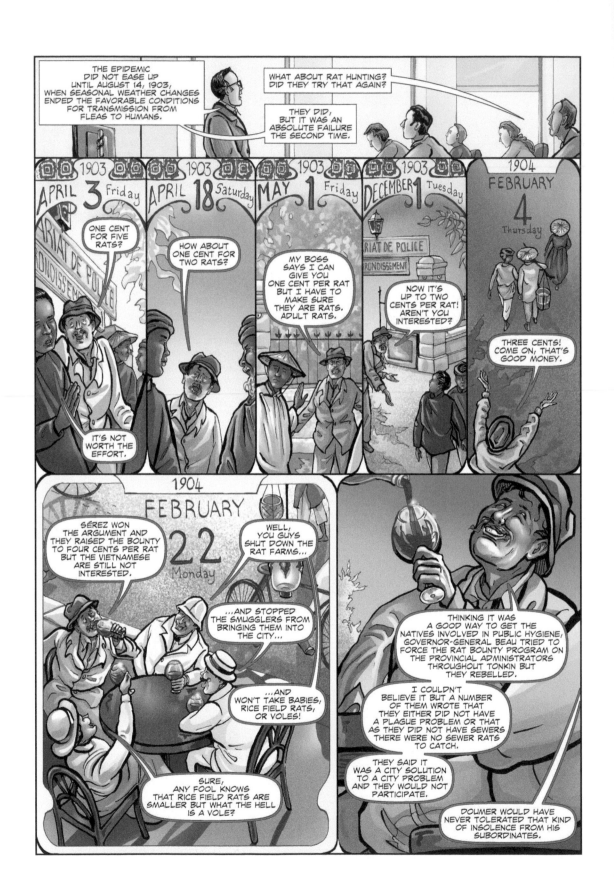

THE EPIDEMIC DID NOT EASE UP UNTIL AUGUST 14, 1903, WHEN SEASONAL WEATHER CHANGES ENDED THE FAVORABLE CONDITIONS FOR TRANSMISSION FROM FLEAS TO HUMANS.

WHAT ABOUT RAT HUNTING? DID THEY TRY THAT AGAIN?

THEY DID, BUT IT WAS AN ABSOLUTE FAILURE THE SECOND TIME.

1903 APRIL 3 Friday

ONE CENT FOR FIVE RATS?

IT'S NOT WORTH THE EFFORT.

1903 APRIL 18 Saturday

HOW ABOUT ONE CENT FOR TWO RATS?

1903 MAY 1 Friday

MY BOSS SAYS I CAN GIVE YOU ONE CENT PER RAT BUT I HAVE TO MAKE SURE THEY ARE RATS. ADULT RATS.

1903 DECEMBER 1 Tuesday

NOW IT'S UP TO TWO CENTS PER RAT! AREN'T YOU INTERESTED?

1904 FEBRUARY 4 Thursday

THREE CENTS! COME ON, THAT'S GOOD MONEY.

1904 FEBRUARY 22 Monday

SÉREZ WON THE ARGUMENT AND THEY RAISED THE BOUNTY TO FOUR CENTS PER RAT BUT THE VIETNAMESE ARE STILL NOT INTERESTED.

WELL, YOU GUYS SHUT DOWN THE RAT FARMS...

...AND STOPPED THE SMUGGLERS FROM BRINGING THEM INTO THE CITY...

...AND WON'T TAKE BABIES, RICE FIELD RATS, OR VOLES!

SURE, ANY FOOL KNOWS THAT RICE FIELD RATS ARE SMALLER BUT WHAT THE HELL IS A VOLE?

THINKING IT WAS A GOOD WAY TO GET THE NATIVES INVOLVED IN PUBLIC HYGIENE, GOVERNOR-GENERAL BEAU TRIED TO FORCE THE RAT BOUNTY PROGRAM ON THE PROVINCIAL ADMINISTRATORS THROUGHOUT TONKIN BUT THEY REBELLED.

I COULDN'T BELIEVE IT BUT A NUMBER OF THEM WROTE THAT THEY EITHER DID NOT HAVE A PLAGUE PROBLEM OR THAT AS THEY DID NOT HAVE SEWERS THERE WERE NO SEWER RATS TO CATCH.

THEY SAID IT WAS A CITY SOLUTION TO A CITY PROBLEM AND THEY WOULD NOT PARTICIPATE.

DOUMER WOULD HAVE NEVER TOLERATED THAT KIND OF INSOLENCE FROM HIS SUBORDINATES.

104

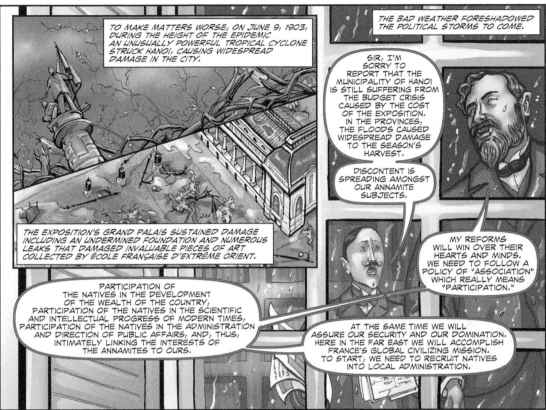

TO MAKE MATTERS WORSE, ON JUNE 9, 1903, DURING THE HEIGHT OF THE EPIDEMIC AN UNUSUALLY POWERFUL TROPICAL CYCLONE STRUCK HANOI, CAUSING WIDESPREAD DAMAGE IN THE CITY.

THE EXPOSITION'S GRAND PALAIS SUSTAINED DAMAGE INCLUDING AN UNDERMINED FOUNDATION AND NUMEROUS LEAKS THAT DAMAGED INVALUABLE PIECES OF ART COLLECTED BY ÉCOLE FRANÇAISE D'EXTRÊME ORIENT.

THE BAD WEATHER FORESHADOWED THE POLITICAL STORMS TO COME.

SIR, I'M SORRY TO REPORT THAT THE MUNICIPALITY OF HANOI IS STILL SUFFERING FROM THE BUDGET CRISIS CAUSED BY THE COST OF THE EXPOSITION. IN THE PROVINCES, THE FLOODS CAUSED WIDESPREAD DAMAGE TO THE SEASON'S HARVEST.

DISCONTENT IS SPREADING AMONGST OUR ANNAMITE SUBJECTS.

MY REFORMS WILL WIN OVER THEIR HEARTS AND MINDS. WE NEED TO FOLLOW A POLICY OF "ASSOCIATION" WHICH REALLY MEANS "PARTICIPATION."

PARTICIPATION OF THE NATIVES IN THE DEVELOPMENT OF THE WEALTH OF THE COUNTRY, PARTICIPATION OF THE NATIVES IN THE SCIENTIFIC AND INTELLECTUAL PROGRESS OF MODERN TIMES, PARTICIPATION OF THE NATIVES IN THE ADMINISTRATION AND DIRECTION OF PUBLIC AFFAIRS, AND, THUS, INTIMATELY LINKING THE INTERESTS OF THE ANNAMITES TO OURS.

AT THE SAME TIME WE WILL ASSURE OUR SECURITY AND OUR DOMINATION. HERE IN THE FAR EAST WE WILL ACCOMPLISH FRANCE'S GLOBAL CIVILIZING MISSION. TO START, WE NEED TO RECRUIT NATIVES INTO LOCAL ADMINISTRATION.

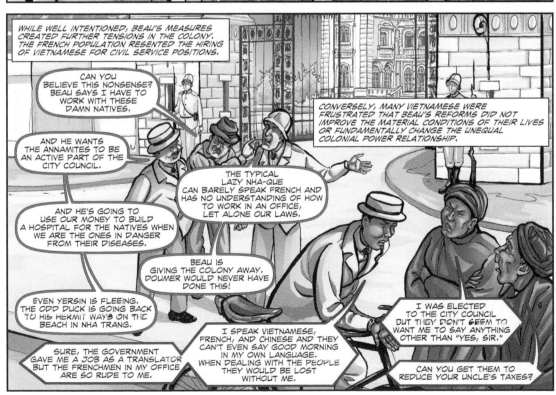

WHILE WELL INTENTIONED, BEAU'S MEASURES CREATED FURTHER TENSIONS IN THE COLONY. THE FRENCH POPULATION RESENTED THE HIRING OF VIETNAMESE FOR CIVIL SERVICE POSITIONS.

CAN YOU BELIEVE THIS NONSENSE? BEAU SAYS I HAVE TO WORK WITH THESE DAMN NATIVES.

AND HE WANTS THE ANNAMITES TO BE AN ACTIVE PART OF THE CITY COUNCIL.

AND HE'S GOING TO USE OUR MONEY TO BUILD A HOSPITAL FOR THE NATIVES WHEN WE ARE THE ONES IN DANGER FROM THEIR DISEASES.

THE TYPICAL LAZY NHA-QUE CAN BARELY SPEAK FRENCH AND HAS NO UNDERSTANDING OF HOW TO WORK IN AN OFFICE, LET ALONE OUR LAWS.

BEAU IS GIVING THE COLONY AWAY. DOUMER WOULD NEVER HAVE DONE THIS!

EVEN YERSIN IS FLEEING. THE ODD DUCK IS GOING BACK TO HIS HERMIT WAYS ON THE BEACH IN NHA TRANG.

SURE, THE GOVERNMENT GAVE ME A JOB AS A TRANSLATOR BUT THE FRENCHMEN IN MY OFFICE ARE SO RUDE TO ME.

I SPEAK VIETNAMESE, FRENCH, AND CHINESE AND THEY CAN'T EVEN SAY GOOD MORNING IN MY OWN LANGUAGE. WHEN DEALING WITH THE PEOPLE THEY WOULD BE LOST WITHOUT ME.

CONVERSELY, MANY VIETNAMESE WERE FRUSTRATED THAT BEAU'S REFORMS DID NOT IMPROVE THE MATERIAL CONDITIONS OF THEIR LIVES OR FUNDAMENTALLY CHANGE THE UNEQUAL COLONIAL POWER RELATIONSHIP.

I WAS ELECTED TO THE CITY COUNCIL BUT THEY DON'T SEEM TO WANT ME TO SAY ANYTHING OTHER THAN "YES, SIR."

CAN YOU GET THEM TO REDUCE YOUR UNCLE'S TAXES?

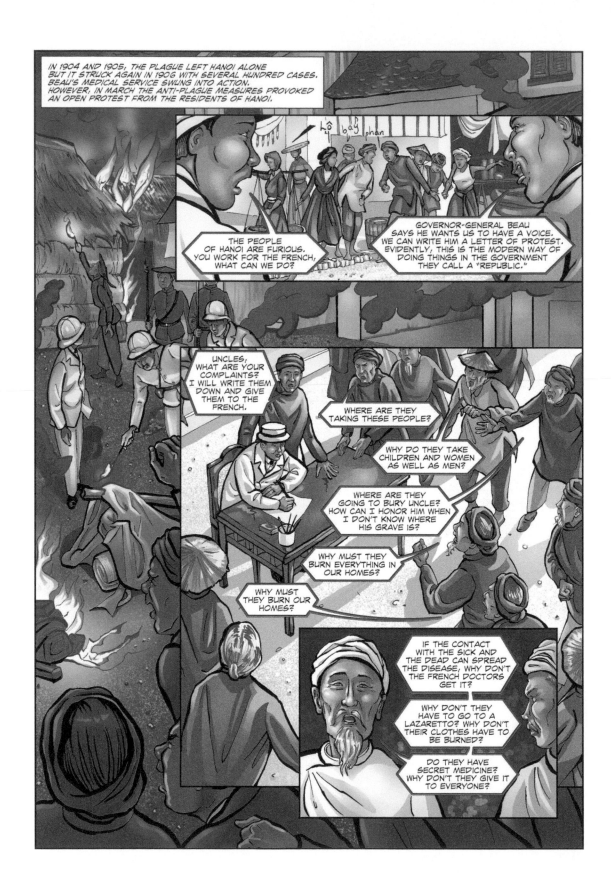

IN 1904 AND 1905, THE PLAGUE LEFT HANOI ALONE BUT IT STRUCK AGAIN IN 1906 WITH SEVERAL HUNDRED CASES. BEAU'S MEDICAL SERVICE SWUNG INTO ACTION. HOWEVER, IN MARCH THE ANTI-PLAGUE MEASURES PROVOKED AN OPEN PROTEST FROM THE RESIDENTS OF HANOI.

THE PEOPLE OF HANOI ARE FURIOUS. YOU WORK FOR THE FRENCH, WHAT CAN WE DO?

GOVERNOR-GENERAL BEAU SAYS HE WANTS US TO HAVE A VOICE. WE CAN WRITE HIM A LETTER OF PROTEST. EVIDENTLY, THIS IS THE MODERN WAY OF DOING THINGS IN THE GOVERNMENT THEY CALL A "REPUBLIC."

UNCLES, WHAT ARE YOUR COMPLAINTS? I WILL WRITE THEM DOWN AND GIVE THEM TO THE FRENCH.

WHERE ARE THEY TAKING THESE PEOPLE?

WHY DO THEY TAKE CHILDREN AND WOMEN AS WELL AS MEN?

WHERE ARE THEY GOING TO BURY UNCLE? HOW CAN I HONOR HIM WHEN I DON'T KNOW WHERE HIS GRAVE IS?

WHY MUST THEY BURN EVERYTHING IN OUR HOMES?

WHY MUST THEY BURN OUR HOMES?

IF THE CONTACT WITH THE SICK AND THE DEAD CAN SPREAD THE DISEASE, WHY DON'T THE FRENCH DOCTORS GET IT?

WHY DON'T THEY HAVE TO GO TO A LAZARETTO? WHY DON'T THEIR CLOTHES HAVE TO BE BURNED?

DO THEY HAVE SECRET MEDICINE? WHY DON'T THEY GIVE IT TO EVERYONE?

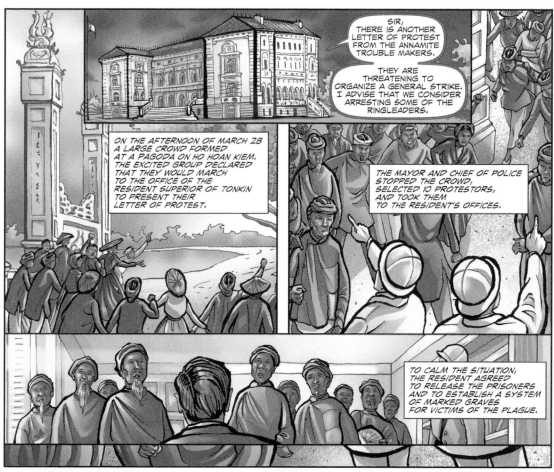

SIR, THERE IS ANOTHER LETTER OF PROTEST FROM THE ANNAMITE TROUBLE MAKERS.

THEY ARE THREATENING TO ORGANIZE A GENERAL STRIKE. I ADVISE THAT WE CONSIDER ARRESTING SOME OF THE RINGLEADERS.

ON THE AFTERNOON OF MARCH 28 A LARGE CROWD FORMED AT A PAGODA ON HO HOAN KIEM. THE EXCITED GROUP DECLARED THAT THEY WOULD MARCH TO THE OFFICE OF THE RESIDENT SUPERIOR OF TONKIN TO PRESENT THEIR LETTER OF PROTEST.

THE MAYOR AND CHIEF OF POLICE STOPPED THE CROWD, SELECTED 10 PROTESTORS, AND TOOK THEM TO THE RESIDENT'S OFFICES.

TO CALM THE SITUATION, THE RESIDENT AGREED TO RELEASE THE PRISONERS AND TO ESTABLISH A SYSTEM OF MARKED GRAVES FOR VICTIMS OF THE PLAGUE.

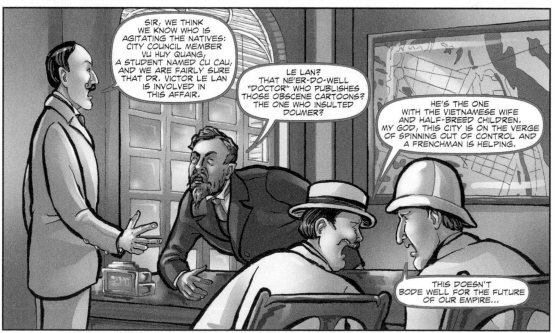

SIR, WE THINK WE KNOW WHO IS AGITATING THE NATIVES: CITY COUNCIL MEMBER VU HUY QUANG, A STUDENT NAMED CU CAU, AND WE ARE FAIRLY SURE THAT DR. VICTOR LE LAN IS INVOLVED IN THIS AFFAIR.

LE LAN? THAT NE'ER-DO-WELL "DOCTOR" WHO PUBLISHES THOSE OBSCENE CARTOONS? THE ONE WHO INSULTED DOUMER?

HE'S THE ONE WITH THE VIETNAMESE WIFE AND HALF-BREED CHILDREN. MY GOD, THIS CITY IS ON THE VERGE OF SPINNING OUT OF CONTROL AND A FRENCHMAN IS HELPING.

THIS DOESN'T BODE WELL FOR THE FUTURE OF OUR EMPIRE...

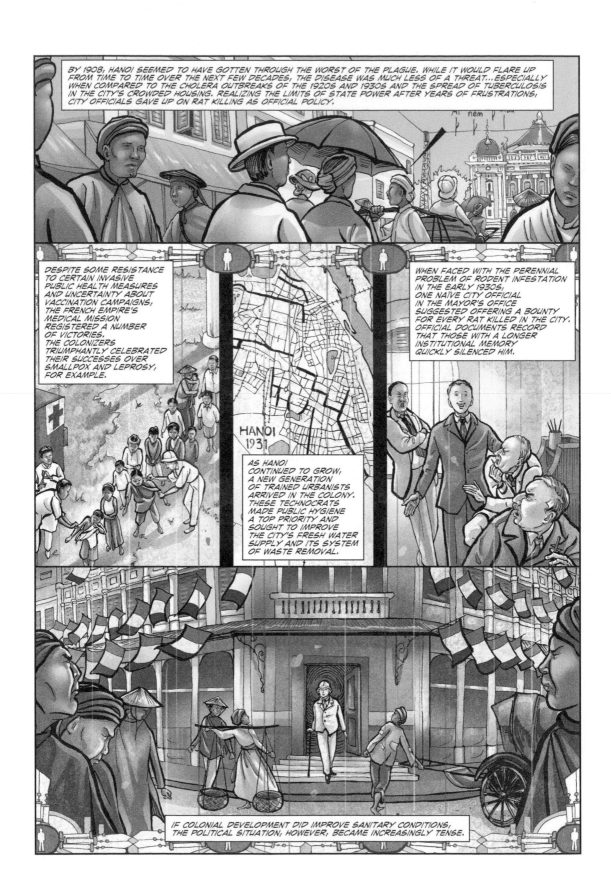

BY 1908, HANOI SEEMED TO HAVE GOTTEN THROUGH THE WORST OF THE PLAGUE. WHILE IT WOULD FLARE UP FROM TIME TO TIME OVER THE NEXT FEW DECADES, THE DISEASE WAS MUCH LESS OF A THREAT...ESPECIALLY WHEN COMPARED TO THE CHOLERA OUTBREAKS OF THE 1920S AND 1930S AND THE SPREAD OF TUBERCULOSIS IN THE CITY'S CROWDED HOUSING. REALIZING THE LIMITS OF STATE POWER AFTER YEARS OF FRUSTRATIONS, CITY OFFICIALS GAVE UP ON RAT KILLING AS OFFICIAL POLICY.

DESPITE SOME RESISTANCE TO CERTAIN INVASIVE PUBLIC HEALTH MEASURES AND UNCERTAINTY ABOUT VACCINATION CAMPAIGNS, THE FRENCH EMPIRE'S MEDICAL MISSION REGISTERED A NUMBER OF VICTORIES. THE COLONIZERS TRIUMPHANTLY CELEBRATED THEIR SUCCESSES OVER SMALLPOX AND LEPROSY, FOR EXAMPLE.

HANOI 1931

WHEN FACED WITH THE PERENNIAL PROBLEM OF RODENT INFESTATION IN THE EARLY 1930S, ONE NAÏVE CITY OFFICIAL IN THE MAYOR'S OFFICE SUGGESTED OFFERING A BOUNTY FOR EVERY RAT KILLED IN THE CITY. OFFICIAL DOCUMENTS RECORD THAT THOSE WITH A LONGER INSTITUTIONAL MEMORY QUICKLY SILENCED HIM.

AS HANOI CONTINUED TO GROW, A NEW GENERATION OF TRAINED URBANISTS ARRIVED IN THE COLONY. THESE TECHNOCRATS MADE PUBLIC HYGIENE A TOP PRIORITY AND SOUGHT TO IMPROVE THE CITY'S FRESH WATER SUPPLY AND ITS SYSTEM OF WASTE REMOVAL.

IF COLONIAL DEVELOPMENT DID IMPROVE SANITARY CONDITIONS, THE POLITICAL SITUATION, HOWEVER, BECAME INCREASINGLY TENSE.

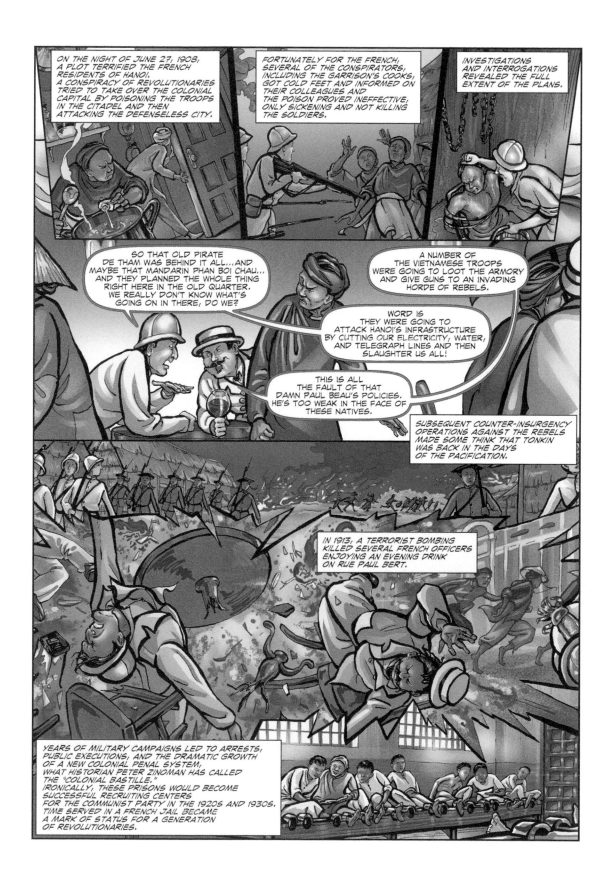

ON THE NIGHT OF JUNE 27, 1908, A PLOT TERRIFIED THE FRENCH RESIDENTS OF HANOI. A CONSPIRACY OF REVOLUTIONARIES TRIED TO TAKE OVER THE COLONIAL CAPITAL BY POISONING THE TROOPS IN THE CITADEL AND THEN ATTACKING THE DEFENSELESS CITY.

FORTUNATELY FOR THE FRENCH, SEVERAL OF THE CONSPIRATORS, INCLUDING THE GARRISON'S COOKS, GOT COLD FEET AND INFORMED ON THEIR COLLEAGUES AND THE POISON PROVED INEFFECTIVE, ONLY SICKENING AND NOT KILLING THE SOLDIERS.

INVESTIGATIONS AND INTERROGATIONS REVEALED THE FULL EXTENT OF THE PLANS.

SO THAT OLD PIRATE DE THAM WAS BEHIND IT ALL...AND MAYBE THAT MANDARIN PHAN BOI CHAU... AND THEY PLANNED THE WHOLE THING RIGHT HERE IN THE OLD QUARTER. WE REALLY DON'T KNOW WHAT'S GOING ON IN THERE, DO WE?

A NUMBER OF THE VIETNAMESE TROOPS WERE GOING TO LOOT THE ARMORY AND GIVE GUNS TO AN INVADING HORDE OF REBELS.

WORD IS THEY WERE GOING TO ATTACK HANOI'S INFRASTRUCTURE BY CUTTING OUR ELECTRICITY, WATER, AND TELEGRAPH LINES AND THEN SLAUGHTER US ALL!

THIS IS ALL THE FAULT OF THAT DAMN PAUL BEAU'S POLICIES. HE'S TOO WEAK IN THE FACE OF THESE NATIVES.

SUBSEQUENT COUNTER-INSURGENCY OPERATIONS AGAINST THE REBELS MADE SOME THINK THAT TONKIN WAS BACK IN THE DAYS OF THE PACIFICATION.

IN 1913, A TERRORIST BOMBING KILLED SEVERAL FRENCH OFFICERS ENJOYING AN EVENING DRINK ON RUE PAUL BERT.

YEARS OF MILITARY CAMPAIGNS LED TO ARRESTS, PUBLIC EXECUTIONS, AND THE DRAMATIC GROWTH OF A NEW COLONIAL PENAL SYSTEM, WHAT HISTORIAN PETER ZINOMAN HAS CALLED THE "COLONIAL BASTILLE." IRONICALLY, THESE PRISONS WOULD BECOME SUCCESSFUL RECRUITING CENTERS FOR THE COMMUNIST PARTY IN THE 1920S AND 1930S. TIME SERVED IN A FRENCH JAIL BECAME A MARK OF STATUS FOR A GENERATION OF REVOLUTIONARIES.

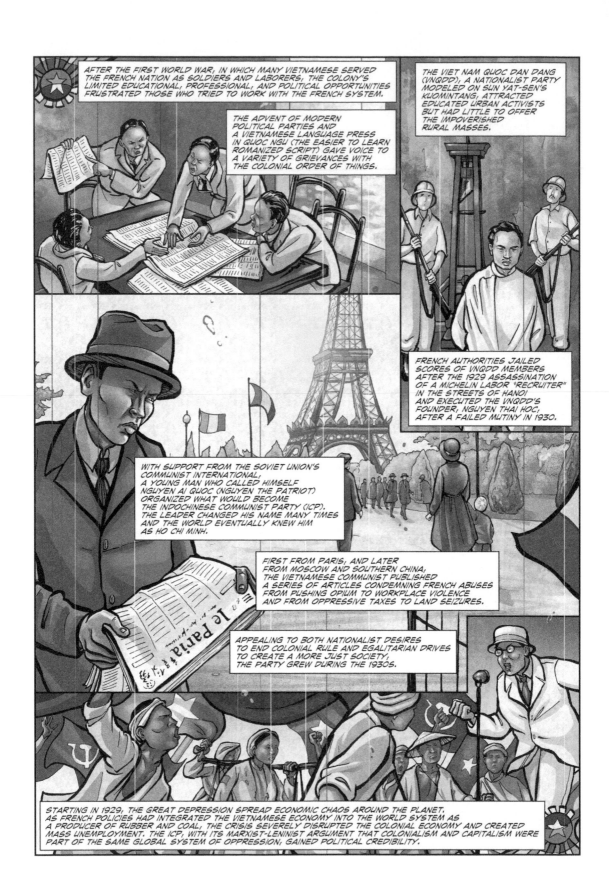

AFTER THE FIRST WORLD WAR, IN WHICH MANY VIETNAMESE SERVED THE FRENCH NATION AS SOLDIERS AND LABORERS, THE COLONY'S LIMITED EDUCATIONAL, PROFESSIONAL, AND POLITICAL OPPORTUNITIES FRUSTRATED THOSE WHO TRIED TO WORK WITH THE FRENCH SYSTEM.

THE ADVENT OF MODERN POLITICAL PARTIES AND A VIETNAMESE LANGUAGE PRESS IN QUOC NGU (THE EASIER TO LEARN ROMANIZED SCRIPT) GAVE VOICE TO A VARIETY OF GRIEVANCES WITH THE COLONIAL ORDER OF THINGS.

THE VIET NAM QUOC DAN DANG (VNQDD), A NATIONALIST PARTY MODELED ON SUN YAT-SEN'S KUOMINTANG, ATTRACTED EDUCATED URBAN ACTIVISTS BUT HAD LITTLE TO OFFER THE IMPOVERISHED RURAL MASSES.

FRENCH AUTHORITIES JAILED SCORES OF VNQDD MEMBERS AFTER THE 1929 ASSASSINATION OF A MICHELIN LABOR "RECRUITER" IN THE STREETS OF HANOI AND EXECUTED THE VNQDD'S FOUNDER, NGUYEN THAI HOC, AFTER A FAILED MUTINY IN 1930.

WITH SUPPORT FROM THE SOVIET UNION'S COMMUNIST INTERNATIONAL, A YOUNG MAN WHO CALLED HIMSELF NGUYEN AI QUOC (NGUYEN THE PATRIOT) ORGANIZED WHAT WOULD BECOME THE INDOCHINESE COMMUNIST PARTY (ICP). THE LEADER CHANGED HIS NAME MANY TIMES AND THE WORLD EVENTUALLY KNEW HIM AS HO CHI MINH.

FIRST FROM PARIS, AND LATER FROM MOSCOW AND SOUTHERN CHINA, THE VIETNAMESE COMMUNIST PUBLISHED A SERIES OF ARTICLES CONDEMNING FRENCH ABUSES FROM PUSHING OPIUM TO WORKPLACE VIOLENCE AND FROM OPPRESSIVE TAXES TO LAND SEIZURES.

APPEALING TO BOTH NATIONALIST DESIRES TO END COLONIAL RULE AND EGALITARIAN DRIVES TO CREATE A MORE JUST SOCIETY, THE PARTY GREW DURING THE 1930S.

STARTING IN 1929, THE GREAT DEPRESSION SPREAD ECONOMIC CHAOS AROUND THE PLANET. AS FRENCH POLICIES HAD INTEGRATED THE VIETNAMESE ECONOMY INTO THE WORLD SYSTEM AS A PRODUCER OF RUBBER AND COAL, THE CRISIS SEVERELY DISRUPTED THE COLONIAL ECONOMY AND CREATED MASS UNEMPLOYMENT. THE ICP, WITH ITS MARXIST-LENINIST ARGUMENT THAT COLONIALISM AND CAPITALISM WERE PART OF THE SAME GLOBAL SYSTEM OF OPPRESSION, GAINED POLITICAL CREDIBILITY.

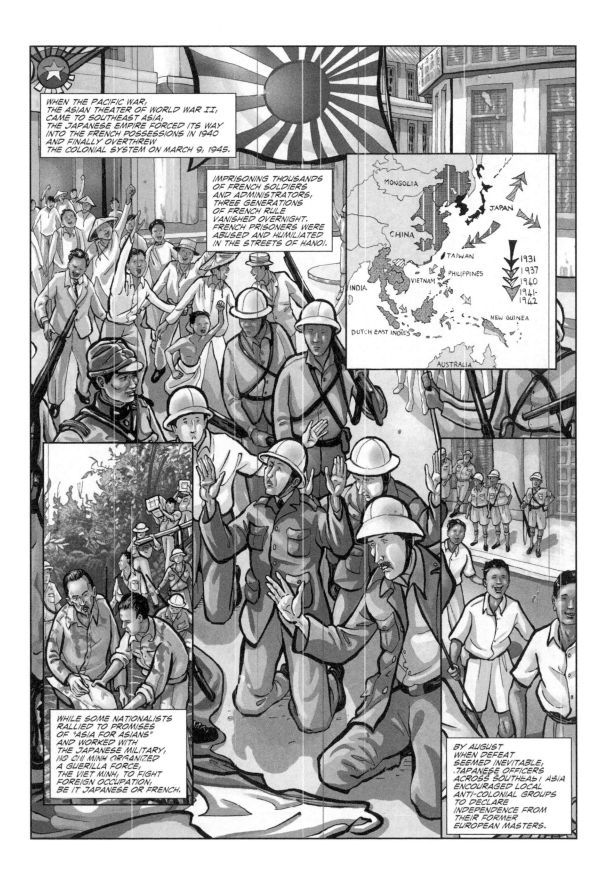

WHEN THE PACIFIC WAR,
THE ASIAN THEATER OF WORLD WAR II,
CAME TO SOUTHEAST ASIA,
THE JAPANESE EMPIRE FORCED ITS WAY
INTO THE FRENCH POSSESSIONS IN 1940
AND FINALLY OVERTHREW
THE COLONIAL SYSTEM ON MARCH 9, 1945.

IMPRISONING THOUSANDS
OF FRENCH SOLDIERS
AND ADMINISTRATORS,
THREE GENERATIONS
OF FRENCH RULE
VANISHED OVERNIGHT.
FRENCH PRISONERS WERE
ABUSED AND HUMILIATED
IN THE STREETS OF HANOI.

WHILE SOME NATIONALISTS
RALLIED TO PROMISES
OF "ASIA FOR ASIANS"
AND WORKED WITH
THE JAPANESE MILITARY,
HO CHI MINH ORGANIZED
A GUERILLA FORCE,
THE VIET MINH, TO FIGHT
FOREIGN OCCUPATION,
BE IT JAPANESE OR FRENCH.

BY AUGUST
WHEN DEFEAT
SEEMED INEVITABLE,
JAPANESE OFFICERS
ACROSS SOUTHEAST ASIA
ENCOURAGED LOCAL
ANTI-COLONIAL GROUPS
TO DECLARE
INDEPENDENCE FROM
THEIR FORMER
EUROPEAN MASTERS.

MONGOLIA

JAPAN

CHINA

TAIWAN

PHILIPPINES

INDIA

VIETNAM

1931
1937
1940
1941-
1942

DUTCH EAST INDIES

NEW GUINEA

AUSTRALIA

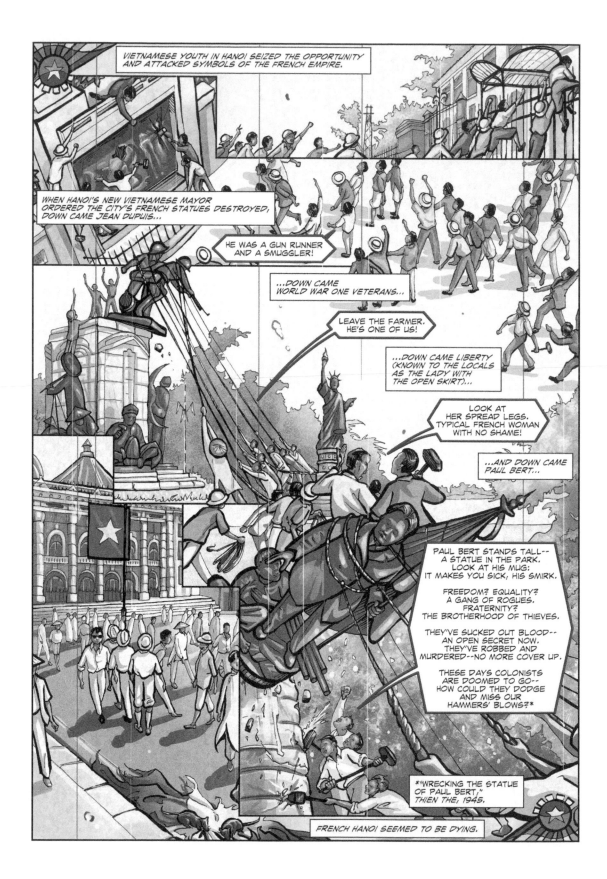

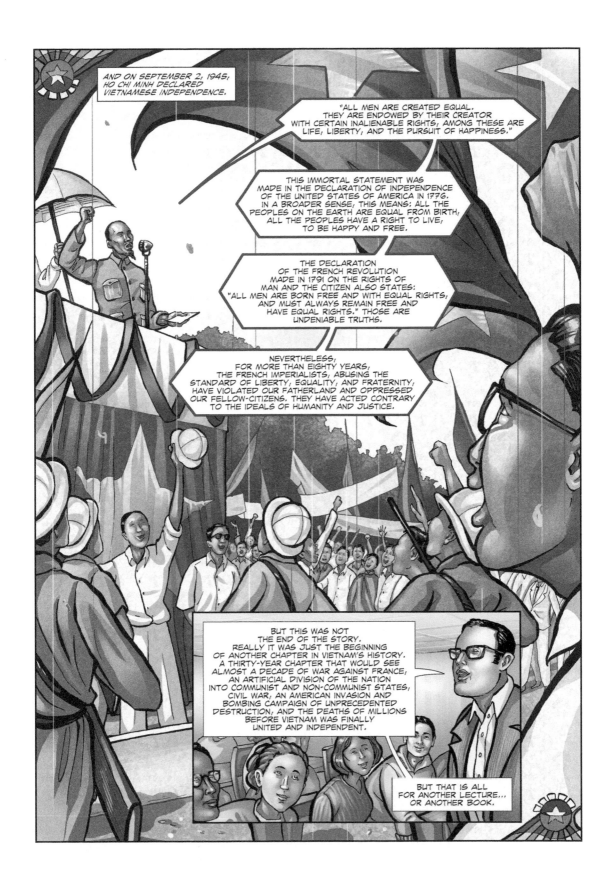

AND ON SEPTEMBER 2, 1945, HO CHI MINH DECLARED VIETNAMESE INDEPENDENCE.

"ALL MEN ARE CREATED EQUAL. THEY ARE ENDOWED BY THEIR CREATOR WITH CERTAIN INALIENABLE RIGHTS, AMONG THESE ARE LIFE, LIBERTY, AND THE PURSUIT OF HAPPINESS."

THIS IMMORTAL STATEMENT WAS MADE IN THE DECLARATION OF INDEPENDENCE OF THE UNITED STATES OF AMERICA IN 1776. IN A BROADER SENSE, THIS MEANS: ALL THE PEOPLES ON THE EARTH ARE EQUAL FROM BIRTH, ALL THE PEOPLES HAVE A RIGHT TO LIVE, TO BE HAPPY AND FREE.

THE DECLARATION OF THE FRENCH REVOLUTION MADE IN 1791 ON THE RIGHTS OF MAN AND THE CITIZEN ALSO STATES: "ALL MEN ARE BORN FREE AND WITH EQUAL RIGHTS, AND MUST ALWAYS REMAIN FREE AND HAVE EQUAL RIGHTS." THOSE ARE UNDENIABLE TRUTHS.

NEVERTHELESS, FOR MORE THAN EIGHTY YEARS, THE FRENCH IMPERIALISTS, ABUSING THE STANDARD OF LIBERTY, EQUALITY, AND FRATERNITY, HAVE VIOLATED OUR FATHERLAND AND OPPRESSED OUR FELLOW-CITIZENS. THEY HAVE ACTED CONTRARY TO THE IDEALS OF HUMANITY AND JUSTICE.

BUT THIS WAS NOT THE END OF THE STORY. REALLY IT WAS JUST THE BEGINNING OF ANOTHER CHAPTER IN VIETNAM'S HISTORY. A THIRTY-YEAR CHAPTER THAT WOULD SEE ALMOST A DECADE OF WAR AGAINST FRANCE, AN ARTIFICIAL DIVISION OF THE NATION INTO COMMUNIST AND NON-COMMUNIST STATES, CIVIL WAR, AN AMERICAN INVASION AND BOMBING CAMPAIGN OF UNPRECEDENTED DESTRUCTION, AND THE DEATHS OF MILLIONS BEFORE VIETNAM WAS FINALLY UNITED AND INDEPENDENT.

BUT THAT IS ALL FOR ANOTHER LECTURE... OR ANOTHER BOOK.

AFTERWORD

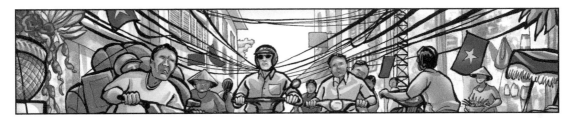

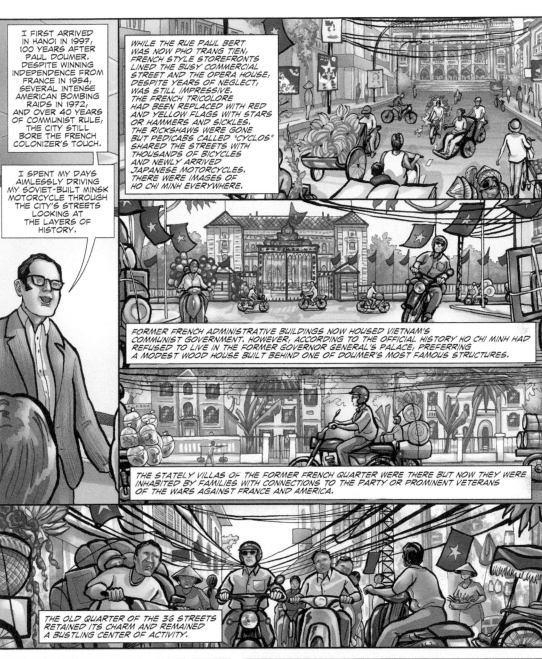

I FIRST ARRIVED IN HANOI IN 1997, 100 YEARS AFTER PAUL DOUMER. DESPITE WINNING INDEPENDENCE FROM FRANCE IN 1954, SEVERAL INTENSE AMERICAN BOMBING RAIDS IN 1972, AND OVER 40 YEARS OF COMMUNIST RULE, THE CITY STILL BORE THE FRENCH COLONIZER'S TOUCH.

I SPENT MY DAYS AIMLESSLY DRIVING MY SOVIET-BUILT MINSK MOTORCYCLE THROUGH THE CITY'S STREETS LOOKING AT THE LAYERS OF HISTORY.

WHILE THE RUE PAUL BERT WAS NOW PHO TRANG TIEN, FRENCH STYLE STOREFRONTS LINED THE BUSY COMMERCIAL STREET AND THE OPERA HOUSE, DESPITE YEARS OF NEGLECT, WAS STILL IMPRESSIVE. THE FRENCH TRICOLORE HAD BEEN REPLACED WITH RED AND YELLOW FLAGS WITH STARS OR HAMMERS AND SICKLES. THE RICKSHAWS WERE GONE BUT PEDICABS CALLED "CYCLOS" SHARED THE STREETS WITH THOUSANDS OF BICYCLES AND NEWLY ARRIVED JAPANESE MOTORCYCLES. THERE WERE IMAGES OF HO CHI MINH EVERYWHERE.

FORMER FRENCH ADMINISTRATIVE BUILDINGS NOW HOUSED VIETNAM'S COMMUNIST GOVERNMENT. HOWEVER, ACCORDING TO THE OFFICIAL HISTORY HO CHI MINH HAD REFUSED TO LIVE IN THE FORMER GOVERNOR GENERAL'S PALACE, PREFERRING A MODEST WOOD HOUSE BUILT BEHIND ONE OF DOUMER'S MOST FAMOUS STRUCTURES.

THE STATELY VILLAS OF THE FORMER FRENCH QUARTER WERE THERE BUT NOW THEY WERE INHABITED BY FAMILIES WITH CONNECTIONS TO THE PARTY OR PROMINENT VETERANS OF THE WARS AGAINST FRANCE AND AMERICA.

THE OLD QUARTER OF THE 36 STREETS RETAINED ITS CHARM AND REMAINED A BUSTLING CENTER OF ACTIVITY.

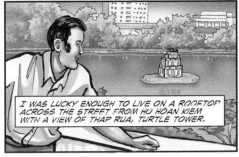

I WAS LUCKY ENOUGH TO LIVE ON A ROOFTOP ACROSS THE STREET FROM HO HOAN KIEM WITH A VIEW OF THAP RUA, TURTLE TOWER.

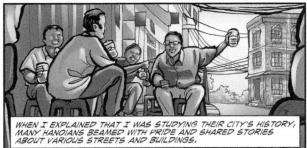

WHEN I EXPLAINED THAT I WAS STUDYING THEIR CITY'S HISTORY, MANY HANOIANS BEAMED WITH PRIDE AND SHARED STORIES ABOUT VARIOUS STREETS AND BUILDINGS.

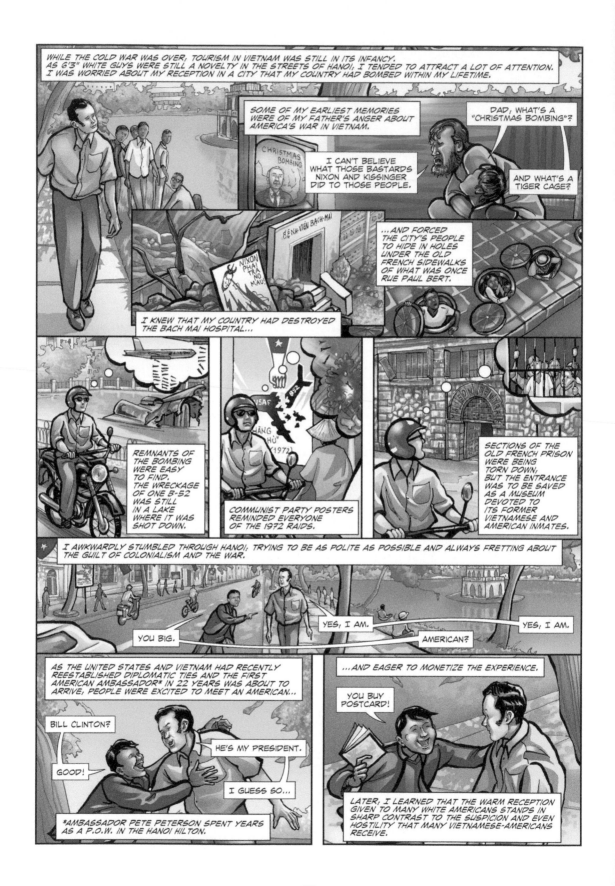

WHILE THE COLD WAR WAS OVER, TOURISM IN VIETNAM WAS STILL IN ITS INFANCY.
AS 6'3" WHITE GUYS WERE STILL A NOVELTY IN THE STREETS OF HANOI, I TENDED TO ATTRACT A LOT OF ATTENTION.
I WAS WORRIED ABOUT MY RECEPTION IN A CITY THAT MY COUNTRY HAD BOMBED WITHIN MY LIFETIME.

SOME OF MY EARLIEST MEMORIES WERE OF MY FATHER'S ANGER ABOUT AMERICA'S WAR IN VIETNAM.

DAD, WHAT'S A "CHRISTMAS BOMBING"?

CHRISTMAS BOMBING

I CAN'T BELIEVE WHAT THOSE BASTARDS NIXON AND KISSINGER DID TO THOSE PEOPLE.

AND WHAT'S A TIGER CAGE?

BỆNH-VIỆN BẠCH-MAI

NIXON PHẢI TRẢ NỢ MÁU!

...AND FORCED THE CITY'S PEOPLE TO HIDE IN HOLES UNDER THE OLD FRENCH SIDEWALKS OF WHAT WAS ONCE RUE PAUL BERT.

I KNEW THAT MY COUNTRY HAD DESTROYED THE BACH MAI HOSPITAL...

REMNANTS OF THE BOMBING WERE EASY TO FIND. THE WRECKAGE OF ONE B-52 WAS STILL IN A LAKE WHERE IT WAS SHOT DOWN.

COMMUNIST PARTY POSTERS REMINDED EVERYONE OF THE 1972 RAIDS.

SECTIONS OF THE OLD FRENCH PRISON WERE BEING TORN DOWN; BUT THE ENTRANCE WAS TO BE SAVED AS A MUSEUM DEVOTED TO ITS FORMER VIETNAMESE AND AMERICAN INMATES.

I AWKWARDLY STUMBLED THROUGH HANOI; TRYING TO BE AS POLITE AS POSSIBLE AND ALWAYS FRETTING ABOUT THE GUILT OF COLONIALISM AND THE WAR.

YOU BIG.

YES, I AM.

AMERICAN?

YES, I AM.

AS THE UNITED STATES AND VIETNAM HAD RECENTLY REESTABLISHED DIPLOMATIC TIES AND THE FIRST AMERICAN AMBASSADOR* IN 22 YEARS WAS ABOUT TO ARRIVE, PEOPLE WERE EXCITED TO MEET AN AMERICAN...

...AND EAGER TO MONETIZE THE EXPERIENCE.

YOU BUY POSTCARD!

BILL CLINTON?

HE'S MY PRESIDENT.

GOOD!

I GUESS SO...

*AMBASSADOR PETE PETERSON SPENT YEARS AS A P.O.W. IN THE HANOI HILTON.

LATER, I LEARNED THAT THE WARM RECEPTION GIVEN TO MANY WHITE AMERICANS STANDS IN SHARP CONTRAST TO THE SUSPICION AND EVEN HOSTILITY THAT MANY VIETNAMESE-AMERICANS RECEIVE.

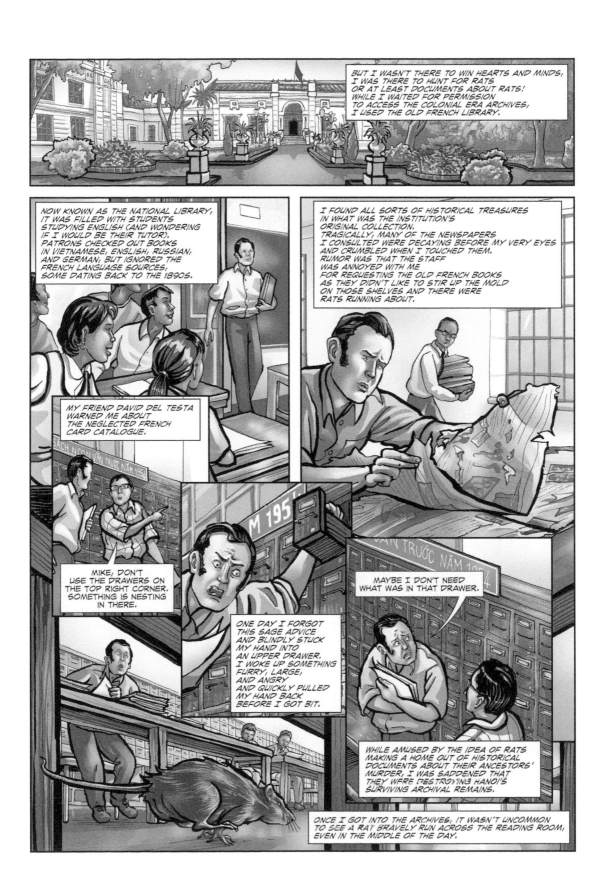

BUT I WASN'T THERE TO WIN HEARTS AND MINDS, I WAS THERE TO HUNT FOR RATS OR AT LEAST DOCUMENTS ABOUT RATS! WHILE I WAITED FOR PERMISSION TO ACCESS THE COLONIAL ERA ARCHIVES, I USED THE OLD FRENCH LIBRARY.

NOW KNOWN AS THE NATIONAL LIBRARY, IT WAS FILLED WITH STUDENTS STUDYING ENGLISH (AND WONDERING IF I WOULD BE THEIR TUTOR). PATRONS CHECKED OUT BOOKS IN VIETNAMESE, ENGLISH, RUSSIAN, AND GERMAN, BUT IGNORED THE FRENCH LANGUAGE SOURCES, SOME DATING BACK TO THE 1890S.

I FOUND ALL SORTS OF HISTORICAL TREASURES IN WHAT WAS THE INSTITUTION'S ORIGINAL COLLECTION. TRAGICALLY, MANY OF THE NEWSPAPERS I CONSULTED WERE DECAYING BEFORE MY VERY EYES AND CRUMBLED WHEN I TOUCHED THEM. RUMOR WAS THAT THE STAFF WAS ANNOYED WITH ME FOR REQUESTING THE OLD FRENCH BOOKS AS THEY DIDN'T LIKE TO STIR UP THE MOLD ON THOSE SHELVES AND THERE WERE RATS RUNNING ABOUT.

MY FRIEND DAVID DEL TESTA WARNED ME ABOUT THE NEGLECTED FRENCH CARD CATALOGUE.

SÁCH NGOẠI VĂN TRƯỚC NĂM 1954

M 1954

MIKE, DON'T USE THE DRAWERS ON THE TOP RIGHT CORNER. SOMETHING IS NESTING IN THERE.

VĂN TRƯỚC NĂM 1954

MAYBE I DON'T NEED WHAT WAS IN THAT DRAWER.

ONE DAY I FORGOT THIS SAGE ADVICE AND BLINDLY STUCK MY HAND INTO AN UPPER DRAWER. I WOKE UP SOMETHING FURRY, LARGE, AND ANGRY AND QUICKLY PULLED MY HAND BACK BEFORE I GOT BIT.

WHILE AMUSED BY THE IDEA OF RATS MAKING A HOME OUT OF HISTORICAL DOCUMENTS ABOUT THEIR ANCESTORS' MURDER, I WAS SADDENED THAT THEY WERE DESTROYING HANOI'S SURVIVING ARCHIVAL REMAINS.

ONCE I GOT INTO THE ARCHIVES, IT WASN'T UNCOMMON TO SEE A RAT BRAVELY RUN ACROSS THE READING ROOM, EVEN IN THE MIDDLE OF THE DAY.

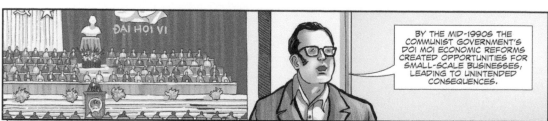

BY THE MID-1990S THE COMMUNIST GOVERNMENT'S DOI MOI ECONOMIC REFORMS CREATED OPPORTUNITIES FOR SMALL-SCALE BUSINESSES, LEADING TO UNINTENDED CONSEQUENCES.

I LEARNED THAT COMMUNIST PARTY OFFICIALS WERE WORRIED ABOUT THE CITY'S GROWING RAT POPULATION.

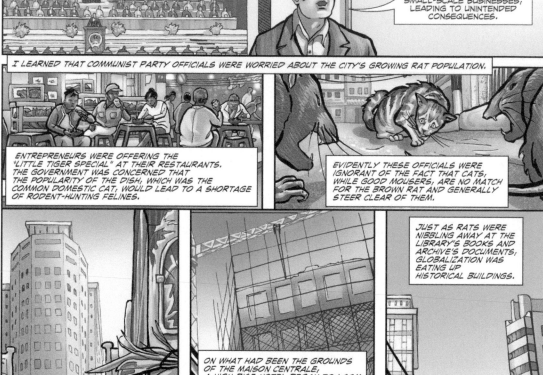

ENTREPRENEURS WERE OFFERING THE "LITTLE TIGER SPECIAL" AT THEIR RESTAURANTS. THE GOVERNMENT WAS CONCERNED THAT THE POPULARITY OF THE DISH, WHICH WAS THE COMMON DOMESTIC CAT, WOULD LEAD TO A SHORTAGE OF RODENT-HUNTING FELINES.

EVIDENTLY THESE OFFICIALS WERE IGNORANT OF THE FACT THAT CATS, WHILE GOOD MOUSERS, ARE NO MATCH FOR THE BROWN RAT AND GENERALLY STEER CLEAR OF THEM.

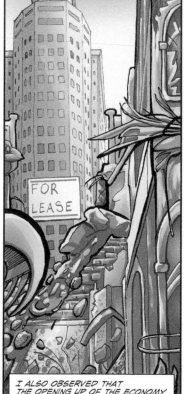

FOR LEASE

I ALSO OBSERVED THAT THE OPENING UP OF THE ECONOMY TO DIRECT FOREIGN INVESTMENT THREATENED HANOI'S HISTORY. IN 1995, THE COUNTRY JOINED THE ASSOCIATION OF SOUTHEAST ASIAN NATIONS, THE REGIONAL TRADE ORGANIZATION. AS CAPITAL FROM SOUTH KOREA, JAPAN, EUROPE, AND THE UNITED STATES OF AMERICA BEGAN TO FLOW INTO VIETNAM, COLONIAL ERA BUILDINGS WERE BEING TORN DOWN TO MAKE WAY FOR SHINY NEW HIGH RISES.

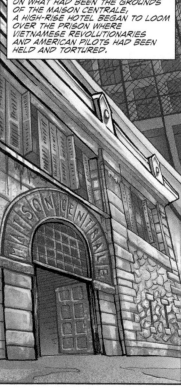

ON WHAT HAD BEEN THE GROUNDS OF THE MAISON CENTRALE, A HIGH-RISE HOTEL BEGAN TO LOOM OVER THE PRISON WHERE VIETNAMESE REVOLUTIONARIES AND AMERICAN PILOTS HAD BEEN HELD AND TORTURED.

MAISON CENTRALE

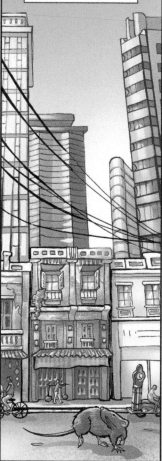

JUST AS RATS WERE NIBBLING AWAY AT THE LIBRARY'S BOOKS AND ARCHIVE'S DOCUMENTS, GLOBALIZATION WAS EATING UP HISTORICAL BUILDINGS.

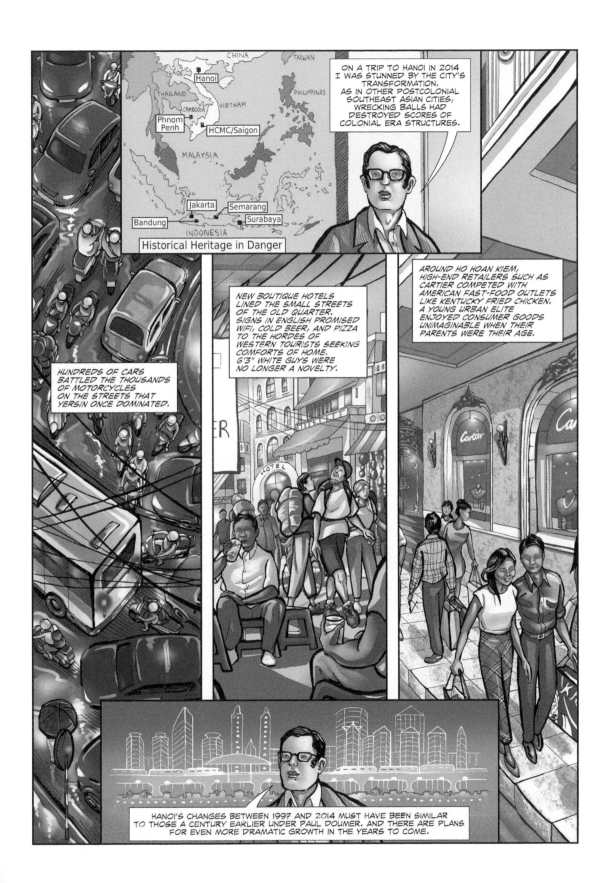

ON A TRIP TO HANOI IN 2014 I WAS STUNNED BY THE CITY'S TRANSFORMATION. AS IN OTHER POSTCOLONIAL SOUTHEAST ASIAN CITIES, WRECKING BALLS HAD DESTROYED SCORES OF COLONIAL ERA STRUCTURES.

Historical Heritage in Danger

NEW BOUTIQUE HOTELS LINED THE SMALL STREETS OF THE OLD QUARTER. SIGNS IN ENGLISH PROMISED WIFI, COLD BEER, AND PIZZA TO THE HORDES OF WESTERN TOURISTS SEEKING COMFORTS OF HOME. 6'3" WHITE GUYS WERE NO LONGER A NOVELTY.

AROUND HO HOAN KIEM, HIGH-END RETAILERS SUCH AS CARTIER COMPETED WITH AMERICAN FAST-FOOD OUTLETS LIKE KENTUCKY FRIED CHICKEN. A YOUNG URBAN ELITE ENJOYED CONSUMER GOODS UNIMAGINABLE WHEN THEIR PARENTS WERE THEIR AGE.

HUNDREDS OF CARS BATTLED THE THOUSANDS OF MOTORCYCLES ON THE STREETS THAT YERSIN ONCE DOMINATED.

HANOI'S CHANGES BETWEEN 1997 AND 2014 MUST HAVE BEEN SIMILAR TO THOSE A CENTURY EARLIER UNDER PAUL DOUMER. AND THERE ARE PLANS FOR EVEN MORE DRAMATIC GROWTH IN THE YEARS TO COME.

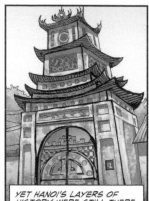

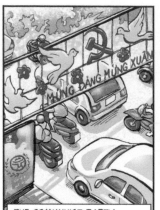

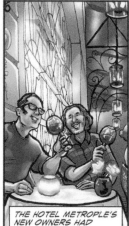

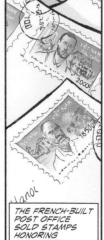

YET HANOI'S LAYERS OF HISTORY WERE STILL THERE. RECOGNIZING THE CITY'S CULTURAL LEGACY, THE GOVERNMENT RESTORED MANY OF THE BEST EXAMPLES OF FRENCH, CONFUCIAN, AND BUDDHIST ARCHITECTURE.

THE COMMUNIST PARTY PROMOTED PEACE, PROSPERITY, AND EVEN A GREEN HANOI IN STREET DECORATIONS THAT MIXED HAMMERS AND SICKLES WITH PEACEFUL DOVES.

THE HOTEL METROPLE'S NEW OWNERS HAD RESTORED ITS ONCE LOST LUXURY. FLÂNEURS DRANK WINE ON ITS SIDEWALK CAFÉ.

THE FRENCH-BUILT POST OFFICE SOLD STAMPS HONORING ALEXANDRE YERSIN.

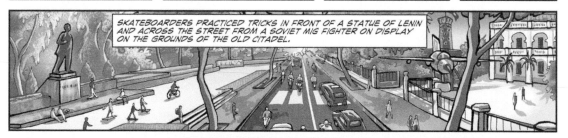

SKATEBOARDERS PRACTICED TRICKS IN FRONT OF A STATUE OF LENIN AND ACROSS THE STREET FROM A SOVIET MIG FIGHTER ON DISPLAY ON THE GROUNDS OF THE OLD CITADEL.

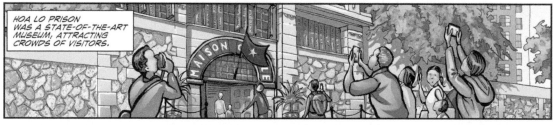

HOA LO PRISON WAS A STATE-OF-THE-ART MUSEUM, ATTRACTING CROWDS OF VISITORS.

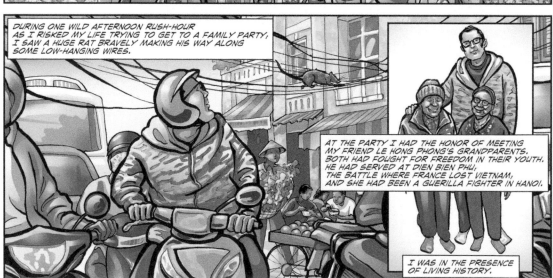

DURING ONE WILD AFTERNOON RUSH-HOUR AS I RISKED MY LIFE TRYING TO GET TO A FAMILY PARTY, I SAW A HUGE RAT BRAVELY MAKING HIS WAY ALONG SOME LOW-HANGING WIRES.

AT THE PARTY I HAD THE HONOR OF MEETING MY FRIEND LE HONG PHONG'S GRANDPARENTS. BOTH HAD FOUGHT FOR FREEDOM IN THEIR YOUTH. HE HAD SERVED AT DIEN BIEN PHU, THE BATTLE WHERE FRANCE LOST VIETNAM, AND SHE HAD BEEN A GUERILLA FIGHTER IN HANOI.

I WAS IN THE PRESENCE OF LIVING HISTORY.

ENDNOTES

Page 11   Doumer, Paul. *Indo-Chine française (souvenirs)* (Paris: Vuibert et Nony, 1905), 286.

Page 60   Anonymous, "Poem on True Heroism (ca. 1900)," in Trung Buu Lam, *Patterns of Vietnamese Response to Foreign Intervention: 1858–1900* (New Haven: Yale University Press, 1967), 143.

Page 62   Centre des Archives d'Outre-Mer, AF, carton 9 dossier 51 & 54: "Rapport sur la situation politique et économique de l'Indochine" (1905).

Page 63   Anonymous, "The Asian Ballad (~1905–1906)," in Trung Buu Lam, *Colonialism Experienced: Vietnamese Writings on Colonialism, 1900–1931* (Ann Arbor: University of Michigan Press, 2000), 89. "'Le Petit Parisien' en Indochine," *Le Petit Parisien*, 31 May, 1930: 2.

Pages 90–91, 94, 96, 104   Centre Archives d'Outre-Mer, Gouvernement-Général de l'Indo-Chine 6675, Commissaire Central, "Note de Service: Destruction des animaux, Hanoi-Ville" (1902).

Page 101   Nguyen Khuyen, "At an exposition (n.d.)," in Huynh Sanh Thong (ed. and trans.), *An Anthology of Vietnamese Poetry* (New Haven: Yale University Press, 1996), 95.

Page 112   Thien Thu, "Wrecking the Statue of Paul Doumer (1945)," in Huynh Sanh Thong (ed. and trans.), *An Anthology of Vietnamese Poetry* (New Haven: Yale University Press, 1996), 139.

Page 113   Ho Chi Minh, "Declaration of Independence of the Democratic Republic of Vietnam (September 2, 1945)," in *Down with Colonialism!* (London: Verso, 2007), 51.

PART II
PRIMARY SOURCES

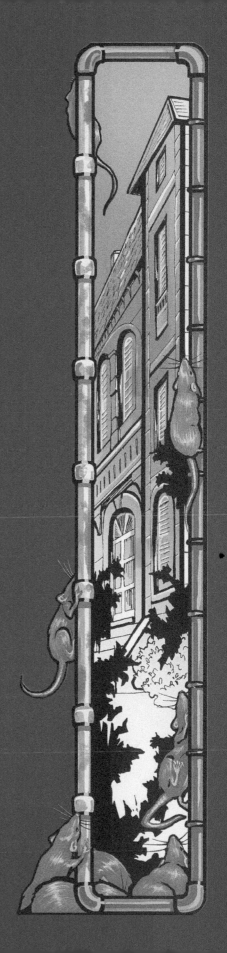

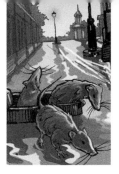

Primary sources are what historians use to write their work. They are essentially voices from the past. They are documents from the time period being studied, as opposed to secondary sources, which are written after the events in question. Think of primary sources as a witness's testimony. Like an attorney, the role of a historian is to build an argument based upon such evidence. We historians spend much of our time in archives and libraries reading, analyzing, and organizing such sources. As no one source is ever complete, and frequently two sources might contradict each other, historians do their best to triangulate such primary sources.

This chapter discusses some of the source materials I used to write the story of the Great Hanoi Rat Hunt. While it contains nowhere near all of the documents I consulted, this sample should give you an idea of the wide variety of things that can serve as primary sources. As you read through these documents, try to keep a critical eye. Always ask yourself if you can trust these sources. Pay attention to the author's name, as that can be a clue toward any potential bias. Be on the lookout for documents that contradict other documents. Consider why two observers of the same event might disagree.

URBAN LIFE

In this collection of documents, consider the various ways in which the French and other Europeans represented colonial Hanoi. Most white observers praised Hanoi's new architecture and infrastructure and a few embraced the exotic Orientalism of the so-called Native Quarter. While many observers praised the city as embodying the positive values of modernity and the benefits of Western urbanization, others called into question the structural inequalities of city life. Many whites racialized the potential health threats posed by turn-of-the-century cities, often singling out Chinese as a dangerous category of people.

1. JOSEPH CHAILLEY-BERT, *PAUL BERT AU TONKIN*

Paul Bert was a morning person. He began his day at six A.M. Dressed in white, a large helmet over his shaved head, a baton in hand, always jolly, he left, before the strong heat of the day, and wandered about some quarter of the city, which would soon be, with its river and lakes, the pearl of the Orient. These were always important visits; he would go to inspect or prepare construction projects; and, very frequently, he brought a tradesman with him. One day, it was the river, which when flooding, threatening the concession; another day, the swampy area around the rue des Incrusteurs, across which he planned to build new streets; or the houses around the small lake, destined to be the Résidence d'Hanoï, the Tribunal, the Commission Municipale, etc.; and finally the customs houses, rendered inaccessible to boats by a sand bar, etc. etc.

Source: Joseph Chailley-Bert, *Paul Bert au Tonkin* (Paris: Charpentier, 1887), 154–55. Translated by Michael G. Vann.

2. "HANOÏ: STATUE DE PAUL BERT," PIERRE DIEULEFILS POSTCARD

The postcard on the right shows the memorial dedicated to Paul Bert, Hanoi's first civilian administrator and urban planner. A hero of the French Third Republic, the statue shows French optimism and faith in the progressive values of the Enlightenment. However, with a barefoot, subservient Vietnamese man cowering at Bert's feet as the well-dressed Frenchman holds out a hand to protect him, the statue also depicts Bert and France's paternalist attitude towards colonial subjects. The two Vietnamese men staring at the photographer display an ambiguous attitude towards the statue.

Source: Michael G. Vann.

3. *L'AVENIR DU TONKIN*

April 23, 1887

We wonder what will become of the beautiful statue of *Liberty lighting the world* that was erected on a lovely plant covered pedestal in the Exposition garden. This statue, made of hammered copper, is one-sixteenth the size of Bartholdi's colossal statue in New York. The Parisian firm Gaget-Gauthier and Company sent it to us. We don't think it should be sent back, it should be installed somewhere in the city of Hanoi.

November 26, 1887

The city of Hanoi is becoming more beautiful every day. European construction is gradually replacing grass huts in the main streets.

The European quarter, whose center was initially Jean-Dupuis Street, has spread in the past two years towards Paul-Bert Street. Paul-Bert Street now offers a lively atmosphere, especially in the evenings.

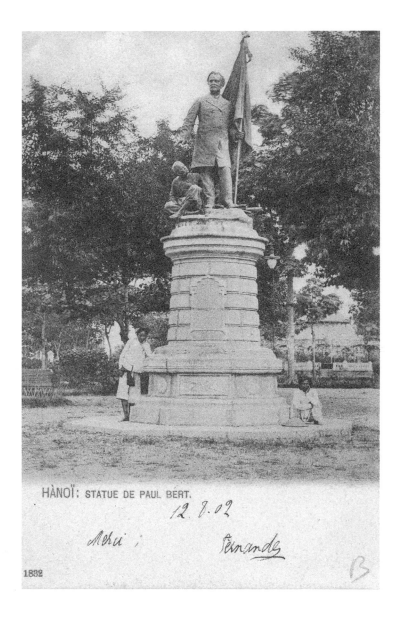

HÀNOÏ: STATUE DE PAUL BERT.

12. 8. 02

1832

This neighborhood will become more important thanks to the recently approved construction projects that will soon be started. Work on buildings around a square has commenced. While at the moment the four buildings seem to be haphazardly thrown between the levee and the boulevard, there will be an entirely different ambiance when there is an English style garden with much greenery and decorative planting.

This square will be crossed by a street running parallel to Paul-Bert Street and ending at the levee. The levee must be kept as it is an indispensable defense against floodwaters from the river.

Another avenue is planned to skirt the new buildings and will hit the rue Paul-Bert at almost a right angle.

If one takes a quick look at the map of Hanoi, we can see that the European city will soon stretch towards the Little Lake and that a new quarter will arise in a triangle formed by the Street of Cards, the extension of the Street of Embroiders, and Exposition Avenue.

Source: *L'Avenir du Tonkin*, April 23, 1887, and November 26, 1887. Translated by Michael G. Vann.

4. MARIUS BOREL, *SOUVENIRS D'UN VIEUX COLONIALIST*

[. . .] three hundred masons, two hundred coolies for ditch digging, three hundred women to bring bricks and mortar to the masons. There were sixty carpenters for woodworking and scaffold building and removal. Finally, there were numerous coolies for various small jobs.

The total was close to a thousand individuals to watch over. I say watch over as they were generally rather intelligent, so one had to be firm and very fair with them.

Source: Marius Borel, *Souvenirs d'un vieux colonialiste* (Rodez: Imprimerie Subervie, 1963), 62–63. Translated by Michael G. Vann.

5. VICTOR LE LAN, "THE OLD QUARTERS," FEBRUARY 5, 1898

The Old Quarters

Through the interminable streets,
The curved or pointed roofs,
With their acute or obtuse angles,
Rise up in the crisp light.

Below the peaks with sharp edges,
Small uncomfortable slums
Alternating with pagodas,
Temples, walls, and towers.

And there are those lonely dreamers,
Contemplating debris from the past
In front of the closed shutters and lowered blinds
Of houses full of mysteries.

Source: Victor Le Lan, "The Old Quarters," in *La Vie Indochinoise*, February 5, 1898. Translated by Michael G. Vann.

6. VICTOR LE LAN, "OPIUM," JANUARY 16, 1897

Opium

In sweet dreams, in crazy dreams,
Sleep inducing opium, killer of suffering,

Takes his heart, his crazy but gentle heart,
To the illusive world of fantasies.

He wanders, he walks in golden visions
In the gay revelries of a frolicking dance.
As Kong-phu-tseu still ponders
The cadence of verses with a sacred rhythm.

He tells himself that the soul is but a whiff of air, nothing,
A lock of hair in a light breeze;
That it is fine to die, but that living is good, too,
And that opium kills the misery.

Source: Victor Le Lan, "Opium," in *La Vie Indochinoise*, January 16, 1897. Translated by
Michael G. Vann.

7. "HANOÏ-TONKIN-MUSÉE," PIERRE DIEULEFILS POSTCARD

This postcard shows the main hall of the Hanoi Exposition after it was
repurposed as the city's museum. The imposing Neo-Classical architecture
conveys the French sense of order, power, and permanence. The pond in the
foreground shows how Hanoi was built in the Tonkin basin's wetlands.

Source: Michael G. Vann.

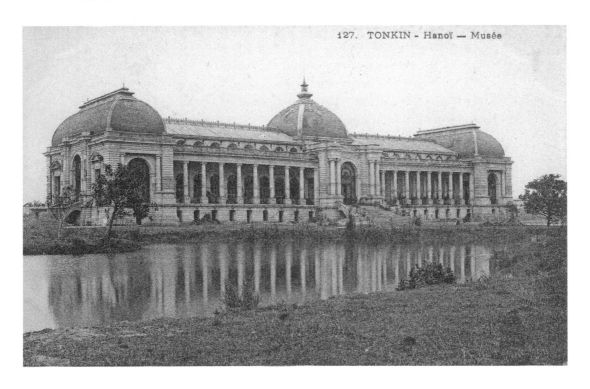

127. TONKIN - Hanoï — Musée

8. "RAPPORT PÉRIODIQUE SUR LA SITUATION INTÉRIEURE DE L'INDO-CHINE (1901)"

[. . .] the bridge over the Red River, exhibition hall, palace of justice, the Governor General's palace, construction of sewers and of sidewalks, etc. All these work projects daily occupy numerous workers and contribute to the maintenance of tranquility in the country.

Source: Paul Doumer, Centre des Archives Section d'Outre-Mer, AF carton 9, dossier A 20 (50): "Rapport périodique sur la situation intérieure de l'Indo-Chine (1901)."

9. ALFRED CUNNINGHAM, *THE FRENCH IN TONKIN AND SOUTH CHINA*

An English war correspondent, Mr. James G. Scott, who visited Hanoi in 1884 during the Tonkin campaign, in recording his impressions of the native capital in his interesting work *France and Tongking* wrote as follows: "There can be no dispute that Hanoi will eventually far surpass Saigon, fine town as it is, just as it is eventually destined to supplant Saigon as the chief town of the French possessions in the 'Far East.'"

Although it is questionable whether in some respects Hanoi as a city is superior at present to the capital of Cochin-China, yet under M. Doumer's regime the prophecy of Mr. Scott has been fulfilled, for to-day Hanoi is the capital of Indo-China, comprising the countries of Chochin-China, Annam, Laos, Cambodia and Tonkin. It is well worthy of the honour.

Hanoi, as a city built up amid Asiatic surroundings, is superior to any in the Far East. Shanghai may claim more business; Hongkong may proudly refer to its Peak residential quarter and its roads cut from solid rock; Manila to its ancient city, and Singapore to its splendid breadth, but in *tout ensemble* Hanoi is undoubtedly the superior. In the matter of spacious and well-kept roads, open spaces and detached residences, Singapore is in places quite equal to Hanoi; but after sundown Singapore slumbers whilst Hanoi is at its best.

The average Continental conception of British colonial life, is that, with the exception of the Anglo-Saxon passion for out-door sport in any temperature—which they cannot understand—the colonists contrive to make themselves publicly as miserable as possible. The Anglo-Saxon conception of French colonial life is, that our neighbours spend their public money on making themselves as comfortable as possible. In many respects this is correct, and whoever has visited a French colony must admit that French colonial life has much to commend it, and is infinitely more attractive than ours. The French colonist is loathe to sacrifice the pleasure of his home life, and there is surely no reason why he should.

Social life in Tonkin is characterised by absence of inconvenient formality, by complete freedom from our society restraints, with the consequence that while the British lead to a great extent an artificial social existence, the French are entirely at their ease, and when business is concluded yield themselves unreservedly to recreation and enjoyment. Our fine social distinctions are not there in evidence. We take our recreation seriously and often make a business of it; the French do not, and are quite unconventional.

Imagine, ye gods, in Hongkong, the wife of a leading fonctionnaire tripping along the streets in the midday heat of summer in white topee and loose morning gown, dropping in at the hotel to lunch and a subsequent chat. Or a military or naval officer of high rank seated, with his wife, after dinner, at a small table on the pavement outside a cafe, sipping liqueur, conversing; and gazing at the occupants of passing carriages!

As a contrast, picture a concert room in an Easter British colony, with the audience gravely seated, arrayed in full evening dress, everything to the Gallic mind, as stiff, as formal and as uncomfortable as it can possibly be. The Anglo-Saxon makes a duty of his pleasures; our neighbours make a pleasure of their duties.

One evening in Hanoi we dined with an important military officer and his friend the constructor of the Hanoi bridge. His house was a mansion full of beautiful things. The dinner was excellent, our host was in his every-day uniform, with putties, his friend in a closely-buttoned white suit!

Again, when up country, we were delightfully entertained at the Chief Residency of the provinces. Twelve of us sat down to a sumptuous repast, which was none the less enjoyable though no one was in evening dress. It is impossible to imagine this in an English colony.

Yet, although we are apt to scoff at the French, their social customs, and methods of colonisation, we are the first to use and appreciate these when we visit their colonies. One cannot, however, go so far as to suggest that the English lady visitor would walk the streets in the heat of the day in a topee and morning-gown. She would be horrified at the idea!

The late Prince Henri d'Orleans remarked: "When we French men colonise, we often manifest great inexperience and want of foresight; but side by side with these defects are certain good qualities which we carry with us all over the globe. In the first place we have a knack of clearing a native town and of constructing by the side of it something at once clean and elegant, utilising the smallest detail so as to make the whole effect pleasing to the eye. The good taste of the Montmartre grisette is to be traced in the work of the Californian pioneer and the Cochin-China non-commissioned officer, that subtle and intangible something which is derived from our temperament and is of our very essence, accounting for the fact that, at a small outlay in money, we have cleared out and partially reconstructed two of the most beautiful towns in the Far-East—Hanoi and Saigon. Compare them with the English-built towns of Bombay and Calcutta in India, or of Hongkong in China, and you will find in the latter large and massive buildings, denoting forte and power, but heavy; whereas in the French built towns there is always some little resemblance to Paris."

Most travellers will acknowledge the correctness of his opinion. After a visit to Hanoi one is curious to learn what the French would have done with Hongkong if they had possessed it. The work of the English has in many respects been marvellous, yet the development of the island colony has been more due to private enterprise than to official labour. In the matter of commercial buildings Hongkong is far ahead of Hanoi; there are no gigantic business houses there as here. There is no need for them, for, as in Singapore, land is plentiful, is flat and cheap.

In Municipal administration Hanoi is far more advanced than Hongkong is or ever will be, while it is a crown colony. The functions of the Hongkong Government are Municipal rather than Imperial; its sphere of action being limited to a few square miles of territory. Outside of Municipal affairs the Military are quite capable alone of carrying on the government. It is a costly machine as it is at present, and its Municipal administration has been disastrous. In Hongkong we suffer continually from the shortsighted and clumsy policy of our early officials, and the Government of to-day instead of recognizing this stultifies itself in endeavouring to vindicate past blunders by a patch-work policy of administration, opposes freedom of action, shirks wholesome expenditure on public works, and avoids a modern municipal system. Government departments are cut down to as fine a point as possible, nearly every branch is undermanned and consequently incapable of doing the work which so rapidly a growing city demands. The ambition of the Governor is to show an annual surplus—accumulated at the expense of essential public works and of sanitary improvements. In Hanoi everything that the Administration can do in effecting public improvements, beautifying and perfecting the city, they do. They are as willing to spend money as we are to hoard it. No residents complain of oppressive Municipal taxation but all appreciate the magnificent work of their city engineers.

The striking feature of French city building, as exemplified at Hanoi, and nearer at Kwang-chau-wan, is the foresight they display. They design and build for the future and in this respect they are strikingly superior to the British. Whether their engineers are superior to ours in a matter of training is a question worthy of consideration; they certainly show better results.

For instance, Hongkong has recently suffered from a plethora of epidemics, plague, cholera and small-pox, the result experts have declared of overcrowding, and, the community also add, of unsuitable drains and a water famine. This reveals a want of administrative ability in past Governors, in not estimating the rapid development of the port, and their failure to keep pace with it. It also shows that our engineers were not equal to their real work, or if they were they were unable to enforce their opinions. At present public means of cheap and rapid transit to relieve terribly congested districts are non-existent, and no public ferry provides the necessary connection between the island and the mainland, such being left to the exclusive service of a local company. However, an electric tramway service is promised, and one official has suggested a bridge across the harbour, but public steam ferries, large enough to carry a tram, would be less expensive and more practicable.

Although the colony has had such a fearful object lesson in such misgovernment, in spite of that at Kowloon are being perpetrated the same blunders, the same evils. Land, every foot of it that can be sold, for building purposes is disposed of by the Government. The roads, which are rapidly becoming main roads into the New Territory, are narrow and in width are but equal to the average street in the native quarters of Hanoi. Lofty Chinese houses, many jerry built, ugly and insanitary, are being daily erected, abutting in some cases on to the very edge of these roads, and the actual foreign houses, standing detached in their own grounds, and suitable for occupation in a tropical climate, are few indeed. Landlords have been permitted to erect terraces of dwellings for foreign occupation, which would challenge an exploited London suburb, and are utterly unsuitable for the place and when vacant lots are built upon and Chinese flock into the centre and overcrowd it, a repetition of the Hongkong epidemics will probably ensue. In August 1902, Sir William Gascoigne opened a small park, previous to which there was no provision for open spaces.

There is every reason to believe that if the French had laid out Kowloon it would have been a beautiful settlement, with gardens and fine boulevards, hills would have been cut down and residences spread over a larger area with public means of communication. The Chinese would have their special quarter and remain there. The future health and happiness of his compatriots would have been the ideal of the French engineer.

There are numerous hotels, cafes and pensions in Hanoi to accommodate visitors, the most important being the Hotel Metropole and the Hanoi Hotel. The former is a splendid building, recently erected, and is situated on the Boulevard Henri Riviere, immediately opposite the Residence Superieure. The hotel is elegantly furnished, each bed-room has a bathroom adjoining; and there is a public hall, *salons de conversations*, reading room. The sanitary arrangements are perfect, and the general accommodation leaves nothing to be desired. The service is good, the servants in the dining-room being Chinese and the room boys are Annamites. The cuisine is what one would expect in a French town, and the charges vary from $6 to $7.50 a day or $125 to $155 a month. For two persons $10 to $12 a day and $210 to $250 a month, and according to custom a bottle of white or red wine, and liqueur, is free at both meals, tiffin and dinner. The Hanoi Hotel is also a large well-conducted place, is likewise extensively patronised, and possesses a very popular cafe.

Hanoi is a very convenient city to travel about in. There are numerous *pousse-pousses*, as they term the jinrickishas, with Annamite pullers. An electric tramway traverses the town and suburbs for a distance of eight miles, and is well patronized by foreigners and natives alike. The principal public buildings are the Mairie, Post and Telegraph office, Residence Superior, Treasury, Military and other offices. The Public Schools, which cost 175,000 francs, form a magnificent block of buildings, with separate sections for boys and girls, lecture hall, etc. A new palace for the Governor-general is in course of erection near the Public Gardens, also a new Palace of Justice. The superb centre block of the Exposition buildings, now being completed, will be ultimately turned into an archaeological and philogical institute.

A new theatre to seat 800 people, is being erected by the municipality within a few yards of the pretty little French Protestant church. The roads are wide, well shaded by trees, and in excellent condition. They are all macadamized and their total length, including suburban thoroughfares, amounts to over fifty miles.

The large and well-filled stores constitute a striking feature of Hanoi life, and the numerous millinery and drapery establishments will delight the hearts of lady visitors during the Exposition. In fact, the view afforded of several streets of first-class stores of all descriptions, with their coloured canvass sun awnings, their temptingly arrayed windows, the foreign bakers' and butchers' shops, all run by French and not Asiatics, is an attractive picture which recalls pleasing visions of home life. As in Chinese cities the native stores are confined to special quarters. The copper and brass smiths have one section, the scroll makers have another, and so on. The best native work produced is mother-of-pearl inlaid in native black-wood, of which remarkably handsome specimens may be obtained in the form of screens, cabinets, trays, boxes, etc. The home of this work is really the town of Bac-ninh. Some very elegant embroideries on silk may also be procured.

In the centre of the town is situated the Petit Lac, with its small island and rustic bridge at one end, and in the middle the quaint Annamite pagoda, surmounted by a bronze statue of Liberty. The money for this statue was collected in small amounts from numerous native subscribers. The lake is nearly half-a-mile square, the path round it makes a pleasant promenade, and if the pedestrian grows tired, he may rest at the cafe of the Hotel de Lac, and gaze on the view before him. Adjoining the lake is the fine Roman Catholic Cathedral, and on the other side, by the Post and

Telegraph Office, is a small public garden with a band-stand and a bronze statue of Paul Bert.

From the Petit Lac the visitor may take a tram to the Citadel, the interesting old Annamite fortress of Hanoi, the walls of which still exist. Here the various branches of the military are quartered. On the grounds of this citadel a Paris company is now busy constructing an estate of well-designed European residences, with market and other conveniences attached. Further on the tram passes the ancient city with its small quaint houses, a locality which the French have thoroughly drained and improved and the streets are now wide, clean and well kept.

The tram then emerges into the suburbs, on one side are scattered pretty detached villa residences of all sizes to suit all purses, whilst on the right stretch the lake of Truc Bac and the Grand Lake of Tay Ho. There are numerous native temples and pagodas, the chief being that of the Grand Bouddha, on the shore of the Grand Lake, which contains an enormous bronze idol.

Near here are the Jardins Botaniques which are really the finest and most picturesque public gardens in the Far East. The gardens are beautifully laid out, and are intersected with carriage drives shaded by trees. Here in the cool of the evening the residents of Hanoi ride in their carriages, and those who prefer to walk find many charming retreats. There is a small but good collection of animals, and some fine specimens of Tonkin tigers, panthers and bears are on view. The gardens, which cover an area of 23 hectares, contain over 3,000 specimens of plants.

Further on, the Race Course is reached, and appears to be well patronised. Races were held on the Sunday we were there, and the scene was a festive one. The mounts are Tonkin ponies, spirited little animals, something like though somewhat larger than the Deli pony of the Straits. They are not big enough for Europeans to ride so the jockeys are diminutive Annamites, and together they put up some good racing. The jockeys seem very proud of their office, and strut about arrayed in their owners' colours, objects of native admiration. The ponies are plentiful and cheap, and as there are many delightful drives, the majority of people keep a carriage and pair. The scenes on the roads through the gardens recall visions of the Lunetta in Manila in the Spanish days, especially when a band is playing.

Then is the time to see the French lady at her best. She has doffed the light loose dress of the earlier part of the day, and may be seen arrayed in elegant Parisian costume, in her carriage drawn by a pair of ponies, with coachman and "tiger" with arms folded, smart uniform, and top boots.

The scene is one of brilliance, vivacity and pleasure; the stream of carriages moving through beautiful drives, with handsomely attired occupants. Hanoi is indeed a city possessing many beautiful women.

At 7 p.m., the community dines, and after 8 the cafes commence to fill. Parties arrive and seat themselves at the small marble tables: sip cognac or liqueurs, smoke and converse. Beer is a favourite beverage. A clap of the hands, a short order in pidgin French, and the white-clad Annamite "boy" brings a small mat, which is placed on the middle of the table, and a game of cards follows, in which the ladies join. Cafe life is very temperate, very enjoyable and very popular. An Englishman, unless he be an abstainer, would probably need stronger drinks and more excitement; a glass of beer or a small liqueur suffices the Frenchman for the evening.

The military are much in evidence, the officers of all ranks being compelled to always appear in uniform. As the usual French military tunic is generally of black cloth, with red, gold or silver facings, the effect on the wearer and the observer is not quite so trying as the red coat of an English officer would be, if he were compelled to appear continually in regimentals. Khaki is extensively worn—especially up country, and putties of the English design are coming into fashion.

Soirees, balls, concerts and theatricals make up the social enjoyments of the Hanoi existence.

There is a large and steadily increasing business transacted at Hanoi, which would, of course, vastly develop if the country were only thrown open to foreign trade. Several local industries have been created, amongst these being a brewery, cotton yarn mill, paper factory, distilleries of native spirits, and match factories.

Neither Hanoi nor Haiphong has yet reached the stage when local money is invested in public companies, and people with surplus cash invest it in their own business, or send it to France. The share market as it exists in Hongkong or Shanghai is unknown, but as one or two public companies have been formed to run several of the few industries which exist, such an institution is possible in the future.

The principal enterprise is the Electric Tramway Company, which they explained to us was partly private and partly a public company, whatever that may mean. The works were constructed in 1900, and a most excellent service of trams is provided, the length of the line being about eight miles. The cars are well-built and comfortable, divided into first-class and second-class, and are of French make. Attached to the car is a small open waggon with canvas side blinds, in which the passenger may prefer to sit in hot weather. The tramway is run on the trolley system, by a current varying from 500 to 600 volts. The generating plant consists of three powerful engines of 250 horse-power, and there are 22 cars. The conductors and drivers are Annamites, the entire staff being about 100 men, of whom 8 are French. The trams are well patronised by Europeans and natives alike, and the company is said to be earning good returns. The maximum fare is

5 cents first-class, and 3 cents second class, and the passenger has a delightful ride for forty minutes for a very cheap fare.

A handsome railway-station has been constructed on the Boulevard Gambetta, where the whole of the network of Tonkin railways will soon converge. From the magnificent bridge across the Red River the railway crosses a stone viaduct 600 metres long, and then passes through the town.

In 1897, 384 foreign residences existed in the urban centre of Hanoi, from then till 1901 their number was increased to 608. Of native brick residences 1,225 constructed in the same period. There are several well-built markets, and others are being erected as required. The Municipal authorities deserve great credit for the splendid system of drainage they have provided at unlimited expense, as the country is flat and marshy, and many lakes had to be filled in which existed in the town and suburbs. The Waterworks were constructed in 1895-6, the water being conveyed by a canal, 25 kilometers long, from large wells, which supply 5,000 cubic metres a day. The water is laid on in the foreign houses, and there are 85 Borne fountains and 85 branches for native supply.

The town is well lighted with electricity, there being 523 incandescent lamps, and 55 arc lights in the foreign quarters. Outlying native districts are lighted with petroleum lamps. The place is well policed but the police are very unobtrusive. The estimated Municipal budget for 1902 amounts to $844,304, made up with other lesser items of taxes on rent $29,000; patents $60,000; capitation of foreign Asiatics $17,484; personal tax on Annamites $9,458. The income from markets in 1901, was $71,497; abattoirs $18,682; jinrikishas $43,370.

The population of Hanoi is 160,000, of whom 1,500 are Europeans, exclusive of the large garrison, and 4,000 Chinese. The city is remarkably healthy, and the maximum temperature in summer, which begins in April, is 35° centigrade (95° F.) and the minimum in winter, which commences in October, 6° cent. (42.8° F.) The railway now enables residents to reach the hills in a few hours, where the heat of the summer may be evaded, and where delightful residences may be built.

At present the community is enthusiastically interested in the Exposition which will be opened in Hanoi in November 1902, which will attract visitors from all parts, and a description of which has been reserved for another chapter.

It is said that when Monsieur Doumer, the Governor-General, went home to raise his last loan of two hundred million francs for the development of Indo-China, the French financiers naturally hesitated. They desired to know something of the resources of the country they were asked to promote.

The reply of the Governor-General was characteristic of the man. They wished to know something of Indo-China? They should have a very practical illustration. He would build an exhibition as an object lesson in French colonial enterprise. He at once formulated a scheme for an exposition of native products and colonial undertakings, which would constitute a gigantic advertisement of France's possessions in the Far East. This would inspire confidence in French minds which knew only Indo-China by name, and that very indistinctly, and would also illustrate convincingly to the natives the resources of France and her greatness.

To-day the Exposition at Hanoi is almost completed; in November, 1902, it will be opened. When the time drew near of M. Doumer's departure for France, some one, in a moment of happy inspiration, suggested it might form a fitting farewell act if he were to be directly associated with the building before leaving. Consequently, on the 26th February, 1902, inaugurative ceremonies were held in the Palais Central, a magnificent erection which will form the centre of the Exposition buildings; and which will ultimately be preserved as the headquarters of the French Institute for the study of the Philology and Archaeology of Eastern Asia.

The spectacle was one of magnificence never before seen in Hanoi, and was attended by the King and Queen of Annam, M. Doumer, General Dodds, and other high officials. M. Thomé, the able administrator of the Exposition, in welcoming M. Doumer, on behalf of the colonists, pointed out their regret at his impending departure, after his having taken such an active part in the colony's affairs for the previous five years, and having by his energy and ability given the colony an impulsion that would definitely guarantee its prosperity. They were as confident as he in the future of the colony, and would always realise that he would remain attached to it after having prepared the way for its advance.

"Flourishing in the interior," said M. Thomé, "strong on the frontiers, this great colony, made up of numerous states, is solidly and definitely united to continue that programme of progress to which you have again devoted the last few days you remain with us.

"I salute you, sir, the Governor-General, the first artisan of French Indo-China."

Source: Alfred Cunningham, *The French in Tonkin and South China* (Hong Kong: Hongkong Daily Press, 1902), 65–93.

10.   "HANOÏ-TONKIN-PAGODON DU PETIT LAC," PIERRE DIEULEFILS POSTCARD

This postcard celebrates French colonial urbanism. An electric street car passes a pousse-pousse, or rickshaw, on a wide boulevard that separated the French Quarter from Ho Hoan Kiem, the Lake of the Returned Sword. Powerlines and gas lighting illustrate the city's modernization, while barefoot coolies-pousses pull their passengers down the road and women carry baskets loaded with goods. A French department store stands in sharp contrast to the lone Sino-Vietnamese guardhouse in the foreground.

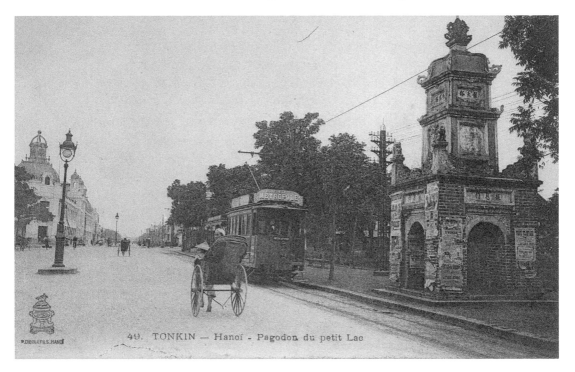

49. TONKIN — Hanoï - Pagodon du petit Lac

Source: Michael G. Vann.

11. "CHINATOWN IS A MENACE TO HEALTH," *THE SAN FRANCISCO CALL*, NOVEMBER 23, 1901

TELLS OF UNSANITARY STATE OF CHINATOWN

Dr. Williamson of the Board of Health Reads an Interesting Paper to Delegates.

Supervisor Charles Wesley Reed suggested that the Rev. Peter C. Yorke be invited to address the convention. The suggestion was greeted with applause and Mr. Reed was appointed a committee to bring the clergyman to the convention. Dr. Williamson, of the San Francisco Board of Health, then read the following paper:

> In presenting views upon the subject assigned by the committee of arrangements, the writer feels it incumbent upon himself as a representative of the municipal government, to limit his remarks as closely as possible to the influences exerted by the Chinese upon the general health of this community. At the same time an attempt will be made to show in what principal respects the race in question is an undesirable element, especially when colonized in cities and towns. Industrial or

social conditions will not be considered, as these features can be more thoroughly dealt with by those whose study and research of the problems involved have qualified them to discuss the subject with both intelligence and understanding.

What may be said concerning the Chinese of San Francisco will apply with almost an equivalent amount of force to any community upon the Pacific Coast in which people of the Chinese race may be found, and it can be accepted by those interested as one of the contributing factors to the many reasons which justify and even demand the re-enactment of the exclusion act.

Taking the habits and customs of the Chinese of San Francisco as typical of those exhibited by them when grouped in any American community, it can be alleged without danger of contradiction that the section of the city inhabited by them has given more concern to the authorities than all the rest of the city combined. Violations of sanitary laws and indecencies of many descriptions are no sooner suppressed or abated than they are almost invariably repeated. The Chinese, exclusive of the official and mercantile classes, appear to revel in dirt and wallow in filth in preference to becoming and remaining clean, even when the cleanliness is provided and paid for by the landlord, the city or the State.

During the past five years the holders of real estate in San Francisco's Chinatown have been compelled to spend many thousands of dollars for sanitary plumbing to replace that of antique and inefficient character which has been condemned to the health officials. It is an acknowledged fact that unless a strict daily watch is maintained some of the occupants of the premises where improved plumbing has been placed will exhibit their disapproval of such innovation by willfully breaking and damaging the same.

Property owners in Chinatown, who would otherwise be perfectly willing to follow the directions of the Board of Health, have often complained against being forced to put forth large expenditures for modern plumbing, claiming that as soon as it is installed it will be ruined beyond repair.

In the Chinese quarter of San Francisco open sewers have been found running through underground living apartments. After these have been closed by the authorities they have been repeatedly reopened by the persons living in the premises, who seem to regard an open sewer as a convenience instead of a nuisance. In the subterranean strata there are places where tunnels have been dug leading from inhabited basements beneath the street as far as the main sewer, which has been opened in order to afford ready access, for what particular purpose the Chinese alone can say. On one tour of inspection tiers of bunks occupied by sleeping Chinese were found in a tunnel just on the verge of an open sewer.

The utter contempt for the simplest principles of sanitation has resulted in the deliberate breaking or obstructing of drain pipes which unless discovered by inspectors have been permitted to discharge their output into cellars and other excavations, where it saturates the soil and continually gives forth offensive exhalations.

Opium smoking, once a purely Oriental vice, has received so much attention In the past that little reference is necessary, except it be to point with disgust and chagrin to the readiness with which the habit has been adopted by a considerable number of whites who after reaching their appropriate level of degradation find in the crowded and unhealthy purlieus of Chinatown a haven of uncleanliness admirably adapted to their debased instincts.

Police vigilance has minimized to a great extent the prostitution in the quarter which served as a notorious distributing center for venereal diseases and It Is not long since the district was cleared of many white girls who plied this calling among the Chinese exclusively.

As a result of poorly ventilated and overcrowded apartments, the utter disregard of ordinary principles of cleanliness and the universal infatuation for dirt, disease is active.

In the fiscal year ending June 30, 1899, 548 deaths occurred among the Chinese. Estimating the population at 13,000, this number gives a death rate of 30.44 per thousand; the city's death rate was 19.72 per thousand. In the following year 562 deaths were credited to the Chinese, or 31.22 per thousand; the city's death rate was 18.81 per thousand. During the last fiscal year 418 deaths were reported, or 23.22 per thousand, while the city's rate was 19.48 per thousand. These figures show the death rate among these people to be vastly in excess of the general death rate in the city of San Francisco. The diminution during the last fiscal year is due without question to the fact that many sick Chinese left the city during the quarantine excitement and their death took place at different points of the interior.

Source: "Chinatown Is a Menace to Health," *The San Francisco Call*, November 23, 1901.

12. GOUVERNEMENT-GÉNÉRAL DE L'INDO-CHINE, *VILLE DE HANOI (TONKIN): HISTORIQUE, DÉVELOPPEMENT FINANCIER, RÈGLEMENTATION ADMINISTRATIVE ET FONCTIONNEMENT DES DIVERS SERVICES MUNICIPAUX DE LA VILLE DE HANOI*, 1905 (PP. 17–19)

The city of Hanoi, located at 21.58° north, and 103.29 ° east, occupies an area of 945 hectares, 25 acres, and 49 centiares.

It extends on the right bank of the Red River over a length of about 4 kilometers, creating an isosceles triangle whose base would be the concession and the summit the pagoda of the Great Buddha.

It is surrounded by a suburban belt which makes a 9 kilometer arc ending at the river and creates a buffer zone between the city and the neighboring provinces of Sontay to the North, Ha-Dong to the South-West, and Bac-Ninh to the East.

Hanoi seems to have been first mentioned in the ninth century CE. Founded by the Kinh-Duong-Vuong dynasty on the site of a village called Long-Ao. The Ha Khao pagoda was built there but was since moved to Rue des Pavillons Noirs, to make room for the Royal Palace.

Hanoi was then called Gia-Chi-Bo or Ke-So which translates as Big Market. Cao-Biên built a citadel and surrounded it with a rampart which he called Dai la Thanh (865). Later in 1028, King Thay-Ton of the Ly dynasty built a palace on a mound of earth called Thang-Long, and which gave its name to the city. Thang-Long Palace used to be on the site currently occupied by the racetrack at the corner of the Parreau dike and the adjacent road leading to the Paper Village Bridge. During construction on the road connecting the Parreau dike to the racetrack, artifacts were discovered on this site. Recovered ruins, vases, and coins indicate the existence of a large city in the era of Chinese occupation, some ten centuries ago. In an effort to expand their trade connections, the Dutch established a trade post at Hung Yen.

Traveling by river, Hanoi is 150 kilometers from the sea. However, the Cua Hoc La river mouth is unfortunately too shallow for major commercial shipping. The capital nevertheless remains in communication with all the provinces by divergent branches of the river and the railway lines that link Hanoi to Haiphong, the Chinese border, to the Border, Vinh, and Lao-Kay.

Gia-Long (1801–1820) was the true founder of the present city, which was situated in the vicinity of Paper Village Bridge. Towards the twelfth year of his reign, that is to say, in 1802, Gia-Long ordered a citadel constructed with Vauban style fortifications designed by a French officer: Colonel Olivier. Minh-Mang, Gia-Long's son, who succeeded him from 1821 to 1841, gave the name of Hanoi to the capital of Tonkin.

With an area of 156 hectares 25 acres, this enormous citadel was the largest in Tonkin until its 1894 demolition (Bazin's firm had the contract). Today only a large walled gate and the citadel tower are still standing.

Hanoi lost its status as capital. Due to various political revolutions, the seat was transported successively to Sontay and Ninh-Binh. With each change of king there was the construction of a palace in a new capital. However, since Gia-Long, it has remained the capital of Tonkin. Today it is the capital of Indo-China and headquarters government and all administrative services.

Hanoi's population breaks down as follows:

Roughly 3000 Europeans
2150 Chinese
60 Japanese
50 Indians
100,000 Annamites

Historical or remarkable Annamese monuments that deserve mention include such sites as the Quan-Thanh Pagoda of the Great Buddha which contains a colossal bronze statue of the sacred Tran Vu and the Van-Mieu royal temple of literature (Europeans call it Cave Pagoda) where there are memorials to the literary examinations held in Hanoi from the reign of Le-Thai-Tê to the revolt of Tay Son at the end of the last century. There are 82 steles, covered with inscriptions, each on a stone turtle. The pagoda of the Truong sisters, the two Tonkinese Joans of Arc who rescued their country from the yoke of the Chinese in 38 CE. The pagoda of Bach Ma in the street of Sails, dedicated to the Chinese general Cao Bien, who reigned in Hanoi in 860. The Ninth Century Mat pagoda, which the scholars call Lotus, erected on a single column of stone, located near the Botanical Garden behind the powder magazine. Jade Island pagoda (Ngoc Son) in the middle of Hanoi's small lake, which is connected to boulevard Francis Garnier by an arched wood footbridge. The spirit of this pagoda is Van Xuong, god of the literati who lives in the Big Bear constellation. For 500 years this site has been a meeting place for Tonkin's scholars. At the entrance, one will notice a monumental inkwell and paintbrush statue under which many bones are buried.

Among the European monuments that give Hanoi a big city ambiance, we must mention the train station, whose importance has just been considerably increased by the addition to the main body of two wings serving as offices and the construction of workshops, shops and housing for employees.

A short distance away on the same boulevard are the offices of the Indo-China and Yunnan Railway Company. This three-story building faces the Great Exhibition Hall, one of the most beautiful monuments of the city.

Then, in the city center, we must mention a group of four older buildings: the Town Hall, the Treasury, the Post Office, and the Superior Resident's offices which surround the square Paul-Bert.

There are also the Paul-Bert elementary school with its vast courtyards, the Chambers of Commerce and Agriculture, formerly the Palace of Kinh

Luoc, the Gendarmerie, the civil prison, the Hôtel Métropole, the officers of the Indo-Chinese Trade Union, and the Hanoi cathedral, with its Romanesque style, is the oldest of the monuments the city.

Other buildings are nearing completion: the High Court with its grandiose proportions, the new palace of the General Government near the Botanical Garden, and finally the Municipal Theater, a piece of modern architecture situated at the of Paul-Bert, the city's main street.

Source: Gouvernement-Général de l'Indo-Chine, *Ville de Hanoi (Tonkin): Historique, Développement financier, Règlementation administrative et Fonctionnement des divers services municipaux de la Ville de Hanoi* (Hanoi: Taupin, 1905), 17–19. Translated by Michael G. Vann.

13. ALFRED MEYNARD, "TONKIN," IN JOSEPH FERRIÈRE, GEORGES GARROS, ALFRED MEYNARD, AND ALFRED RAQUEZ, *L'INDO-CHINE,* 1906

In any case, life in Tonkin will never have the same character as in Cochinchina, as Saigon's proximity to sea-lanes brings in new energy. Hanoi, the economic center of Northern Indo-China, is in the interior: one does not pass by, one has to go there. There is even less sense of contact with distant Europe than in Saigon; life is much more self-absorbed there and more provincial. And as this natural isolation is compounded by the region's chilly winters, it is understandable why the Hanoians made their city feel more western.

In Hanoi we can find something lacking in the great English cities of India: intimacy. Though it is a large city with wide avenues and houses spaced at some distance from each other, one can immediately feel at home. In the native part does not have that immense and anonymous swarming of the Hindoo crowds. Rather, each quarter has its own activity, its particular classification. The French city and the Annamite city form a harmonious duality, and if hygiene is poor in the Old Quarter, the picturesque makes up for it. The houses of Hanoi are grouped around the Lake of the Sword, its clear glistening waters surrounded by green foliage and the ancient pagoda of Literature rising up in the middle. This lake and these monuments of Annamite art give the white city a unique aspect, the still living but slowly dying face of history.

Around this limpid jewel circulate pleasant alleys, home to gardens, monuments, shops, and comfortable houses lost in the red shade of the Flamboyant trees' summertime blossoms. There is the Philharmonic Society, the General Secretariat of Indo-China, the headquarters of the Post and Telegraph, and Paul-Bert Square, all buried under the shade, where, on warm evenings, the townsfolk listen to live music. In addition to the major streets, there is Paul-Bert Street, less broad than its brothers, the modern boulevards, but forming, by itself, the original center of the city. It is the street of cafes, hotels and shops. At the end of it stands the massive (but not very elegant) construction site for the New Theater on the grounds of the former French concession where the first military buildings and the Governor General's Palace were built.

From the top of the New Theater, the view extends over this city spread out on the bank of the river. Scattered monuments poke out of the greenery verdure and the low private dwellings. You can see the Superior Residence, the Hotel Metropole, the former palace of the Kinh-Luoc (viceroy) now transformed into Chamber of Commerce, the train station, the barracks of the native troops, the Union club, hospitals, the cathedral and its two towers, the Office of Public Works, the Doumer Bridge, and so on. In the distance, isolated in a less dense neighborhood, there is the newly built and imposing high court, whose awkward construction seems to be just as ugly as the recently completed General Governor's palace.

Hanoi now has the appearance of a large city with a firmly established community, with a strong revue base, with an equal number of luxurious and utilitarian buildings. If it has cafes and theaters, it also has sewers, water and electricity plants, a brewery, a spinning mill, a distillery, a ceramic factory, two match factories, a tobacco factory, many workshops, mechanics, active and diverse indigenous industries, and large and luxurious food, furniture, jewelry and hardware stores.

Visitors to the distant city will find it similar to life back in the metropole, but will also realize how brand new it all is. Indeed, in 1897, there were twenty-three European houses in Hanoi; there are now 831. And the growth is constant. Currently, Hanoi is already one of the most beautiful cities of the Far East. Majestically framed by a two-kilometer arc of the Red River, with its Petit-Lac and the abundant greenery (in spite of typhoons), it will not only be an economic center, railway hub, and government seat, it will increasingly become the elegant and stately capital of Indo-China. As head of the countries of the Union, it will resurrect the intellectual grandeur of the Annamese people.

[. . .]

Despite acts of municipal vandalism, Hanoi has not lost its historic grace. The remains of the ancient city, even in the middle of the European city, retain the religious spirit of the Annamese race. With the coquetry of a domesticated foreign woman who still hints at her origins, amongst various utilitarian structures Hanoi reveals harmonious steles, an old and memorable gate (the Jean-Dupuis gate recently escaped demolition), and a dreamy little pagoda. All that remains of the famous citadel is only a high stone watchtower, now assigned to wireless telegraphy.

The native and Chinese city, in spite of the electric tramway's disruptive traffic, has lost none of its integrity. With the liveliness of its merchant life, the perpetual activity of its inhabitants, the whole of its existence takes place in the streets. With crowded theaters, countless boutiques, wandering food vendors, smiling Cong Gaï, Boys playing, and interpreters with their fancy umbrellas, the neighborhood is a spectacle of an incredible and ever surprising diversity. There the childish, playful, and quarrelsome character of the Annamite comes out. Their true nature is often hidden in when dealing with Europeans. The street is an interminable and familiar playground where every passer-by has something to say, from the rickshaw coolie pulling a passenger to the merchant carrying his wares on protruding bamboo poles to the dignified mandarin going to his office.

There is nothing more vibrant, nothing more alive and picturesque than the noise of this disorderly but always harmonious crowd. No one is a stranger to another. There is constant friendly communication and none of the blind rudeness of European mobs.

Life here is not a constant dull struggle that creates individual selfishness; rather, it is slow and carefree with a simple society and few private lusts for wealth. Necessity is the real issue and thus shops only carry the wide variety of Annamese foods and the merchants stock ordinary objects, cloths, or tobacco.

Eating, laughing, smoking, and sleeping, that is the existence of the poor Annamite, and the poor are 99% of the population. Hence, the very soul of the race can be found relaxing amidst in the hustle and bustle of the street.

The Chinese have adjusted to the smiling indifference of the Annamites by maintaining their practical sense of business. Everywhere in the Annamese quarter are seen the fantastic signs of their stores; they are jewelers, silk and opium merchants, but above all they sell the curiosities of Shanghai and Canton, and the other ancient knickknacks, to satisfy the profitable European curiosity. Some Hindus and some Japanese supplement this commercial abundance. As for the indigenous workers, they manufacture and sell their modest trinkets, the varied and meticulous productions from various regions of Annam.

The coppersmiths, the stone carvers, the wood carvers, the lacquerers, the embroiderers, have their own particular streets where they live and work. There are also the more modest vendors of mats, coffins, bamboos, objects made of zinc, cotton, fans, and umbrellas.

The Annamite city looks like an immense and complex anthill. Each of its houses is a shop and each of its streets offers you an unexpected new activity. These allegedly lazy people work all day long and in such a way that they seem to do it for their own pleasure.

Source: Alfred Meynard, "Tonkin," in Joseph Ferrière, Georges Garros, Alfred Meynard, and Alfred Raquez, *L'Indo-Chine, 1906* (Levallois-Perret: Welihoof et Roche, 1906), 34–35. Translated by Michael G. Vann.

14. HANOI TOWN HALL, DOSSIER: 38: "NOTE ON THE DEVELOPMENT OF THE CITY OF HANOI FROM 1 JANUARY 1902 TO 30 JUNE 1907"

The last five years of the city's economic development have been, in general, less than brilliant when compared to the preceding period [1897–1902].

Hanoi, as the commercial center of Tonkin, has suffered from the repercussions of the various difficulties that have been felt in all the countries of the Far East. Added to this are the rather severe local crises (typhoons and bad harvests) that have hit Tonkin especially hard.

Despite everything, however, the situation has remained propitious and has even progressed in a satisfactory manner, seen in the continuing construction, a sure sign of an increase in the public wealth.

Source: Hanoi Town Hall, Dossier: 38: "Note on the development of the City of Hanoi from 1 January 1902 to 30 June 1907." Vietnam National Archives I. Translated by Michael G. Vann.

15. BRIEUX, *VOYAGE AUX INDES ET EN INDO-CHINE: SIMPLES NOTES D'UN TOURISTE*

We are, it is true, the masters in title, but the Chinese are the true masters. They are two hundred thousand and we are ten thousand. We send soldiers and they send merchants. [. . .] We administer the colony while they exploit it.

Source: Brieux, *Voyage aux Indes et en Indo-Chine: Simples notes d'un touriste* (Paris: Librarie Ch. Delagrave, 1910), 154–55. Translated by Michael G. Vann.

16. MICHAEL MY, *LE TONKIN PITTORESQUE: SOUVENIRS ET IMPRESSIONS DE VOYAGE 1921–1922*

For travelers coming from Haiphong by ferry, Hanoi is announced by the great Doumer Bridge, a fitting honor to the man, a gigantic work which impresses the new arrival and which testifies to the strength of the French genius.

This 1,800-meter-long bridge, not including two kilometers of viaducts and access ramps, is the most beautiful artwork executed in the colony. It spans the Red River, powerfully pushing its feet through the alluvial sand and Phuc-Xa island which the annually high waters submerge. After the Pont Doumer, trains almost immediately enter the station.

At one end of the Boulevard Gambetta, the train station crowns the street. It occupies some 1,200 meters. Traffic is intense. More than thirty trains come and go every day. Hanoi is the central hub for the lines heading to Haiphong; to Nam-Dinh and Thanh-Hoa, and Vinh; to Yunnan (by way of Lao-Kay); and towards eastern China (by Langson). Thousands of travelers from these four provinces are served by the network, arriving or leaving Hanoi at all hours of the day and even at night. This traffic signals intense and constant movement.

French trade is very important in Hanoi. Almost all the large Indochinese firms have branch offices, if not their headquarters, in the city. There are companies with substantial capital that operate large department stores comparable to those in the big cities of France.

U. C. I. A., in particular, runs Réunis which occupy an entire square between Rue Paul-Bert and the Boulevards Dong-Khanh and Rollandes, the most modern corner of the city, where I suggest my readers begin their visit to various neighborhoods of the Indochinese capital.

With regard to native trade every family engages in all of its forms, with the exception of a few rich landlords and senior officials but even their wives and children engage in some speculation. The Tonkinese is born a merchant, just as the Cochinchinese is, by nature, a farmer. From the most tender age, children are initiated into commerce as a means of earning money. This is necessary as the soil is not fertile enough to support the population.

Hanoi's industrial base is worth mentioning. In addition to the water works and the power station, which are indispensable to every large city, there are a large number of French industries in Hanoi: breweries, spinning mills, cotton, silk weaving workshops, soap factories, a ceramic factory, match factories, button makers, the famous Fontaine distillery, the Indochina Tobacco Factory, pottery factories, large printing presses, food canners, cabinet workshops, construction companies, etc. . . .

The natives embrace all branches of economic activity. The Tonkinese, perfect imitators, manufacture everything that the population needs for daily use or to supply households. Indigenous craftsmen are grouped into streets named for their craft, and they can be quite picturesque.

As in all major cities, Hanoi's hotel industry is very prosperous. Throughout the city there are large hotels and modest garnished to accommodate passenger of all budgets.

Source: Michael My, *Le Tonkin pittoresque: Souvenirs et impressions de voyage, 1921–1922* (Saigon: Imprimerie J. Viet, 1925), 32–36. Translated by Michael G. Vann.

17. HANOI'S MUNICIPAL THEATER

Due to a number of delays and cost overruns, Hanoi's municipal theater was completed long after Governor General Paul Doumer's departure. Its stunning architecture was modeled on Paris's opera house at one end of rue Paul Bert. Considered the crowning jewel of Hanoi's French Quarter, the French designed building was built with low cost Vietnamese and Chinese "coolie" labor and paid for with tax revenue collected from the city's Asian residents. Until the Vietnamese struggle for national liberation, the theater staged Western productions for white audiences.

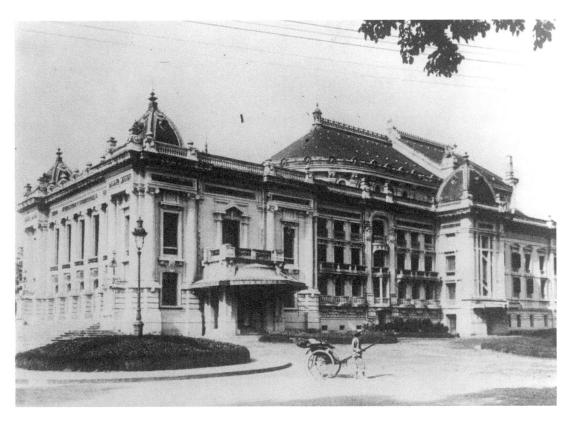

Source: Hanoi's Municipal Theater, CAOM 30FI119 1658.

18.   M. GEORGES MASPERO, *UN EMPIRE COLONIAL FRANÇAIS: L'INDOCHINE*

Of all the geographical transformations brought to Indochina by its French colonization, urban development is probably the most apparent. In this overwhelmingly rural country, which lacks significant of communications infrastructure and industry, urban organization has been rather mediocre and stunted for decades. In the land of the Annamites, cities are comprised of an official center surrounded by walls, with mandarins, a garrison, official offices, rice and salt granaries, and a commercial town composed of a jumble of straw huts, some sort of permanent "market" where neighbors opened shops to sell the agricultural and manufactured products from their home villages. For the Tonkin region, *Description of the Kingdom of Tonkin* (1685) by a curious English Baron offers a first-hand account of Hanoi in the seventeenth century: then as today each street only sold one product or type of merchandise, "But these streets," wrote the Baron, "are divided up between one or more villages, whose inhabitants alone have the privilege of keeping a shop there." In this ancient state, administrative towns and commercial towns had a rather precarious existence; the suppression of the former could cause the decline of the latter. Thus, with the fall of a dynasty or the rise of a new sovereign, the administrative districts and their headquarters, that is to say, the official cities, are often changed. It can be said that the rural village was the main competent of old Annam, providing with a strong communal organization. The city was the unstable element and changing, whose organization has always remained rudimentary.

The French have been great builders in Indochina. Rejecting the clay, bamboo, and woven grass of the natives, they used brick and iron, reinforced cement, sometimes stone. They built solid structures for the future. Native cities have been sanitized and expanded, rather luxurious European neighborhoods have been created, large public buildings have been built, and banks, trading houses, and theaters have been erected. Then industrial establishments were set up, drawing more workers into the city. And when these administrative and economic centers are linked into a railway network or augmented by a modern port, and endowed with a perfected municipal organization, the city becomes something stable and permanent. There are many examples of this evolution.

Source: M. Georges Maspero, *Un empire colonial français: L'Indochine* (Paris: Les Éditions G. Van Oest, 1929), 48–49. Translated by Michael G. Vann.

19. CLAUDE FARRÈRE, *LES CIVILISÉS*

Chapter 14

The smoking-room at Torral's house was dark, because the shades with large slats blocked the sun after two in the afternoon. The opium lamp yellowed the ceiling, and brown spirals rolled heavily in the air impregnated with the drug. The sizzling pipe bowl alternated with silence. Torral was smoking, his sleeping boys at his feet.

It was the torrid hour of a dreamless siesta. Saigon slept, and the murderous sun reigned in the empty streets. Smokers can live in the bottom of a closed world, and the thread of their thought, miraculously softened by opium, can stretch beyond the human world, extending to the calm and lucid regions that Confucius tried to explain to his disciples.

Lying on the left side, his right hand touching the needle to the lamp's flame, Torral was preparing his sixth pipe. He had placed Cambodian cushions made of fresh rice straw under him. His unbuttoned pajamas revealed his brown chest, too narrow for his big head. His torso, at once robust and sickly, the torso of a civilized man who constantly works his inherited intelligence but scornfully gives up his body to debauchery. Torral then smoked his sixth pipe.

He drank in the black smoke without taking breath, and suffocated rather than reject it. His head fell to the ground, knocked a cushion, and he stiffened voluptuously, his senses vibrating like a bowstring. The warm smell of the drug satisfied his nostrils, and the smoky lamp intoxicated his metallic eyes. The light breath of the sleeping boys quivered in his ears like an exquisite violin complaint.

Outside, far away in the street as silent as the Sahara, there were footsteps, and no one but a smoker could have heard it at first. Torral listened curiously to the man who was coming—a man, for it was a wide and careful stride—the acute perceptions of the smoker were improved by the game. The man stopped, then walked again. At the edge of the sidewalk, Torral guessed the walker's short hesitation, forced to cross the street to abandon the shadow of the trees. The footsteps ceased before the door and Torral immediately recognized Fierce, although Fierce was not one to walk the streets at this time of the day.

Torral struck his foot on the pile of sleeping brown flesh. The boys stretched out, disentangled. They were like little fallen statues. Sao stood up, opium swelling his red eyes. He looked for his white linen shirt, thrown into a corner for the siesta. Fierce impatiently struck him as well. The boy then went naked to another room, tying his long hair under his black turban.

Fierce entered, dropped his hat, and sat down, silent.

"What?" Asked the smoker.

"Nothing."

As he stretched out to the right of the lamp, Torral offered a pipe to Fierce who shook his head. Torral smoked alone, and then lay drowsy. The boys had gone back to sleep.

Source: Claude Farrère, *Les Civilisés* (Paris: Flammarion, 1905), 98–99.

20. CHARLES BAUDELAIRE, "THE EYES OF THE POOR"

Ah! you want to know why I hate you to-day. It will probably be less easy for you to understand than for me to explain it to you; for you are, I think, the most perfect example of feminine impenetrability that could possibly be found.

We had spent a long day together, and it had seemed to me short. We had promised one another that we would think the same thoughts and that our two souls should become one soul; a dream which is not original, after all, except that, dreamed by all men, it has been realised by none.

In the evening you were a little tired, and you sat down outside a new cafe at the corner of a new boulevard, still littered with plaster and already displaying proudly its unfinished splendours. The cafe glittered. The very gas put on all the fervency of a fresh start, and lighted up with its full force the blinding whiteness of the walls, the dazzling sheets of glass in the mirrors, the gilt of cornices and mouldings, the chubby-cheeked pages straining back from hounds in leash, the ladies laughing at the falcons on their wrists, the nymphs and goddesses carrying fruits and pies and game on their heads, the Hebes and Ganymedes holding out at arm's-length little jars of syrups or parti-coloured obelisks of ices; the whole of history and of mythology brought together to make a paradise for gluttons. Exactly opposite to us, in the roadway, stood a man of about forty years of age, with a weary face and a greyish beard, holding a little boy by one hand and carrying on the other arm a little fellow too weak to walk. He was taking the nurse-maid's place, and had brought his children out for a walk in the evening. All were in rags. The three faces were extraordinarily serious, and the six eyes stared fixedly at the new cafe with an equal admiration, differentiated in each according to age.

The father's eyes said: "How beautiful it is! how beautiful it is! One would think that all the gold of the poor world had found its way to these walls." The boy's eyes said: "How beautiful it is! how beautiful it is! But that is a house which only people who are not like us can enter." As for the little one's eyes, they were too fascinated to express anything but stupid and utter joy.

Song-writers say that pleasure ennobles the soul and softens the heart. The song was right that evening, so far as I was concerned. Not only was I touched by this family of eyes, but I felt rather ashamed of our glasses and decanters, so much too much for our thirst. I turned to look at you, dear love, that I might read my own thought in you; I gazed deep into your eyes, so beautiful and so strangely sweet, your green eyes that are the home of caprice and under the sovereignty of the Moon; and you said to me: "Those people are insupportable to me with their staring saucer-eyes! Couldn't you tell the head waiter to send them away?"

So hard is it to understand one another, dearest, and so incommunicable is thought, even between people who are in love.

Source: Charles Baudelaire, "The Eyes of the Poor," in T. R. Smith (ed.), *Baudelaire: His Prose and Poetry* (New York: Boni and Liveright Publishers, 1919). http://archive.org/stream/baudelairehispro00baudiala/baudelairehispro00baudiala_djvu.txt.

21. PHAN VAN HY, "THE RICKSHA MAN"

The Ricksha man

The ricksha man does quite a simple job:
he who can hardly walk pulls him who can.
He'll fake the slave for now and bide his time:
he may yet throw the bigwig who sits there.
He fights his way through streets against the cars;

the wind blows dust and smudges up his face.

Both he who pulls and he who's pulled are men:

between the two the difference lies in luck.

Source: Phan Van Hy, "The Ricksha man," in Huynh Sanh Thong (ed. and trans.), *An Anthology of Vietnamese Poems: From the Eleventh through Twentieth Centuries* (New Haven: Yale University Press, 1996), 127.

22. LAURENT JOSEPH GAIDE AND PIERRE MARIE DUROLLE, *LA TUBERCULOSE ET SA PROPHLYLAXIE EN INDOCHINE FRANÇAISE*

Vietnamese homes in cities and in the countryside, often grass shacks, have scarcely been modified for centuries. However, they can be cleaned up. Areas with filthy and overcrowded dwellings are to be found above all in neighborhoods populated with Chinese.

There is less poverty in the countryside. Social factors play a major part in the cities and large concentrations of people, but they are not negligible in the countryside. Rural homes are often cluttered and deprived of air and light. The inhabitants sleep on cots and the ignorance of hygienic precautions is as frequent as in the big cities.

Source: Laurent Joseph Gaide and Pierre Marie Durolle, *La tuberculose et sa prophlylaxie en Indochine française* (Hanoi: IDEO, 1930), 27. Translated by Michael G. Vann.

THE THIRD PLAGUE PANDEMIC

The bubonic plague epidemic that started in nineteenth-century Yunnan became a global pandemic at the turn of the century. Traveling on the newly industrialized maritime transportation networks of the European and American empires, the disease quickly moved from port city to port city. These documents show how Western medicine struggled to understand the disease and its rapid propagation. Frequently resorting to racist explanations, Europeans and Americans often singled out overseas Chinese communities as the source of the disease.

1. "BLACK PLAGUE IN HAWAII. BREAKS OUT IN TWO ISLANDS— SITUATION IN HONOLULU IMPROVES," *PORTSMOUTH HERALD*, FEBRUARY 24, 1900

Honolulu, Feb. 15, via San Francisco, Feb. 23.—The black plague has broken out at both Kahului, on the island of Maui, and Hilo, on the island of Hawaii. The latest advices report seven deaths at Kahului, all Chinese, and one at Hilo, a Portuguese woman, the wife of A.G. Seneo. The news was received here Feb. 10 in a letter from Sheriff Baldwin.

Chinatown in Kahului, which had about 300 inhabitants, has been destroyed by fire. The sanitary conditions were worse than in Honolulu. The towns of Lahaine [Lahaina] and Hauhua have established quarantine against other portions of Maui. An unfortunate feature of the case is the proximity to Kahului of several large plantations with their thousands of laborers. It is thought that the plague reached Kahului through the shipment of Chinese new year goods.

In Honolulu the health situation is better than at any time since the outbreak of the plague. Not a case has developed in the last ten days. Although the board of health is confident that the trouble is over, vigilance will not be relaxed. Up to Feb. 6, the date of the last case, there had been 50 deaths from the plague in this city. The board of health has passed a resolution prohibiting the landing of all merchandise from countries where the bubonic plague exists.

Saturday, Feb. 17, has been set apart as "rat killing" day, and a great slaughter of the rodents is expected.

Source: "Black Plague in Hawaii. Breaks Out in Two Islands—Situation in Honolulu Improves," *Portsmouth Herald*, February 24, 1900.

2. "THE SCOURGE OF THE CENTURY," *LINCOLN COUNTY LEADER*, MAY 11, 1900

HUNDREDS OF INFECTED COOLIES SHOT DOWN, THOUSANDS OF HOMES LAID WASTE BY FIRE, IN EFFORTS TO STAMP OUT EPIDEMICS.

Though Many Times Declared to be Suppressed the Bubonic Cure Continues Its Terrible March around the Globe.

BUBONIC plague—the dreaded "black death" of the Orient—will never get a foothold in the United States, or in any other civilized country where modern methods of sanitation prevail. This is the assertion of Surgeon General Wyman of the United States army and it is endorsed by medical experts generally. So far as known only two cases of genuine bubonic plague have been found in the United States. These were brought into New York last fall on a steamer from Santos, Brazil, where the disease is now epidemic. There was considerable alarm when the fact of the presence of the plague was known, but this quickly passed off when it became evident that the quarantine regulations in this country are such that it is almost impossible for a disease of this nature to spread. Since then vessels have been continually arriving from Santos, but no new cases of the plague have developed.

"So far as the United States is concerned," says Surgeon General Wyman, "there is absolutely no danger of a bubonic plague invasion. The plague is essentially a dirt disease; it cannot thrive where the people are cleanly, and well-nourished; or where modern methods of sanitation prevail. It is found in its worst stages in lands like India and China, whore the natives are dirty in their personal habits; where the very soil is saturated with filth; where there is an utter lack of anything like sanitation even of the crudest kind, and where the people's bodies, weakened and emaciated by lack of proper food, invite disease."

Most Deadly of Diseases.

Under the conditions obtaining in the Orient, the bubonic plague is the most virulent and deadly of diseases. The symptoms manifest themselves in from twelve hours to twelve days after the system absorbs the disease; the usual period being about four days. At first the patient complains of high fever, a swelling of the glands of the thigh and groin, and sometimes of the neck, and finally becomes delirious. The crisis is reached in from two to eight days, generally in forty-eight hours. If life can be prolonged for five or six days the chances of successful treatment are greatly increased. As a rule, however, little can be done to save the natives of the countries where the plague is epidemic. A few of the well-nourished ones escape; of the rest death claims an average of from 50 to 100 per cent, of the total number of cases. This fearful mortality is best shown in the following figures, furnished by Dr. Wyman: Bombay, cases 220,907, deaths 164,083; Hong-Kong, cases 1,600, deaths 1,541; Formosa, cases 2,408, deaths1,866. Strangely enough this death rate varies greatly according to nationalities. From statistics obtained during the prevalence of the plague in Hong Kong the following official showing is made, the percentage being based on the total number of cases reported: Chinese, 93 deaths out of every 100 persons attacked with the disease; East Indians 77 out of every 100; Japanese, 60; Eurasians, 100; Europeans, 18. This small relative percentage of mortality among Europeans is attributed to better blood and stamina, and to the success of treatment in the early stages of the disease, the intelligence of the European leading him to call in a physician at the first sign of trouble, while the ignorance and prejudice of the Orientals prompt them to conceal themselves and reject medical aid.

An interesting suggestion as to the cause for the great prevalence and mortality of the plague in India and China is offered by Dr. Charles W. Dabney, Jr., who attributes it to the fact that the people, when fed at all, live almost entirely upon rice and other grains which contain very little protein, meat or fish being rare articles of diet, while wheat, oats, Indian corn and rye, all of which are richer in protein than rice, are unknown. In other words, the bodies of these natives lack proper nourishment.

Methods of Contracting Plague.

Medical scientists have determined that bubonic plague may be contracted in three ways—by inoculation through an external wound or abrasion, by respiration (breathing air laden with the plague germs), and by introduction into the stomach of food or water that has become infected. Contrary to the general belief, the disease is not infectious or contagious in the ordinary manner. A person might even sleep in a bed occupied by a plague victim, or wear clothing taken from his body, and yet escape infection, provided there were no wounds or abrasions on the skin in which the disease germs could get lodgment. Even the breath of a patient is not necessarily poisonous, the greatest source of danger being in the discharges from the swellings. All this being granted, the question will naturally arise. Why, then, should the disease rage so among the Orientals? The assertion that the plague is not usually infectious or contagious in the ordinary way applies only to people who are ordinarily cleanly in their habits. To those acquainted with the Oriental no further explanation is necessary. Once the plague gets a foothold among East Indians or Chinese coolies it is almost impossible to check it, except with the extermination of the population affected. Russia has adopted heroic methods in dealing with the plague in its Chinese colonies. All those affected are taken out and shot. "It saves trouble and other people's lives," the Russian grimly remarks.

The conditions of environment favorable to the plague are similar to those that encourage typhus fever, namely, density of population, bad ventilation and drainage, impure water, imperfect nourishment, and inattention to sanitary requirements.

It is said of this disease, as of yellow fever, that human habitations and the soil may become so thoroughly infected as to establish endemicity, or regular recurrence of the disease. The bacillus will infect food and water, though how long it will retain its virility in water is as yet undetermined.

Heat and moisture, darkness, and the presence of organic matter, vegetable or animal, especially if in a state of decomposition, furnish the ideal conditions for the propagation of the plague bacilli. Light, dryness and heat are fatal to the germs. The bacilli are killed by direct sunlight in three or four hours, and in a dry room at ordinary temperature in three or four days. A temperature of 170 degrees Fahrenheit kills the germs in five minutes, and solutions of corrosive sublimate, sulphuric acid, or hydrochloric acid have the same effect.

Treatment of Plague Patients.

The consulting committee of public health of the French Government has framed the following rules for the treatment of patients:

A patient stricken with plague should be isolated and kept in a state of the utmost cleanliness, the persons charged with his care alone to have access to him. The attendants should observe the following precautious: To take neither food nor drink in the sick-room; never to take food without washing the hands with soap and a disinfecting solution; to rinse the mouth from time to time, and always before eating, with a disinfecting solution; carpets, curtains, rugs and other furniture to be removed from sick-room; cloths, coverings and mattresses to be disinfected by steam or boiling at the conclusion of the case, or as often as they accumulate; the floor of the room to be washed daily with a disinfecting solution.

To a French physician, Dr. Yersen, belongs the honor of having discovered a remedy for the plague. Dr. Yersen was a student of the Pasteur institute and a believer in the serum treatment. At Amoy, China, in 1890, he first put his theories into practice by using the serum from an immunized horse upon cases of a severe type. He treated twenty-three cases in this manner, all of whom recovered excepting two, whose cases were desperate from the outset. Since that time the Yersen method has been tested until its efficacy is now incontestable. A French commission which has been investigating the plague at Oporto, Portugal, reports that in cases treated with the serum the mortality was only 14 per cent, while in those not treated it was at least 70 per cent. In a case in Bombay a European family resided, with a numerous retinue of native servants, in an infected portion of the city. The little daughter of the family was stricken with the pest in a virulent form; was treated with the serum, and made a rapid recovery. As a precautionary measure the whole family were subjected to inoculation, and the same measure of treatment was offered to the native domestics. Some accepted and escaped infection, while six who declined on the ground of religious scruples were all stricken and five died. A more crucial test could not have been devised.

The bubonic plague, Dr. Wyman asserts, is the same old plague that for centuries past has made its appearance at intervals in various countries to claim its tribute of thousands upon thousands of human lives, and which has been known in turn as the Levantine, Oriental and black plague, and black death. The mere index to the literature on the subject—a simple enumeration of titles with authors—covers forty pages in the index catalogue of the library of the surgeon general's office of the United States army.

Fighting the plague with fire and death—quick obliteration of human beings at the gun muzzle and the utter extinction of dead bodies in the ashes of funeral pyres—is an excess of horror in connection with the progress of the dread black bubonic scourge. The custom of the disposal of bodies of plague victims by the Russian army officials in Manchuria is invariably that of incineration. Between July 6 and 15 last over 300 coolies employed on the rail road work near Newchwang, who became infected by contact with coolie laborers shipped from Hong Kong, and who disclosed unmistakable evidences of having the plague in its first stages, were rounded up and shot by the Cossack soldiers employed in guarding the camps. Their bodies were piled on logs, saturated with petroleum and burned.

Source: "The Scourge of the Century," *Lincoln County Leader*, May 11, 1900.

3. "MEMORIAL OF THE EXCLUSION CONVENTION ADDRESSED TO THE PRESIDENT AND CONGRESS," *THE SAN FRANCISCO CALL*, NOVEMBER 23, 1901

MEMORIAL OF THE EXCLUSION CONVENTION ADDRESSED TO THE PRESIDENT AND CONGRESS

To the President and the Congress of the United States: Pursuant to a call officially issued by the city of San Francisco, there assembled in that city the 21st day of November, 1901, for the purpose of expressing the sentiment of the State of California, a convention composed of representatives of County Supervisors, City Councils, trade, commercial and civic organizations to the number of three thousand, and without dissent it was resolved to memorialize the President and the Congress of the United States as follows:

Soon after the negotiation of the Burlingame treaty in 1868 large numbers of Chinese coolies were brought to this country under contract. Their numbers so increased that in 1878 the people of the State made a practically unanimous demand for the restriction of the immigration. Our white population suffered in every department of labor and trade, having in numerous instances been driven out of employment by the competition of the Chinese. The progress of the State was arrested because so long as the field was occupied by Chinese a new and desirable immigration was impossible. After a bitter struggle remedial legislation was passed in 1882 and was renewed in 1892, to run for a period of ten years. Your memorialists, in view of the fact that the present so-called Geary law expires by limitation on May 5 next, and learning that you have been petitioned against its re-enactment, believe that it is necessary for them to repeat and to reaffirm the reasons which, in their judgment, require the re-enactment and the continued enforcement of the law.

The effects of Chinese exclusion have been most advantageous to the State. The 75,000 Chinese resident of California in 1889 have been reduced, according to the last census, to 45,600; and whereas, the white settlement of California by Caucasians had been arrested prior to the adoption of these laws, a healthy growth of the State in population has marked the progress of recent years. Every material interest of the State has advanced and prosperity has been our portion. Were the restriction laws relaxed we are convinced that our working population would be displaced, and the noble structure of our State, the creation of American ideas and industry would be imperiled if not destroyed. The lapse of time has only confirmed your memorialists in their conviction, from their knowledge derived from actually coming in contact with the Chinese, that they are a non-assimilative race and by every standard of American thought undesirable as citizens. Although they have been frequently employed and treated with decent consideration ever since the enactment of the exclusion law in 1882, which was the culmination and satisfaction of California's patriotic purpose, they have not in any sense altered their racial characteristics and have not socially or otherwise assimilated with our people. To quote the Imperial Chinese Consul General in San Francisco: "They work more cheaply than whites; they live more cheaply; they send their money out of the country to China; most of them have no intention of remaining in the United States, and they do not adopt American manners, but live in colonies and not after the American fashion."

Physical Assimilation Impossible.

Until this year no statute had been passed by the State forbidding their intermarriage with the whites, and yet during their long residence but few intermarriages have taken place and the offspring has been invariably degenerate. It is well established that the issue of the Caucasian and the Mongolian does not possess the virtue of either, but develops the vices of both. So physical assimilation is out of the question.

It is well known that the vast majority of Chinese do not bring their wives with them in their immigration because of their purpose to return to their native land when a competency is earned. Their practical status among us has been that of single men competing at low wages against not only men of our own race, but men who have been brought up by our civilization to family life and civic duty. They pay little taxes, they support no institutions—neither school, church nor theater; they remain steadfastly, after all these years, a permanently foreign element. The purpose, no doubt, for enacting the exclusion laws for periods of ten years is due to the intention of Congress of observing the progress of these people under American institutions, and now it has been clearly demonstrated that they cannot, for the deep and ineradicable reasons of race and mental organization, assimilate with our own people and be molded as are other races into strong and composite American stock.

We respectfully represent that their presence excludes a desirable population and that there is no necessity whatever for their immigration. The immigration laws of this country now exclude pauper and contract labor from every land. All Chinese immigration of the coolie class is both pauper and contract labor. It is not a voluntary immigration. The Chinese Six Companies of California deal in Chinese labor as a commodity. Prior to the exclusion they freely imported coolies, provided for them, farmed out their services and returned them, and if they should die their bones, pursuant to a superstitious belief, to their native land.

America is the asylum for the oppressed and liberty-loving people of the world, and the implied condition of their admission to this country is allegiance to its Government and devotion to its institutions. It is hardly necessary to say that the Chinese are not even bona fide settlers, as the Imperial Chinese Consul General admits.

We respectfully represent that American labor should not be exposed to the destructive competition of aliens who do not, will not and cannot take up the burdens of American citizenship, whose presence is an economic blight and a patriotic danger. It has been urged that the Chinese are unskilled and that they create wealth in field, mine and forest, which ultimately redounds to the benefit of the white skilled workingman. The Chinese are skilled and are capable of almost any skilled employment. They have invaded the cigar, shoe, broom, chemical, clothing, fruit canning, matchmaking and woollen [sic] manufacturing industries, and have displaced more than 4000 white men in these several employments in the city of San Francisco. As common laborers they have throughout California displaced tens of thousands of men. But this country is not solely concerned even in a coldly economic sense with the production of wealth.

Grave Danger of Overproduction.

The United States has now a greater per capita of working energy than any other land. If it is stimulated by a non-assimilative and non-consuming race there is grave danger of overproduction and stagnation. The home market should grow with the population. But the Chinese, living on the most meager food, having no families to support, inured to deprivation, and hoarding their wages for use in their native land, whither they invariably return, cannot in any sense be regarded as consumers. Their earnings do not circulate nor are they reinvested—contrary to those economic laws which make for the prosperity of nations. For their services they may be said to be paid twice—first by their employer and then by the community. If we must have protection, is it not far better for us to protect ourselves against the man than against his trade? Our opponents maintain that the admission of the Chinese would cause an enlargement of our national wealth and a great increase of production, but the distribution of wealth and not its production is to-day our most serious public question. In this age of science and invention the production of wealth can well be left to take care of itself. It is its equitable distribution that must now be the concern of the country.

The increasing recurrence of strikes in modern times must have convinced every one that their recent settlement is nothing more than a truce. It is not a permanent industrial peace. The new organization of capital and labor that is now necessary to bring about lasting peace and harmony between those engaged in production will require greater sympathy, greater trust and confidence and a clearer mutual understanding between the employers and the employed. Any such new organization will require a closer union to be formed between them. These requirements can never be fulfilled between the individuals of races so alien to one another as ourselves and the Chinese.

The Chinese are only capable of working under the present unsatisfactory system. All progress then to an improved organization of capital and labor would be arrested. We might have greater growth, but never greater development. It was estimated by the Commissioner of Labor that there were a million idle men in the United States in 1886. Certainly the 76,000 Chinese in California at that time stood for 76,000 white men waiting for employment, and the further influx of Chinese in any considerable numbers would precipitate the same condition again, if not indeed make it chronic. If the United States increases in population at the rate of 12 per cent per decade it will have nearly 230,000,000 people in 100 years. Our inventive genius and the constant improvements being made in machinery will greatly increase our per capita productive capacity. If it be our only aim to increase our wealth so as to hold our own in the markets of the world are we not, without the aid of Chinese coolies, capable of doing it and at the same time preserve the character of our population and insure the perpetuity of our institution? It is not wealth at any cost that sound public policy requires, but that the country be developed with equal pace and with a desirable population which stands not only for industry but for citizenship.

Chinese Crowding Out Americans.

In their appeal to the cupidity of farmers and orchardists the proponents of Chinese immigration have stated that the Chinese are only common laborers, and by this kind of argument they have attempted to disarm the skilled labor organizations of the country; but we have shown you that the Chinese are skilled and are capable of becoming skilled. As agriculturists they have crowded out the native population and driven the country boy from the farm to the city, where he meets their skilled competition in many branches of industry. But shall husbandry be abandoned to a servile class? Shall the boys and girls of the fields and of the orchards be deprived of their legitimate work in the harvest? Shall not our farmers be encouraged to look to their own households and to their own neighbors for labor? Shall the easy methods of contract employment be encouraged? We are warned by history that the free population of Rome was driven by slave labor from the country into the city, where it became a mob and a rabble, ultimately compassing the downfall of the republic. The small farms were destroyed, and under an overseer large farms were cultivated, which led Pliny to remark that "great estates ruined Italy."

The experience of the South with slave labor warns us against unlimited Chinese immigration, considered both as a race question and as an economic problem. The Chinese, if permitted to freely enter this country, would create race antagonisms which would ultimately result in great public disturbance. The Caucasian will not tolerate the Mongolian. As ultimately all government is based on physical force, the white population of this country will not without resistance suffer itself to be destroyed. Economically it was thought wise at one time to employ negro slaves, but the accumulated wealth of the South was wiped out by an appalling expenditure of blood and money, precipitating conditions which bore with terrible force upon a people which were once considered great and prosperous. The cornerstone of their structure was slavery, and the cornerstone of any structure based upon the employment of Chinese coolies is servile labor. It is repugnant to our form of society and to our ideas of government to segregate a labor class and regard it only as its capacity for work. If we were to return to the ante-bellum ideas of the South, now happily discarded, the Chinese would satisfy every requirement of a slave or servile class. They work incessantly, they are docile and they would not be concerned about their political conditions, but such suggestions are repulsive to American civilization. America has dignified work and made it honorable. Manhood gives title to rights, and the Government being ruled by majorities is largely controlled by the very class which servile labor would supersede, namely, the free and independent workingmen of America. The political power invested in men by this Government shows the absolute necessity of keeping up the standard of population and not permitting it to deteriorate by contact with inferior and non-assimilative races.

Question Involves Our Civilization.

But this is not alone a race, labor and political question. It is one which involves our civilization, and that interests the people of the world. The benefactors, scholars, soldiers and statesmen—the patriots and martyrs of mankind—have builded [sic] our modern fabric firmly upon the foundation of religion, law, science and art. It has been rescued from barbarism and protected against the incursions of barbarians. Civilization in Europe has been frequently attacked and imperiled by the barbaric hordes of Asia. If the little band of Greeks at Marathon had not beaten back ten times their number of Asiatic invaders it is impossible to estimate the loss to civilization that would have ensued. When we contemplate what modern civilization owes to the two centuries of Athenian life, from which we first learned our lessons of civil and intellectual freedom, we can see how necessary it was to keep the Asiatic from breaking into Europe. Attila and his Asiatic hordes threatened Central Europe when the Gauls made their successful stand against them. The wave of Asiatic barbarism rolled back and civilization was again saved. The repulse of the Turks, who are of the Mongolian race, before Vienna finally made our civilization strong enough to take care of itself, and the danger of extinction by a military invasion from Asia passed away. But a peaceful invasion is more dangerous than a warlike attack. We can meet and defend ourselves against an open foe, but an insidious foe under our generous laws would be in possession of the citadel before we are aware. The free immigration of Chinese would be for all purposes an invasion by Asiatic barbarians, against whom civilization in Europe has been frequently defended fortunately for us. It is our inheritance to keep it pure and uncontaminated, as it is our purpose and destiny to broaden and enlarge it. We are trustees for mankind.

In an age when the brotherhood of man has become more fully recognized we are not prepared to overlook the welfare of the Chinaman, himself. We need have nothing on our national conscience because the Chinaman has a great industrial destiny in his own country. Few realize that China is yet a sparsely populated country. Let their merchants, travelers and students then come here as before to carry back to China the benefits of our improvements and experiments. Let American ideas of progress and enterprise be planted on Chinese soil. Our commerce with China since 1880 has increased more than 50 per cent. Our consular service reports that "the United States is second only to Great Britain in goods sold to the Chinese. The United States buys more goods from China than does any other nation, and her total trade with China, exports and imports, equals that of Great Britain, not including the colonies, and is far ahead of that of any other country."

Commerce is not sentimental and has not been affected by our policy of exclusion. The Chinese Government, knowing the necessities of the situation, being familiar with the fact that almost every country has imposed restrictions upon the immigration of Chinese coolies, does not regard our attitude as an unfriendly act. Indeed, our legislation has been confirmed by treaty. Nor are the Chinese unappreciative of the friendship of the United States recently displayed in saving possibly the empire itself from dismemberment. So, therefore, America is at no disadvantage in its commercial dealings with China on account of the domestic policy of Chinese exclusion.

Therefore every consideration of public duty, the nation's safety and the people's rights, the preservation of our civilization and the perpetuity of our institutions impel your memorialists to ask for the re-enactment of the exclusion laws which have for twenty years protected us against the gravest dangers, and which, were they relaxed, would imperil every interest which the American people hold sacred for themselves and their posterity.

Source: "Memorial of the Exclusion Convention Addressed to the President and Congress," *The San Francisco Call*, November 23, 1901.

4. CLAUDE BOURRIN, *CHOSES ET GENS EN INDOCHINE: SOUVENIRS DE BONNE HUMEUR, 1898–1908*

I had several weeks leave from my military service at the end of the Exposition. At this time there was a plague epidemic raging in Hanoi. The epicenter was the neighborhood of the exposition hall due to, so it was said, rats who had arrived in crates from India. One night I was awoken by cries coming from the Annamite soldiers' camp. I went to see what was going on and found several men writhing on the ground with suspicious symptoms. I raised the alarm and sent these emergency cases to the hospital.

The next day there were new cases, including fatalities. My young servant boy got sick and became agitated when I spoke of the hospital. I took him myself in a rickshaw to the police station where I repeatedly warned them about him. But that did not prevent the scoundrel from escaping and carrying the disease to his home village where he hid. After which, no doubt happy to have killed some of his own kin, he recovered and survived.

[. . .]

The plague continued to spread and seized hold of the city thanks to the swelling rat population. We hastily removed the collections from the secondary buildings and the firemen, who had been idle during most of the Exposition, set fire to them. A trench was dug around the infested zone and when the rats fled the flames and searched for refuge, they ran into a bed of lime where they were massacred by an army of workers waiting for them.

Despite popular opinion, the Exposition did not create the epidemic, since the city had taken measures to destroy the rats well before the arrival of crates from India. By the decree of April 23, 1902, six months before the opening of the Exposition, there was a reward of four cents for every rat destroyed or captured. A few weeks later they reduced the bounty to a penny a head. This became rather expensive as the natives hunted rats in provinces far from the capital. If the price had stayed at four cents, they would have gone all the way to India to find some big and fat rodents. But at one cent, the business was sufficiently profitable. Our astute protégés began to raise rats within the city to save transportation costs. At the start of June, the price was lowered to half a cent for each rat with a tail. The police would then cut off and burn the tails so that the same cadavers could not be used to collect several rewards, an increasingly common practice. The number of rats brought to the police station each morning did not diminish, indicating the extreme poverty of the Tonkinese population. The administration reduced the price to one cent for five rats on July 10. This was a dangerous decision as the policy designed to destroy the rodents was actually increasing their number.

When, at the end of the dry season in 1903, the epidemic returned with vigor, there had to be a new struggle against the rats. On April 3, faced with the stingy bounty of one cent for five rats, the hunter-farmers sulked. [. . .] Severe penalties were enacted against rat smuggling from the provinces where there was no bounty. To fight against the plague, there should have been bounties in every contaminated province.

Stopping the smuggling put an end to the clandestine activities of the farmers, almost completely ending the nuisance.

Source: Claude Bourrin, *Choses et gens en Indochine: Souvenirs de bonne humeur, 1898–1908* (Saigon: J. Aspar, 1940), 147–149. Translated by Michael G. Vann.

5. COMMISSAIRE CENTRAL, "DESTRUCTION DES ANIMAUX, HANOI-VILLE"

Official reports show a record 20,114 rats killed—or at least their tails collected—on June 12, 1902.

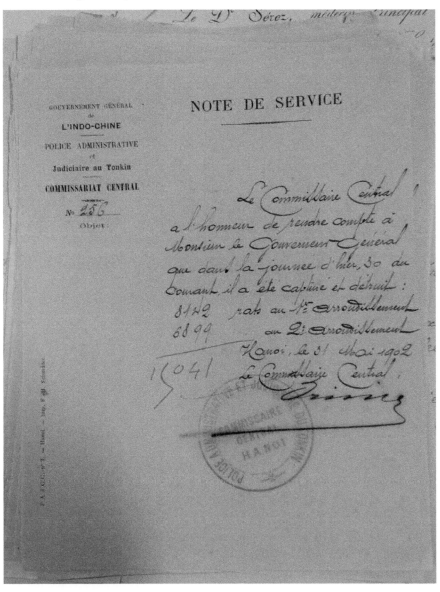

By June 18, 1902, the French authorities claimed to have killed some 413,636 rats, but some doubted the numbers.

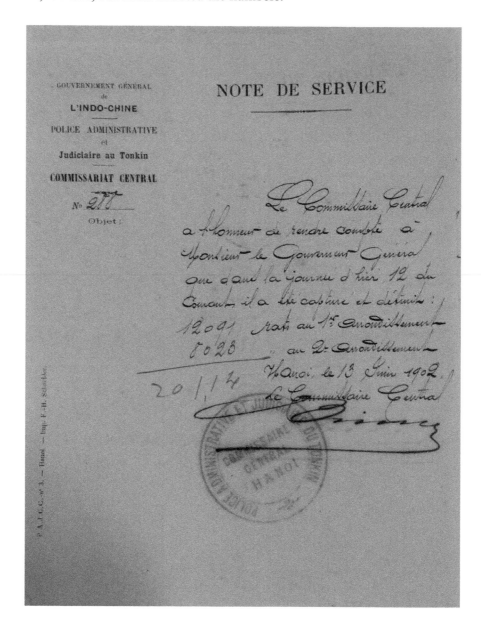

Growing suspicions led to separate entries for adult and baby rats.

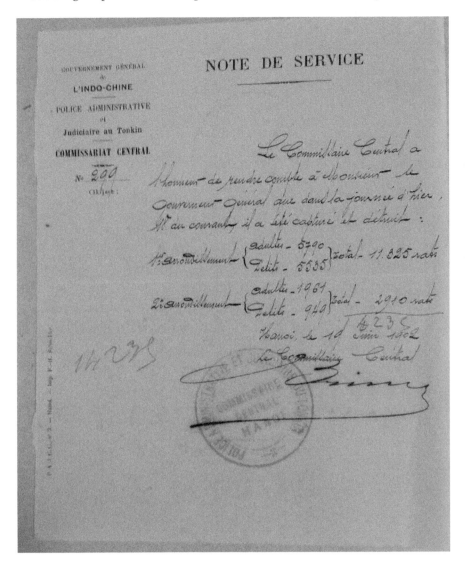

Source: Commissaire Central, "Note de Service," Centre Archives d'Outre-Mer, GGI 6675, "Destruction des animaux, Hanoi-Ville" (1902).

6. DR. LE ROY DES BARRES, *RAPPORT SUR LA MORTALITÉ À HANOI EN 1903*

On the first of January, 1903, for the first time ever the city of Hanoi started a government service to ensure the examination of the bodies of all (Europeans and natives) who had died in the city and to register deaths witnessed in the various hospitals. This service was created at the request of the municipal government, following the plague epidemic of 1902, but did not receive official sanction until almost the end of 1903. Despite this administrative delay, the system has nonetheless functioned well, and the statistics that this report will address are due to the work of the service.

But first of all it is necessary to discuss how the service works.

When a death occurs, the family alerts the native Street Chief; he will issue a declaration form with relevant information regarding the deceased. The closest Police Station will receive this report and give it to a European police agent specifically assigned to this service. This agent, accompanied by a native agent to serve as a translator, will go to the home of the deceased. He will interrogate the family and the neighbors, and other relevant witnesses. The European agent will then add this information and any information from the Street Chief to the file and send it to the Medical Inspector.

With this file and accompanied by a native interpreter, the Medical Inspector will examine the intact nude body and conduct a second interrogation of the family, neighbors, and Street Chief. With this assembled information and after his medical examination he will decide the cause of death. If it seems that the individual died of the plague, a biopsy will be taken and subjected to a microscopic examination. With a final diagnosis established, as best as possible, the Medical Inspector will issue a burial permit.

If the individual is infected, he will make a public declaration according to regulations and advise the Police Station which house is contaminated and needs disinfecting.

In times of an epidemic, there will be a few modifications to this system; one can find a discussion of this in our report on the 1903 Plague epidemic. When bodies are abandoned in the street, they will be brought to the Morgue, recently built near the European cemetery, where they will be examined. During times of Plague or Cholera epidemics, there will be a rise in the number of abandoned corpses from natives trying to avoid having their homes disinfected. In normal times, it is mostly children who are sent to the Morgue in such circumstances.

The City of Hanoi has two native cemeteries at the city limits, situated at opposite ends of the city. The Bach-Mai cemetery is meeting the city's needs, but the Giang-Vu cemetery, as we have previously reported several times, is becoming a health risk and should be shut down. Generally, it is only very poor natives who are buried here. Most families ask for permission to bury their deceased parents on land that belongs to the family located outside of the city limits (burials are not allowed inside the city).

The permission to transport bodies outside of the city limits is granted by the Police Headquarters after a report from the Medical Inspector. Permission is generally granted unless the death was a case of Plague or Cholera. Cadavers from cases of these afflictions must be buried in a specially designated section of the Bach-Mai or Giang-Vu cemeteries, in a grave at least two meters deep and in a coffin filled with lime.

Such is the organization of this service. Now we will discuss the difficulties faced by enacting these policies and the statistics collected in 1903.

At the current moment (January, 1904), with only rare exceptions, all the deaths occurring in Hanoi are known. Possibly in suburban villages, where the distance from the city center makes it difficult to monitor the Street Chiefs, things are not done according to official procedures but this is only a small minority of deaths. It has not always been like this and likely will not be like this in the future. During Plague and Cholera outbreaks, the panicked population hides their dead and secretly buries them; we have already reported on this problem.

There is great concern that should a similar epidemic occur, the natives' behavior will be the same: likely the Police will ensure the implementation of the sanitary regulations and the Administration will have to calm down public opinion, trying to make them understand the importance of these measures.

Source: Dr. Le Roy Des Barres, *Rapport sur la mortalité à Hanoi en 1903* (Hanoi: Imp. Express, 1904), 1–2. Translated by Michael G. Vann.

7. WOOD AND THATCH HOMES

Before the French invasion, Hanoi's residents lived in traditional wood and thatch structures. Typical of construction throughout Southeast Asia, these homes were well suited for the region's heat and humidity and cost very little to erect, maintain, and rebuild. The French viewed them as backwards rural vestiges that had no place in a modern city. The lack of basic urban hygiene infrastructure alarmed Western public health experts.
(see following page)

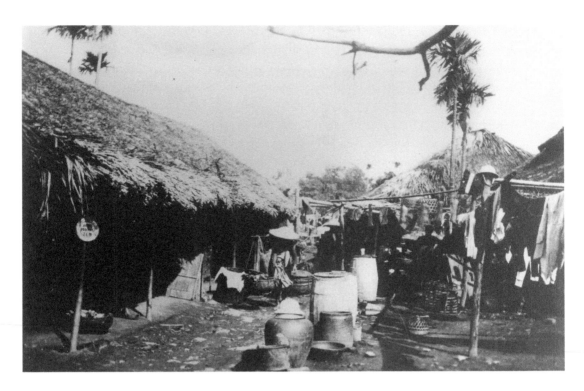

Source: Wood and thatch homes, CAOM 30Fi119 1248.

8. GOUVERNEMENT-GÉNÉRAL DE L'INDO-CHINE, *VILLE DE HANOI (TONKIN): HISTORIQUE, DÉVELOPPEMENT FINANCIER, RÈGLEMENTATION ADMINISTRATIVE ET FONCTIONNEMENT DES DIVERS SERVICES MUNICIPAUX DE LA VILLE DE HANOI*, 1905 (P. 53).

Civil status—births—deaths—contagious diseases

This service was created as a result of Hanoi's 1902–1903 plague epidemic. The reporting of contagious diseases in the colony has been compulsory since the law of 30 November, 1892, and the decree of August 17, 1897. As Annamites had no tradition of civil registration, there were no officially recognized indigenous doctors, and, since there were very few European doctors, it followed that contagious diseases were not reported. To remedy these various loopholes that posed threats to public safety, on April 25, 1903, Doctor Le Roy des Barres was appointed as doctor of civil registration and epidemics. The Mayor tasked him with house calls to record all European and Native deaths, the supervision of the disinfection of contaminated buildings, and administering medical care to natives hospitalized in the Municipal Quarantine in Bach-Mai.

The Bach-Mai Quarantine, completely isolated from the city and neighboring villages, is located in the suburban zone of the city, near the Hue Road police station. It is adjacent to the Military Quarantine. It is made of an iron frame with a thatched straw roof and walls to serve as partitions between various cells. After each epidemic, the walls and roofs are burnt and, after disinfection and reinforcing the metal framework, the cells are immediately reconstructed with materials similar to those incinerated in anticipation of the possibility of a new epidemic.

A disinfecting oven, using the Clayton system, has been installed in the Quarantine.

The Quarantine is near the native cemetery in suburban Bach-Mai, where all deceased natives from the nearby sections of the city are buried. A second suburban cemetery, which was also for burying natives, was created on the opposite side of the town in Giang Vu.

Source: Gouvernement-Général de l'Indo-Chine, *Ville de Hanoi (Tonkin): Historique, Développement financier, Règlementation administrative et fonctionnement des dives services municipaux de la Ville de Hanoi* (Hanoi: Taupin, 1905), 53. Translated by Michael G. Vann.

9. DR. ORTHOLAN, "PESTE EN INDO-CHINE. (HISTORIQUE)"

The plague has always existed in the regions contiguous to Indochina; Yunnan province in particular has always been considered an endemic plague zone and the origins of all recorded epidemics.

History. Until a few years ago, this Chinese province had only fleeting commercial contacts with the French colonial territories; the populated regions of Yunnan and Tonkin were separated from each other by an almost uninhabited and rarely crossed zone. This zone served as a very effective sanitary barrier. This is the same for Laos, Siam, and Burma, which have an identical geographic relationship to Yunnan.

However, this situation is changing since the completion of the Red River Valley railway to Mongtzé will create a heavily trafficked route between Tonkin and Yunnan. This will thus open up these frontier lands to infectious germs of Chinese origin.

From Yunnan, where epidemics have been reported for a long time, the disease has frequently spread along commercial routes towards the east, to Quang Si and Quang Tong; Long Tchéou and the ports of Canton, Pakkoï, and Hong Kong are infected; from there the epidemic entered the French possessions.

Up to now, commercial relations with Indochina have been primarily maritime and only with established ports. There is also a flow of goods and people between Tonkin and Quang Si.

Arrival of the plague in Indochina and the first epidemic surges. Quang Tchéou Wan was the first effected territory and since 1901 there have been numerous reported cases. The population of this colony is Chinese. The land border is only theoretical. The maritime frontier is extensive and it is impossible to establish an effective sanitary surveillance against arrivals from the adjacent territories.

The first recorded epidemic in Indochina proper was in Nhatrang in Annam from June to October, 1898 (72 cases). This outbreak was entirely contained and ran its course without spreading. The infectious germs were probably imported by Chinese junks coming from Canton.

In 1899 and 1900, despite the very numerous cases of plague in Canton, Pakkoï, Hong Kong, and Manila, our colony remained unscathed.

From the first months of 1901, consular reports indicated that there were cases of plague in every port in the Far East. Epidemics struck Singapore, Manila, Amoy, Hong Kong, and throughout the province of Quang-Tong, Canton, Pakkoï, Long Tchéou, etc.

The ports of Indochina were put under rigorous surveillance; the plague spared the colony, except for Quang-Tchéou-Wan, where there were about 4,000 victims (even though the official statistics reported only 376 cases). There were three potential cases recorded in Tonkin: one in Hanoi, one in Lang Song, and one in Haiphong. Doctors focused their attention on the dangers of a possible epidemic, and it is certain that if it had struck, it would not have escaped detection. By the end of the year, all of the outbreaks appeared to have been extinguished.

In 1902, while the plague reawakened with a new intensity in Hong Kong, Pakkoï, and Long Tchéou, it also appeared in Tonkin. In April, 22 cases were reported in Lang Son, Dong Dang, Than Moï, and Hanoi. In May, 11 cases were reported in these same cities. There appeared to be a trail along the railway line between Hanoi and the Chinese border. On the other hand, in Hanoi, the plague appeared to have been introduced by merchandise coming from Hong Kong. After July there were no more cases in Hanoi. The epidemic terminated in August in Pakkoï and in September in Hong Kong.

These events were reproduced in an identical fashion, but with greater intensity, in 1903. From the month of March, the plague reigned epidemically in Hong Kong and Manila. Numerous cases were reported in Quang-Thcéou-Wan and in the same month the epidemic awoke in Hanoi, lasting until August, with 159 officially reported cases. Numerous cases escaped the medical authorities as the local population tried to hide as many as possible. In Dong Dang, Haiphong, and Nam Dinh, there were 52 reported cases.

In 1904, Tonkin was somewhat spared; there were only a dozen cases in Hanoi and Nam Dinh, but the illness continued to ravage Quang-Thcéou-Wan, where it killed some 3,000 natives.

In 1905, the plague was reported in Hong Kong and Bangkok in January; in March it was in Rangoon. Throughout the year, it struck Quang-Thcéou-Wan, where it appeared to become endemic. With only 12 cases in Tonkin, the epidemic did not establish a strong presence.

Epidemics of 1906, 1907, and 1908. [The year] 1906 was marked by a substantial increase. The plague struck from February to July in

Quang-Thcéou-Wan. In Tonkin, there were 165 cases in and around Hanoi, 23 cases in Vinh Yen province, and a few other completely isolated cases. In December, there were three cases in Laokay, a major station on the railway to Yunnan.

In 1906, the plague appeared in Cochinchina for the first time: 3 cases in January and 7 in February in Saigon and its suburbs. It is very likely that this is the first time that the illness has been in this colony.

Since then, a well-organized sanitation service and the relative ease of monitoring all foreign arrivals have successfully protected the area.

Starting in 1907 it seems that the plague can be considered to have taken root in Indochina and created epidemic focal points that will be difficult to extinguish despite possible periods of latency. The disease was present in Quang-Thcéou-Wan for the entire year. In Tonkin there were 362 reported cases with a mortality rate of roughly 1 in 3. These cases happened almost across the entire colony; however the majority (238 cases) were in Haiphong, May had the highest number (99 cases).

In Cochinchina, there were 556 declarations of the plague in Saigon, Cholon, and the suburbs. The largest number of cases was in June (147); this was the same month that the first cases were recorded in Phnom Penh, Cambodia, where from June to November there were 92 recorded cases.

In the first months of 1908 all parts of the Indochinese peninsula were equally affected. In Annam, which had been spared since the local epidemic of 1898, an outbreak developed in the province of Phan Tiet where in March there were already 83 registered cases.

This information is clearly incomplete. It is certain that a rather large number of plague cases escaped the official statistics as the medical services could not be in all parts of these territories. The figures given above should be significantly raised to approach the truth.

All reports from the colony indicate that the mortality rate was about a third amongst the natives. Very few Europeans got sick: only a dozen, of which 3 died.

CONCLUSIONS

In conclusion, the plague is an illness recently brought into Indochina.

In the first period, the introduction seems to have followed the Long-Tchéou-Lang-Son roads. But the cases from this source were few and the outbreaks were quickly suppressed by energetic prophylactic measures.

In the second period starting in 1906, the diffusion was much faster. Maritime routes were certainly the method of the epidemic's penetration. The disease struck the ports and their immediate neighbors in the first months of each year. The thrust of the epidemic did not stop in Tonkin, it went all the way south to Cochinchina, Cambodia, and Annam.

The plague steadily progresses and appears able to settle into areas permanently. This can already be seen in India and China, and our possessions are exposed to the same scourge. It threatens to massively ravage the native population. The European community is not immune to its effects. Furthermore, the plague can cause huge disturbances to international commerce, with each country trying to protect itself from merchandise arriving from infected ports.

Source: Ortholan, M. le Dr. La, "Peste en Indo-Chine. (Historique)," *Annales d'Hygiène et de Médecine Coloniale*, Tome XI (1908): 633–38. Translated by Michael G. Vann.

10. SOUP VENDOR, PIERRE DIEULEFILS POSTCARD

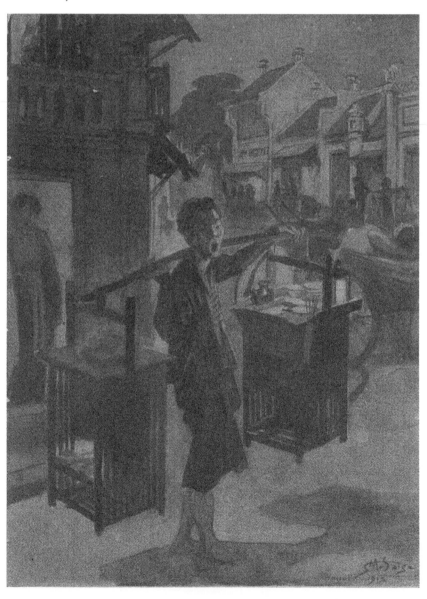

This painting of a soup vendor walking the streets of Hanoi illustrates the vibrancy of Hanoi's Vietnamese neighborhoods. Most of the city's residents ate their meals in the street amid the hustle and bustle of the most densely populated part of the city. Vietnamese urban culture developed a number of delicious offerings including pho, a savory beef broth and rice noodle dish. For Westerns eyes, this painting embodies many of the Orientalist fantasies of an exotic and mysterious Asia.

Source: Michael G. Vann.

11. "BATTLING THE PLAGUE," *LOS ANGELES HERALD*, NOVEMBER 15, 1908

[. . .] The plague has always been fond of sneaking into Manila and sweeping through the entire Filipino archipelago taking toll of the shivering millions by the tens of thousands.

Just across a narrow stretch of water from Manila King Bubonic Plague has his cave, where he appears to have been born and bred. Right in the teeming heart of China, not far from the fens that surround the yellow torrent of the Great Yellow or Yang-ste-Kiang River appear to have been the prehistoric home and breeding place of King Plague.

For countless centuries the Chinese have died like flies from plague. As a result the Chinaman today stands more chance of recovery from bubonic plague than any other race. His blood for centuries has fought, the deadly germ of this disease—a germ that is simply a short, stumpy rod, oval in form, which once in the human body multiplies by the billion and sucks the vitality out of the blood, leaving only a loathsome decaying fluid that carries further death to every bit of human flesh or blood it comes in contact with.

Uncle Sam, however, has never turned tail on any foe. And today, quiet, un assuming men and women, physicians and nurses are waging silent but heroic warfare with the plague bacillus, and if on the ground (that is inside a human body) before the deadly germ, Uncle Sam's physicians with their test tubes and their anti-toxin always defeat King Plague. They can drive him headlong, shriveling and dying from the blood of human beings into which a white clad medical officer has infused a tiny dose of Yersin's toxin. But the antitoxin must get there before the plague.

The terrific virulence of the bubonic germ, its deadliness to human life and the utter helplessness of the human protoplasm or organism when once its vital element is attacked is simply but startlingly told by the death rate. Among Europeans and Americans the rate of mortality is total. That is none recover. Occasionally one here and there out, of thousands may survive, but even in these few isolated instances physicians prefer to doubt that they ever had, the true bubonic plague germ.

DEATH RATE APPALLING

But among the Filipinos one out of four recover. Among the Chinese, however, only every other victim dies. The blood of the Chinaman can better grapple with the bubonic germ because his father and grandfather and many generations back of these have faced and died fighting this dread disease. Hence, the Chinaman's blood inherits certain toxic qualities which counteract the poisonous influences of the germs which swarm in the patient's blood by countless millions. The terrific outbreak of plague and cholera in the Philippines prevented any welcome by the Filipinos to our fleet when the great battleship flotilla finally reached Manila Bay. Just what bubonic plague can do to human beings is told.

[. . .]

The intelligent fighting of the plague, of course, began when the germ was isolated. Yet it was a number of years before the method by which the disease propagates itself was discovered. Bubonic plague, rapidly as it spreads, yet does not spread from one sick man to another. Direct contact is not sufficient to spread the disease. It must enter the human body through the stomach, as in food or by its most usual route by the flea that live on the big oriental rat that swarms in China and the Philippines. Hence the slogan of the American physicians fighting the plague in Manila is:

"Inoculate all suspects who have been near a case of plague."

"Second, kill all the rats that can be caught in the neighborhood of a known case of bubonic plague."

FLIES, FLEAS AND RATS

Flies also spread the disease in the same way that they contribute so largely to the spread of typhoid fever, namely by picking up the germs through walking in filth and flying into human habitations and walking on food material, which is later received into a human stomach. Very simple of course, but that simple fact solved much of the difficulty in the way of beating King Plague once the scientific men found it out and instructed the workers.

But the rats which carry the infected fleas appear in Manila at any rate to be the pest bearers. It must be remembered that in Manila the disease attacks almost entirely the lower classes. Among the population where personal cleanliness is held next to godliness few cases of plague occur. Of course, anyone is exposed to the bite of an infected flea while passing near some Chinaman or Filipino who permits himself to carry about these tiny pests.

As a result of this fact the plague fighters of Uncle Sam in Manila offer rewards for rats dead or alive, no matter where they are caught. This is to attempt to keep down the number of the rodents throughout the Philippines generally. But when a case has developed in a house, the rats are doomed.

Trained rat catchers are sent wearing badges from the health department, which permit them access to any place and a big rat hunt ensues.

Even before the rat catchers arrive, come the medical men with their anti-toxin, and frequently they are compelled to use force in order to compel the ignorant Chinese and Filipinos, to submit to an operation that will practically save their lives. The photograph, showing the physicians injecting, the life-saving anti-toxin into the arm of a Chinese caught in a house where bubonic plague has been found, shows splendidly the sordid surroundings of these natives and gives a fine idea of just what unsanitary conditions the medical men must contend against.

The man himself is an emaciated specimen whose body would offer practically no opposition to the venomous bacillus of the plague unless he were treated by the anti-toxin and his blood made alive with material in itself poisonous to the deadly plague germs. Yet even such a poor specimen of a man can be fortified with anti-toxin and can bid defiance to the plague bacillus, where formerly such a case would be absolutely without hope and not worth carrying to a plague hospital.

Source: "Battling the Plague," *Los Angeles Herald* (Los Angeles), November 15, 1908.

12. LAURENT JOSEPH GAIDE AND HENRI DESIRE MARIE BODET, *LA PESTE EN INDOCHINE*

In the course of this research, we saw the important role of the Chinese in incubating and propagating plague epidemics.

While the Chinese do not seem to be very vulnerable to Cholera, they are frequently victims of Yersin's bacillus, brought to them by rats who frequently live in small shops and rice warehouses.

Source: Laurent Joseph Gaide and Henri Desire Marie Bodet, *La Peste en Indochine* (Hanoi: IDEO, 1930), 5. Translated by Michael G. Vann.

13. JACQUES MAY, *UN MÉDECIN FRANÇAIS EN EXTRÊME-ORIENT*

Between their blood parasites, their intestinal parasites, the insufficiency of their nutrition, and the effort imposed upon them to pull their subsistence from an unproductive soil, the sick were under the yoke of a biological oppression more serious than that of the French occupation. Returning each night from my hospital, I would walk around *le Petit-Lac*. Looking at the pagoda of Lê-Loi, I pleased myself by imagining that I was a new liberator, that my net, thrown in the lake's waters, brought back not a sword but a scalpel with which I would try to liberate the modern Tonkinese from the only oppression which truly put their national existence in danger—that of the parasites living in their bodies.

Source: Jacques May, *Un Médecin français en Extrême-Orient* (Paris: Editions de la Paix, 1951), 229. Translated by Michael G. Vann.

VOICES OF RESISTANCE

From the initial French invasion, through the decades of colonial occupation, and on to the final struggle for national liberation, generations of Vietnamese stood up against French rule. These documents recount elite and popular protests against imperialism, especially taxation. Resistance to invasive public health measures frustrated French officials who were themselves struggling to maintain public order and control the spread of disease.

1. PHAN TRONG QUANG, "A RICKSHA MAN'S IMPROMPTU"

> Born of good parents, you're a filial son.
> Alas, your country knows its darkest hour.
> The wheels of history stoop your back and pull;
> try hard to climb the uphill road ahead.
> The wind and dust may tan your soft-skinned face—
> no thorns or spikes can pierce your iron will.
> The world goes through a play of change and flux—
> this human horse may turn a dragon yet.

Source: Phan Trong Quang, "A Ricksha Man's Impromptu," in Huynh Sanh Thong (ed. and trans.), *An Anthology of Vietnamese Poems: From the Eleventh through the Twentieth Centuries* (New Haven: Yale University Press, 1996), 121.

2. ANONYMOUS, "POEM ON TRUE HEROISM"

> [. . .]
> In the year of I Wei, the seventh year of the reign of Emperor
> Thanh Thai [1895],
> The war indemnities had to be paid in full and at once.
> The official order struck like lightening across the sky.
> They came with summons to this village, with rifles to that hamlet.
> Every place had to declare the number of its inhabitants, houses,
> male adults, rice fields.
> Taxes were increased greatly and were to be paid in money,
> not in kind.
> With each passing year these taxes mounted,
> The cost of all articles rose rapidly, even those of betel, tea, and
> areca nuts.
> The constables, the commissars, the police, the agents of the
> Security Services, all officials competed to harm the people.
> All over the country, city-dwellers
> Paid their taxes on their persons and their houses.

They had to purchase licenses for peddling.

There were taxes on theaters, singers,

Dogs, pigs, and shops selling mutton.

In their exploitation the French did not miss a single item.

There was a monopoly on salt, and alcohol was stored plentifully in the excise offices.

People were obliged to buy and sell

Or they were accused of being smugglers; the situation was simply wretched.

The laws were iron, in a hundred ways,

Every individual was sorrowful, and every family utterly grieved.

Some people sold their wives, some sold their children.

To sell husbands was no longer remarkable.

How is one to recount the sorrow and the suffering?

When one questions Heaven, Heaven remains quite silent.

What debts had our compatriots contracted in their previous lives?

Not only were they exploited by the French, they also suffered a drought.

Of ten crops, more than nine perished.

Then too, there were storms, floods, violent winds, and irregular rains.

Who could tend to his wasted body?

How many died hungry on the sidewalks?

Night and day they were compelled to work for the administration.

No sooner was the younger brother back home than the older brother was at his post,

The administration had a hundred ways of extorting the people's money.

They took collections, they fined and ceaselessly claimed indemnities.

They never checked the truth of their information.

Whenever they heard rumors of unrest anywhere in the country, they immediately sent in their troops.

They governed tyrannically with their laws.

Of superior strength, they oppressed the people.

No one dared complain.

All suffered damage without ever lodging a grievance.

The French gave orders, the Vietnamese obeyed.

Officials of all ranks and of all services slavishly flattered French administrators.

To whom could our people turn to plead their innocence?

They had but Heaven and long nights in which to cry their lament.

Even animals of the same kind know affection for each other,

Those who share blood should know how to help each other.

Are we not aware of this fundamental principle?

Vietnam is the land in which we were born and raised.

Does not our yellow skin tell us that we are compatriots, brothers
and members of the same race?

Why then do we injure ourselves

In our effort to serve the white man, exactly as dogs hunt for prey?

Carriages, horses, umbrellas, parasols, we provide our masters
with them all,

We offer them respect and we revere them as if they were spirits
descended from Heaven.

Had they been of our own race

It would have been understandable that we subject ourselves
slavishly to them.

Source: Anonymous, "Poem on True Heroism" (ca. 1900) in Truong Buu Lam, *Patterns of
Vietnamese Response to Foreign Intervention: 1858–1900* (New Haven: Yale University
Press, 1967), 146–147.

3.   "TONKIN-HANOÏ—LES BORDS DU FLEUVE ROUGE ET LE PONT DOUMER," PIERRE DIEULEFILS POSTCARD

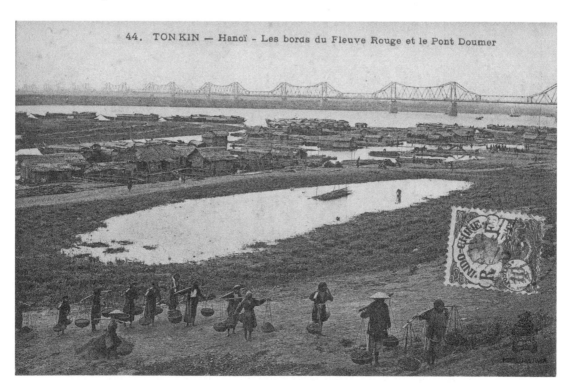

44.   TON KIN — Hanoï - Les bords du Fleuve Rouge et le Pont Doumer

This postcard shows Vietnamese laborers hauling sand from the banks of the Red River as the massive Pont Doumer, the bridge named for the Governor General who ordered its construction, looms behind them. The French residents of Hanoi took tremendous pride in the bridge as a triumph of European engineering. The workers in the foreground and the impoverished neighborhood on the sandbank behind them speak to the dire poverty of many of the city's Vietnamese inhabitants.

Source: Michael G. Vann.

4. ANONYMOUS, "THE ASIAN BALLAD (CHANT TO RAISE THE CONSCIOUSNESS OF THE PEOPLE)"

> All the varieties of taxes;
> They increase them endlessly
> The land tax is hardly paid
> When the tax on buffaloes and cows is due,
> Tax on dogs; tax on pigs
> Tax on matches; tax on alcohol; tax on ferries; tax on cars
> Tax on markets; tax on tea; tax on tobacco
> Tax on licenses; tax on water; tax on lamps
> Tax on houses; tax on pagodas and temples
> Tax on timber from forests; tax on commercial junks
> Tax even on cosmetic products and on city streets
> Tax on emaciated people addicted to drugs
> Tax on hillocks; tax on beaches; tax on dunes
> Tax on dignitaries; tax on actors and musicians
> Tax on oil; tax on honey; tax on paints everywhere
> Tax on rice, vegetable; tax on paddy; tax on cotton
> Tax on silk; tax on iron; tax on bronze
> Tax on birds; tax on fish throughout the three regions
> Nobody can enumerate all the various kinds of taxes
> The most stunning tax is on defection
> It is too painful to talk about all those things
> Shame descends on fathers and sons
> Separation comes between husbands and wives
> At time, we are filled with grudge and anger
> We want to scream and tear off the sky
> We want to draw out swords.

Source: Anonymous, "The Asian Ballad (Chant to Raise the Consciousness of the People)" (1905–1906), in Truong Buu Lam, *Colonialism Experienced: Vietnamese Writings on Colonialism, 1900–1931* (Ann Arbor: University of Michigan Press, 2002), 87–88.

5.   INHABITANTS OF HANOI TO GOVERNOR GENERAL

Hanoi, March 10, 1906
Dear Governor General,

It is our great honor to request an examination of the tragic situation in which many inhabitants of the city of Hanoi currently find themselves.

Since the establishment of the Tonkin Protectorate, it has been our pleasure to enact all orders given us by the administration, or to let it act as it should see fit.

However, following the customs of our country of Annam, all consider of the utmost importance those ceremonies held in honor of the dead, for our elderly relations and young children alike.

The presence in the city of a doctor tasked with examining the dead is causing us great fear and worry. This official had the police arrest all members (young and old) of a family, that by unfortunate circumstances, had a member fallen ill, in order to inoculate all members. Similarly, following the convulsions of a baby or the birth of a child, it is now common to inoculate the whole family. Afterwards, furniture, buildings, personal items, etc., are burned.

There have been several individuals who have fallen ill and then died of fear. In this way, the residents of the city are unable to remain at peace and pursue their occupations.

In this case, we would be deeply grateful should you, Mr. Governor General, please consider putting a cease to the above measures so that we might continue to carry out our business in peace.

Signed,
Inhabitants of the City of Hanoi

Source: Inhabitants of Hanoi to Governor General, Centre des Archives Section d'Outre-Mer, GGI 6739. Translated by Briana S. E. Vann.

6.   CITIZENS OF HANOI TO GOVERNOR GENERAL

Hanoi, March 16, 1906
Dear Governor General,

We, the inhabitants of the city of Hanoi, have the honor of calling your benevolent attention to the following incidents, of which we are victims; incidents for which children and adults alike will not hesitate to demand justice.

The plague has spread through the city of Hanoi since February and March of this year. We suffer from a great misfortune that has fallen upon us not only from nature, but also from the hands of men.

If a case of the plague should be discovered, the Municipal Doctor, after having attended to the afflicted houses, orders the police to monitor these homes, to detain the victim's family members in order to force them under quarantine, and to burn furniture, decorations, leather household items, other types of merchandise, etc.

Not only do the police detain members of the victim's family, but they also detain their neighbors and destroy their belongings as well.

Should the home be a straw hut, the police burn it entirely, along with all household objects.

Should the home be of brick, they burn all decorative elements, along with household objects, without exception.

Thus, if a person dies, his home is demolished and all his belongings destroyed.

It is in this unfortunate state that survivors find themselves, unable to support themselves or to relieve themselves of the tax burden imposed upon them.

We certainly believe that the goal of the French government established here in our land is to protect the interests of the Annamites and to lead them along the proper path, and we remain grateful for this protection. But why must we now be reduced to tolerating this poor treatment?

We present you here with a list of stricken homes that have been burned: homes in the Rue des Éventails, Rue des Voiles, Rue des Changeurs, Ruelle de Ngo-Miêu, Route de Diun-bu, Yeu-Hw Village, Digne de la Rue du Charbon, etc.

The homes and the victims' belongings are thus burned, under the pretense that the plague germs reproduce on the objects, in the home, and even in the neighborhood. This is very surprising to us!

For example, there is the doctor who examines the ill and the coolies who carry the coffins. How is it that the germs do not multiply on the person of the doctor himself, nor on that of the coolies?

Could it be that the doctor has a remedy for the plague for his own personal use? If so, why does he not distribute this effective remedy to the residents of the city, or else allow it to be sold, so that the residents might be able to save their own lives?

If this is not the case, why should the doctor order the police to detain all members of stricken families and to burn whatever is found in their home? It is a great misfortune to find ourselves stripped of all we own.

In the Annamite custom, after a person dies of an illness, the members of the household hasten to burn the bed on which the body has lain; they must also wash and thoroughly clean the room occupied by the deceased, and also heat the room. But they do not feel it necessary to burn all their own belongings, as the police is now doing.

We are the victims of these cruel actions, and we beseech you, Mr. Governor-General, to take pity upon us and to compel the authorities concerned to end these practices so that we might be free of these sad and unfortunate circumstances, and that we might not find ourselves obligated to leave our own country. We would be infinitely grateful.

This affair has attracted the support of all Annamite residents of this city. We have gathered to request the consideration of the Administration, but no one among us dares to be the sole author. We have let this bitter state of affairs continue day in and day out, until now.

Today we have the audacity to address you with this request, and beseech you to take the actions that you deem appropriate, so that we might have the experience of your beneficence.

Your very humble subjects.

Source: Citizens of Hanoi to Governor General, Centre des Archives Section d'Outre-Mer, GGI 6739. Translated by Briana S. E. Vann.

7. SUPERIOR RESIDENT OF TONKIN TO GOVERNOR GENERAL OF INDOCHINA, MARCH 27 AND MARCH 29, 1906

CONFIDENTIAL

Hanoi, March 27, 1906

In Memo No 1847, from March 26 of this year, you endeavor to communicate a complaint lodged by a group of Hanoi residents addressed to the Governor General, protesting daily sanitary measures enacted to halt the spread of the current plague epidemic.

The group's grievances are chiefly concerned with the following:

1. Quarantine and preventative inoculation of individuals having been in contact with plague victims.
2. Incineration of contaminated huts and household items found within.

It is my honor to inform you that the same complaints were brought to the Mayor of Hanoi several days ago. The Chief of Police was tasked with explaining to the natives the necessity of these measures, whose sole purpose is to protect the populace.

On last March 25, Mr. Kersselaers summoned the complainants to his office and tried, in vain, to convince them. They proceeded to issue the same demands as those contained in the letter addressed to the Governor General. Unsuccessful in the goal of their visit, approximately 200–300 protesters amassed at City Hall yesterday morning. The Mayor held an audience with their representatives, and despite his explanations and exhortations, he too was unable to dispel their misconceptions.

This morning, in collaboration with the Mayor of Hanoi, Doctor Leroy Des Barres, epidemiologist, and the Chief of Police, I conducted an inquiry into the appropriateness of possible measures to calm the concerns of the inhabitants of Hanoi.

In the first place, I have advised that any damages owed to interested parties be paid immediately following the incineration of huts or homes, or else of household items. I have additionally advised a large-scale review of the benefits provided under these circumstances. Finally, I have recommended for incineration only those huts and items whose destruction is absolutely necessary to the protection of public health.

I must address the petitioners' erroneous complaints that huts neighboring to contaminated homes are also destroyed. This has only occurred in cases where many families occupy rooms contained in a single building. Clearly in this case the destruction of only one portion of the building would be impossible. To another point, the quarantine, preventative inoculation, and complete disinfection of their living quarters is indispensable in the case of individuals who have been in the proximity of plague victims. Furthermore, Doctor Leroy Des Barres has assured me that none have been held for longer than 24 hours, whereas a strict application of the recommendations would have them held for at least eight days.

All measures currently in place are absolutely legal; they are mandated by documents regulating public health in the Colony. I assure you that these measures are being implemented with the utmost moderation and all appropriate accommodations. Disinfection is carried out by a team of European municipal police officers, who take pains to always inquire whether concerned parties have valuables that should be set aside before incineration, and will not put fire to anything that could be disinfected by heat alone. Doctor Leroy Des Barres himself calls at disinfected sites. This eminent practitioner has informed me of the impossibility of weakening these preventative measures without endangering public health. He assured me, on the contrary, that regulations expressly indicate even greater precaution. He ended by adding that over the course of his constant visits to the native quarters, he had received no serious grievance from the inhabitants and that he consistently noticed calm amongst the inhabitants.

While not yet confirmed by the Administrative and Judicial Police, these observations are most reassuring and serve to demonstrate that the recent complaints brought by some inhabitants of Hanoi were not made spontaneously, but were instigated by a number of agitators.

Among these agitators are two natives: City Council member Vu-Huy-Quang and a student by the name of Cu Cau, living at 4, rue de la Soie, were found to be leaders of the collective demand made by the City of Hanoi's native community. Several sources would also lead us to believe that Dr. Le Lan is not unfamiliar with the protest movements of the past few days.

Following the failure they suffered yesterday morning at City Hall, the protestors are plotting a strike of native employees from a number of European businesses in the city, with the goal of shutting them down. At the current moment, the order to strike has not been given. I have instructed the Chief of Police to ensure that the right to work will not be hindered.

I further directed him to continue his investigation with a view to discovering the leaders of the protests and, if possible, to assemble against them information which would enable them to be prosecuted.

PS: The Mayor of Hanoi just informed me that this afternoon he received a visit from the native City Council members. They informed him that the protests and demonstrations regarding the current sanitation measures came from a tiny fraction of the native community in the city. They added that the same demonstration held at the City Hall would be repeated at the Superior Residence tomorrow. Coordinated measures to avoid any disorderly behavior have been taken by the Mayor's office, the State Prosecutor, and the Chief of Police.

If the situation warrants it, I will give an audience to a delegation of no more than ten inhabitants of the city who can serve as proxies to present their grievances.

Hanoi, March 29 1906

Following upon my letter, number 48c, from March 27 of this year, it is my honor to inform you that yesterday afternoon, a large group of Hanoi residents formed at the Pinceau Pagoda with the goal of airing the grievances of the populace in regards to the sanitary measures necessitated by the current plague epidemic. The Mayor of Hanoi and the Central Commissioner of the administrative and judicial police arrived on the scene aiming to calm the somewhat agitated crowd, and decided to select among the more reputable residents, ten representatives to bring to my offices.

The complaints presented by these upstanding natives were no different than those brought before the Governor General in their last petition. I took great pains to demonstrate to them the absolute necessity of these actions, so that we might avoid a spread of the illness and protect those that have not been stricken. They remained unsatisfied, for the reasons I outlined in the aforementioned letter no. 48. I was, however, able to promise a slight improvement on one point: the natives attach a great importance to knowing the location of their plague-stricken relations' burial sites. Even though the Police has a numerically organized list of tombs and a map of the plague cemetery, I have decided that this information should additionally be available to interested parties at City Hall. Perhaps this location will be less intimidating than the Police Headquarters.

Appealing next to their common sense, I implored them to pay no heed to the misleading advice of agitators who surely seek personal gain from inciting unrest under the current circumstances, and who are unconcerned whether or not their actions are at all advisable or beneficial to the peaceful and honest members of the population.

Finally, I strongly advised them not to repeat the troublesome protests that have recently taken place. I warned them that the Administration would not tolerate them and would disperse the crowds as necessary and without hesitation. Since the office of the Mayor and my office as well is open daily to petitioners, it would be much more convenient to present grievances to the administrative authorities without resorting to these noisy and all too frequent group demonstrations.

As they left, they called for the release of several compatriots who were arrested for battery and resisting the authorities over the course of the previous demonstration. I granted them this favor, on the sole condition that the inhabitants of Hanoi cease the unwarranted protests of late, and that, in the interest of the sick as well as in that of public health, they notify City Hall of any deaths or suspected cases of plague they might encounter.

The delegates of the native population fully consented to these conditions. If, upon leaving my office, they remained unconvinced of the usefulness of the precautionary measures taken by the health authorities, at the very least the resignation with which they met my words was, I hope, a gauge of their future commitment to these indispensable measures and to the cessation of their noisy protests.

I will be sure to inform you should any further incidents occur relating to this matter.

Source: Superior Resident of Tonkin to Governor General of Indochina, Centre des Archives Section d'Outre-Mer, GGI 6739. Translated by Briana S. E. Vann.

8. "TONKIN—POUSSE-POUSSE," PIERRE DIEULEFILS POSTCARD

This postcard shows a French soldier seated in a pousse-pousse, or rickshaw, pulled by a barefoot coolie-pousse outside of a Confucian temple Hanoi. Combining late nineteenth-century industrial technology in its construction and manual labor in its operation, the rickshaw was one of the classic symbols of empire. By combining the confidence and relative wealth of the French man with the impoverishment and shoelessness of the Vietnamese man, the postcard articulates imperialist power relationships and the colonial order of things. *(see following page)*

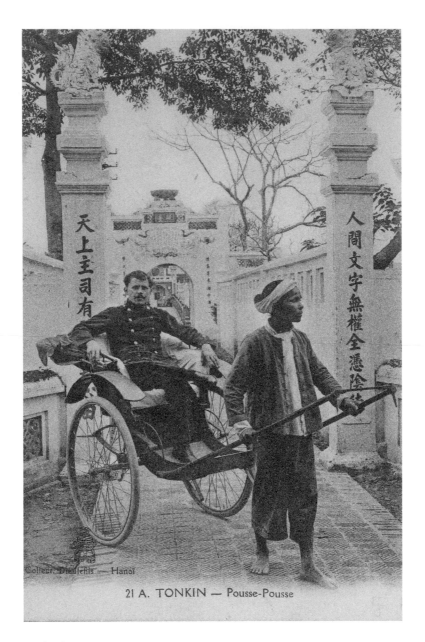

天上主司有   人間文字無權全憑陰

Collect. Dieulefils — Hanoi

21 A. TONKIN — Pousse-Pousse

Source: Michael G. Vann.

9. PHAN BOI CHAU, "THE NEW VIETNAM," 1907

Under the previous dynasties that reigned over our country, taxes the rulers
levied from the people were not heavy, although their collection could not
avoid the following barbarous abuses: (1) the corruption of the mandarins;
(2) the greed of the powerful gentry; and (3) the mismanagement of the
village notables. There were hundreds of ways to oppress the people, who,
consequently suffered a great deal. But that treatment was still somewhat

humane. The French levy every year from our people a head tax of two, three, four, or five piaster. Compared to the price put on a buffalo, a horse, or a chicken, what would be the difference? Alas! Our people have used up their sweat and blood to provide the Frenchmen, their women, their horses, and their dogs each year with so many hundreds , thousands, millions, billions. . . . And yet taxes are levied on everything: on things essential to our survival, on places necessary to our production. Even our bodies, which are created by Heaven and Earth and raised up by our parents with so much pain and care, they also have to be taxed by the French enemy four or five piasters every year. What is the meaning of that? Alas, our bodies are worth less than a buffalo, a horse, or a chicken. How pitiful that is! How pitiful that is! Mistreated in that fashion by the French, how come we have not risen up yet? Taxes, head taxes—that is a form of taxes no other country in the world has, except in our own country. Our people are not made of wood, stone, mud, or ashes: how can we accept being despised to that extent? An animal that is cornered knows how to attack and bite in order to escape; we are human beings, and yet we do not know how to get out of our quandaries. Even a caterpillar knows how to wish that the pine needle would become longer and longer, what then about us? When shall we be able to be proud of ourselves?

After modernization, first we have to get rid of all the wretched old practices that have existed through many dynasties. Second, we shall reform all the inhumane institutions set up by the French. Taxes, corvées, head taxes—none of these will remain after independence. All taxes will be decided upon by Congress. Taxes on this or that commodity have to be agreed upon by our people, and the proceeds must be spent on useful enterprises for the public good. The government can only start implementing its tax policies after the people have given their consent. Our people will not pay even one piaster or one grain of rice, if it is not out of their own will and with enthusiasm. Their patriotism leads them to pay their taxes willingly. No more of the barbarous coercive tactics of yesteryear. Then we shall be as happy as the sky is high and the ocean deep. The day will be warm, the wind harmonious, everybody at peace. How pleasant that will be!

Source: Phan Boi Chau, "The New Vietnam," 1907, in Truong Buu Lam, *Colonialism Experienced: Vietnamese Writings on Colonialism, 1900–1931* (Ann Arbor: University of Michigan Press, 2002), 110–12.

10. PHAN CHU TRINH, "LETTER TO PAUL BEAU," 1907

I, Phan Chu Trinh, former mandarin, am writing to you to describe the critical situation of the Vietnamese country.

Since Vietnam was placed under their protection, the French have built roads and bridges; they have improved communications through the construction of railroads and steamships; they have established post offices and telegraph lines: all these works are indeed very useful to Vietnam, and anybody with ears and eyes can hear and see them. There are, however, a few features I cannot fail to mention to you: they are the abuses perpetrated by the mandarinate, the sufferings accumulated by the people, and the decay of our customs. The French have not only shut their eyes to all these evils that are undermining the future of our nation; they have, furthermore, allowed these evils to spread their evil influence without even bothering to make an inquiry into their destructive effects.

[. . .]

From the time Vietnam became a protectorate of France, bridges, sewers, and roads have been built and repaired; military posts and stations have been erected; salaries and indemnities for the mandarins have accumulated into the millions. And yet, besides the taxes, principally those imposed on land and per head, and not counting customs duties, the government does not know where to go in order to improve its finances.

[. . .]

But now, claiming the mandarins are incompetent and the village people deceitful, the Protectorate applies its own policy. No matter whether the lands are large or small, with good or bad soil, the manpower is big or small in number, rich or poor, they are equally taxed. This year the taxes have been increased by 1 percent; next year it will be another 1 percent. This year an item is added to the tax assets, next year another one. That is the Protectorate's financial policy, which is enforced with utmost energy.

[. . .]

What to say now of the abuses pertaining to forced labor. Every able body, each year, has to give fourteen days of forced labor: four days for public works and ten days of corvée. In addition to these fourteen days the people have to pay for every other public work done by the state in the interest of their community.

[. . .]

The poor people, all year round, run from place to place offering their labor, carrying their products, and yet only one- to two-tenths of the wages due to them reach their pockets. In these miserable circumstances it is difficult to ask the people not to leave everything and become vagabonds.

The fate of the Vietnamese people today is indeed miserable and insecure, indeed not different from buffalos and horses. People can tie them up, whip them at will. They have a mouth but dare not speak. They are about to die without a lament. Weighing down on them is the power of the Protectorate government compounded by the cruelty of the Vietnamese mandarinate. What can one not get out of them through whipping? I am afraid that soon the rich people will be ruined, the poor ones resourceless;

the mild people will become beggars and the tough ones robbers and bandits. A few more years from now villages will be deserted, old and young people will have died, if not of hunger, then of imprisonment or exile; if not from drifting along the highways, then from the oppression of the mandarins. The day will come when rice fields will have no one to tend them; corvée will no longer be honored; taxes no longer paid. Even if you peel their skin or carve their bones, the only good that it will do is to send the Vietnamese people onto the same path as the Red Indians of America. That's all.

[. . .]

Recently, people in the North and South have been entertained by the rumor that the Protectorate is going to change its policy within the government of Vietnam: it will modify its treatment of the Vietnamese people; it will regard the French and Vietnamese in the same way so as to conquer the hearts and minds of the people. I presume all that is to be seen as long-range policy goals. I have read many newspaper articles coming from Hanoi and have learned that the governor-general of Indochina, in speeches delivered in Hanoi, talked of improving the treatment of the Vietnamese, of civilizing the Vietnamese. Many matters are mentioned over and over again—things like reform of the penal code, renovation of the educational system. But with regard to the abuses of the mandarinate, the exactions of taxes and corvée, not a single word has been uttered.

Source: Phan Chu Trinh, "Letter to Paul Beau," 1907, in Truong Buu Lam, *Colonialism Experienced: Vietnamese Writings on Colonialism, 1900–1931* (Ann Arbor: University of Michigan Press, 2002), 126, 134–37.

11. "TONKIN: RAPPORT POLITIQUE GÉNÉRALE POUR L'ANNÉE 1908"

The [native] bourgeoisie of the big cities have become critical and lost all respect for Europeans. Their children know French, read newspapers, cite Voltaire, Jean Jacques Rousseau, and interpret them in their own fashion. To the detriment of other skills, our educational efforts have developed simple memorization amongst the native students who are hardly capable of reasoning, of penetrating the spirit which inspired these orators and writers, of seizing in all their nuances the concepts, so different from those they are brought up with. They have generally just set foot in the world of letters and are taking in the most diverse sociological ideas with the greatest carelessness: it is these semi-scholars, concerned with pride and conceit, from which statements of loyalty imperfectly conceal hostile sentiments which they profess for the nation which has given them the benefits of instruction and of Western civilization.

Source: Centre des Archives Section d'Outre-Mer, GGI, dossier 64179: "Tonkin: Rapport Politique Générale pour l'année 1908" (1908). Translated by Michael G. Vann.

12. LOUIS BONNAFORT, *TRENTE ANS DE TONKIN*

Last night at the Hanoi Hotel in Hanoi, I was quietly sipping my drink, when an explosion shook the air, projecting debris into my glass and releasing a cloud of smoke. A bomb had been thrown onto the terrace. Two old friends from the regiment, Commanders Chapuis and Montgrand, were covered in a sea of blood which flowed onto the sidewalk.

[. . .]

One curious reaction of a young woman seated near the table of Commanders Théry and Montgrand, and whose drink had been contaminated by debris from the walls and other debris:

"Damn country! One can't even drink an absinthe in peace. Boy! Give me another absinthe."

And very calmly she continued.

Source: Louis Bonnafort, *Trente ans de Tonkin* (Paris: Eugène Figuière, 1921), 319–20. Translated by Michael G. Vann.

13. "RAPPORT DE GGI SARRUT AU MINISTRE DES COLONIES"

[. . .] the admirable calm, the perfect *sang-froid*, the spirit of solidarity, and the confidence in the Government given to us by the French of Hanoi and Tonkin have not ceased to strike us and move us as admirable. On the tragic night of 26 April, the European population gave a preview of the sentiments of bravery and of discipline which has since not dissipated. Containing their indignation before the abominable crime, they have kept a noble and virile attitude in front of the native population. All the French, men and women, of Hanoi and the surrounding area, despite the new menaces which threatened them, grouped around the Chief of the Colony at the funerals of Commanders Chapuis and Montgrand, and gave their moving characters' highest significance to this large demonstration.

Source: Centre des Archives Section d'Outre-Mer, Papiers Albert Sarraut, 9 PA, dossier 2: "Rapport de GGI Sarraut au Ministre des Colonies" (1913). Translated by Michael G. Vann.

14. "PAUL BERT'S STATUES TOPPLED AT 9:10 AM YESTERDAY MORNING," AUGUST 2, 1945

The statue commemorating the French Provincial Guard (Soldier in Blue) was knocked down, as well as the statue with a flared dress [Liberty] at the Southern gate. However, even after working all day yesterday, workers are still chiseling the solid statue next to the statue of Jean Dupuis.

A great crowd came to wave and cheer the statues being knocked down.

Tran Lai, the Mayor of Hanoi, along with a group representing the various classes of Hanoi, decided to clear out all of the statues commemorating French people in the city of Hanoi.

This order was carried out in the morning of August 1st (Western calendar), or the 24th day of the 6th month of the year Ất Dậu (1945).

At seven o'clock in the morning several dozen workers attached to the city's Lục Lộ facility broke up into groups and brought ladders to the statue of Paul Bert, the statue commemorating the Provincial Guard, the statue with the flared dress at the Southern gate, and the statue of Jean Dupuis by the Riverside School.

The Mayor and several assembly members of the city came to watch these statues, which took three or four hours to knock down.

The statue of Paul Bert fell at 9:10 AM, the statue at the Southern gate fell at 9:45 AM, and the statue commemorating the Provincial Guard fell at 10:30 AM.

When the statues fell there were iron pilings supporting them from underneath, so trucks were needed to haul them off.

Source: "Paul Bert's Statues Toppled at 9:10 AM Yesterday Morning" Newspaper fragment, August 2, 1945. Translated from Vietnamese by Matthew Berry.

PART III
HISTORICAL CONTEXTS

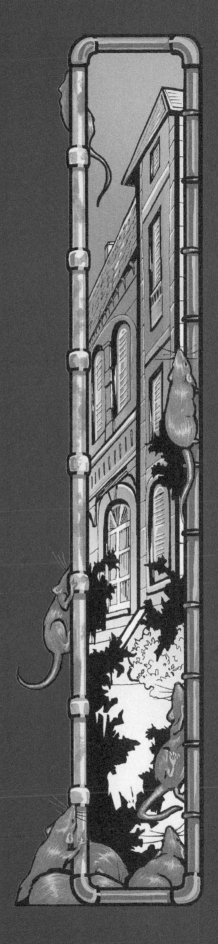

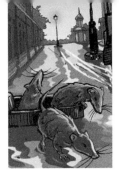

Context is essential for historical understanding. Without knowing how can an event, a piece of art, or a life is the product of a specific economic, political, socio-cultural, and environmental moment in time, we will never really comprehend what was going on. When I initially studied the history of colonial Hanoi, I went about my research as if all history was local. I studied Hanoi in a vacuum. Unfortunately, this is what many beginning urban historians do. Reading William Cronon's award-winning *Nature's Metropolis: Chicago and the Great West* opened my eyes to the reality is that no city is an island (not even Singapore, Mumbai, or Venice!).[1] One of the pioneers of environmental history, Cronon placed the history of Chicago in the larger ecosystem of the Great Plains. Urban systems always have connections to the world around them. Food, water, and fuel come from sources near and far and people constantly move in and out of cities. Thinking about Hanoi, I applied this principle to the historical processes that created the colonial city. Locally, French Hanoi drew in labor, food, and construction material such as wood and stone from Tonkin's Red River delta. Regionally, French Hanoi was still linked to centuries-old trade and migration networks that tied Tonkin to South China. Globally, French Hanoi was connected to metropolitan France but also to the French empire's territories in Africa, the Caribbean, South America, India, China, and the Pacific and Indian Oceans. Trying to make sense of the great rat hunt without these three frameworks would have resulted in an incomplete picture.

The field of world history offers a perspective grounded in understanding the balance between local, regional, and global contexts. World historians reject the idea that the nation-state, with its artificial, changing, and porous boundaries, should be the primary unit of study. This is a break with the conventional practices of the historical profession as established by Leopold von Ranke in the nineteenth century.[2] World historians argue that no nation, be it France or Vietnam, can be understood in isolation.

---

1   William Cronon, *Nature's Metropolis: Chicago and the Great West* (New York: W. W. Norton, 1991).

2   Patrick Manning, *Navigating World History: Historian Create a Global Past* (New York: Palgrave, 2003), 31.

Instead, world history promotes the analysis of various patterns of connection around the globe. Often this is the complex process of economic globalization but it can also be the centuries-old story of cultural interactions. The most important point about world history is that it actively searches for the ways in which groups of people scattered around the world have a shared historical experience. One of the best examples of this is Donald Wright's *The World and a Very Small Place in Africa: The History of Globalization in Niumi, The Gambia*. The book chronicles how a very small region in The Gambia, itself the smallest country in Africa, was steadily enmeshed in a series of global networks that ranged from the Islamic trans-Saharan trade to the British Empire to a post-colonial trade relationship characterized as "dependency" by economic theorists. By exploring Niumi's global connections, Wright demonstrates that Niumi's history cannot be understood without knowing these connections. Numerous historical forces that shaped Niumi's destiny came from thousands of miles away.[3] This is the kind of context that world history offers us. While Niumi was not a city per se, the way in which Wright contextualized the tiny region in the world system was tremendously useful for my thinking about Hanoi. My micro-history of things gone awry in colonial Hanoi took on a much larger significance when I adopted the world historical perspective.

To tell the story of the great rat hunt, I framed the narrative in several world historical contexts, including the age of empire, the Western industrial-capitalist revolution, France's paradoxical political history, the rise of nationalism and communism in Vietnam, and the third bubonic plague pandemic. Without an understanding of these larger processes, micro-histories such as the story of massacring rats in French Hanoi can appear to be a trivial anecdote. With an understanding of these contexts, we can appreciate how global forces impacted the daily life of Hanoi's residents.

THE NEW IMPERIALISM

Historians refer to the colonial expansion of Europe, the United States, and Japan from 1871 to either the First World War (1914–1918) or the start of the Second World War (1939) as the New Imperialism. The era is characterized by Europe exporting many of its conflicts overseas, the rise of nationalism, a certain level of absurdity and irrationality, a dramatic imbalance in global power relationships, and the creation of international boundaries and conflicts that have lasted well into the twenty-first century.

---

3   Donald R. Wright, *The World and a Very Small Place in Africa: A History of Globalization in Niumi, The Gambia* (Armonk: M. E. Sharpe, 2004).

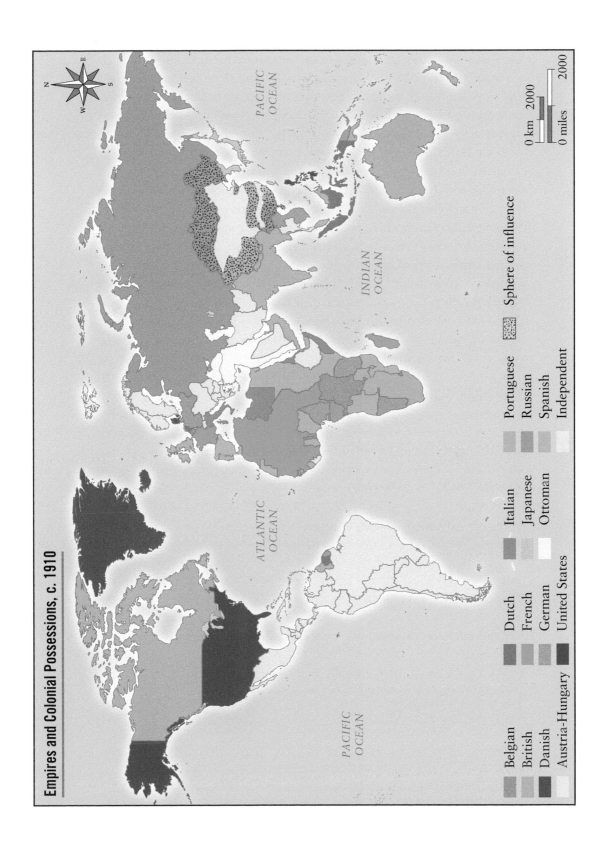

Empires and Colonial Possessions, c. 1910

Belgian
British
Danish
Austria-Hungary

Dutch
French
German
United States

Italian
Japanese
Ottoman

Portuguese
Russian
Spanish
Independent

Sphere of influence

This period of European expansion differed dramatically from earlier colonial empires. Most notably, Europe conquered a huge amount of land in Africa and Asia. While Spain and Britain had done this before in the Americas, the New Imperialism was unaccompanied by the massive migrations that repopulated the New World, creating what Alfred Crosby terms "Neo-Europes."[4] Instead, Europeans seized lands that they rarely visited let alone settled. Biology has an important history in the difference between the "old" and "new" forms of empire. When Europeans came to the Americas, they brought Afro-Eurasian diseases that killed off the vast majority of the previously isolated indigenous population. From New Spain to New England, European colonialism benefited from the germs its people carried. This aspect of what Crosby terms the "Columbian Exchange" devastated isolated populations in the Americas and Polynesia.[5] But when Europeans arrived in Africa, India, and Southeast Asia, they discovered that biology was not in their favor. Much of tropical Africa was home to diseases that so decimated European soldiers, administrators, and merchants that the region was known as "the white man's graveyard."[6] The medical advances of the late nineteenth century helped Europeans survive a little longer than in previous centuries, but a posting in the tropics could still be a death sentence. Thus, this period of expansion was really a form of imperialism, understood as one of many forms of control and intervention over a faraway land, rather than colonialism which entails the conquering country settling its possessions with its own people.[7]

THE IMPERIALIST POWERS

The starting date of the New Imperialism is important and easier to agree upon than when it ended. France's disastrous loss to Prussia in the Franco-Prussian War (1870–1871) signaled a dramatic change in Europe. France, for centuries the great land power, was humiliated by an alliance of German states led by Prussia. To add insult to injury, the peace settlement included the annexation of two eastern French provinces, Alsace and Lorraine. Failure on the battlefield and the loss of territory inflamed French public opinion, resulting in a staunchly anti-German nationalism. Upon its

---

4   Alfred Crosby, *Ecological Imperialism: The Biological Expansion of Europe, 900–1900* (New York: Cambridge University Press, 1986), 2.

5   Alfred Crosby, *The Columbian Exchange: Biological and Cultural Consequences of 1492* (Westport, CT: Greenwood Publishing Co., 1972).

6   Philip D. Curtin, *Death by Migration: Europe's Encounter with the Tropical World in the Nineteenth Century* (Cambridge: Cambridge University Press, 1989).

7   For an excellent discussion of these terms see Heather Streets-Salter and Trevor R. Getz, *Empires and Colonies in the Modern World: A Global Perspective* (New York: Oxford University Press, 2016), 1–20.

victory, the Prussia kingdom united the German states (minus Austria) into the Second German Empire (1871–1918). German unification created an immensely powerful economy, characterized by Chancellor Otto von Bismarck as "an alliance of iron and rye," referring to Germany's industrial and agricultural power. While many French citizens wanted revenge on Germany and the liberation of Alsace-Lorraine, the political and military leadership knew that war with the German Empire would be suicidal. To assuage the national humiliation and feeling of impotence, France turned to Africa and Asia to find military glory in the seizure of vast swathes of land. Glorious campaigns against Africans depicted as brutal savages sold numerous newspapers in Paris and other French cities. French officers, eager for promotion, often pursued aggressive and unauthorized military engagements to further their own careers. While France had a long history of colonialism in the Atlantic, Indian, and Pacific Oceans, and had invaded Algeria in 1831, the speed and scale of French imperialist expansion after 1871 was unprecedented. A diverse group of investors and merchants, geographers and scientists, explorers and adventurers, and politicians and military officers, who came to be known as the "Colonial Lobby," pushed for an expanding empire. They often compared France's colonial holdings with the seemingly efficient, prosperous, and larger British Empire. To the Colonial Lobby's chagrin, France consistently came up lacking. Numerous documents from the era attest to the ways in which they rationalized, justified, and encouraged French imperialism. A culture of imperial boosterism developed at the turn of the century.

Meanwhile, after the success of the war with France, Bismarck was eager to keep the peace in Europe. A careful practitioner of Realpolitik, he actively encouraged French adventures in the tropical world, frowned upon distracting colonial wars, and avoided a costly arms race with other powers. The German economy grew in leaps and bounds over the next decades. By the 1880s, self-confident, if not arrogant, German nationalists began to call for an overseas empire. Bismarck begrudgingly entered the colonial game, but did not play it with much enthusiasm or vigor. When Wilhelm I, the German Emperor or Kaiser, died in 1888, Wilhelm II took the throne. The new Kaiser adopted a much more reckless and daring foreign policy. His behavior was described as that of "a bull in a China shop." Historians have speculated about his motivations, with some pointing to his personal crisis of masculinity stemming from his physical disabilities and shortcomings.[8] He fired the elderly Bismarck in 1890 and his staff began to speak openly about finding "a place in the sun" for Germany to

---

8   Isabel V. Hull, *The Entourage of Kaiser Wilhelm II 1888–1918* (Cambridge: Cambridge University Press, 1982).

colonize. Germany began to compete with France for control of places ranging from Madagascar to Morocco. In the summer of 1900, when the Kaiser addressed troops leaving for China to help suppress the anti-foreigner Boxer Rebellion, he urged them to fight with the infamous violence of Attila the Hun, giving no quarter to surrendering enemies and ensuring that no Chinese would ever dare to even look at a German the wrong way. This bellicose monarch added an unpredictable element to existing imperial rivalries. The French Colonial Lobby called for seizing colonies from Morocco to Madagascar lest they fall into German hands.

Tiny Belgium's entry into the competition for colonies initiated the so-called "Scramble for Africa." When King Leopold II took the throne in 1865 he was frustrated with his small kingdom and its modest wealth. He began to plot a way to build a colonial empire of his own. Leopold contracted the famous British-born American journalist, adventurer, and shameless self-promoter Henry Morton Stanley to explore the heavily forested Congo region in central Africa. Between 1879 and 1885, Stanley persuaded, pressured, or tricked scores of local chiefs to sign treaties that gave Leopold control of their land. It is highly unlikely that any of them understood what they were agreeing to.[9] Leopold then worked with Bismarck to organize the Berlin Conference (1884–1885) in which the European nations agreed to follow certain rules and procedures in the annexation of African territories. Coyly playing the role of the king of a small neutral country, Leopold claimed to be an honest broker who could be a buffer between the great powers. He secured control of almost a million square miles, some eighty times the size of Belgium, and declared it the Congo Free State. Leopold made sure that the African colony was his personal possession and not held by the government of Belgium. He claimed he would govern in the most enlightened and progressive manner and would devote himself to bettering the lives of the supposedly savage Africans. This was a lie. Leopold was one of the most cynical, dishonest, and brutal rulers in history and the Congo Free State is one of the most violent, tragic, and horrifying chapters in the dark history of colonialism. He sent an army of mercenaries to his equatorial empire initially to seize as much ivory as they could. In his novella *The Heart of Darkness*, Joseph Conrad fictionalized the horrific frenzy of violence and rapacious greed that characterized the Belgian Congo. As the ivory ran out in the 1890s, Leopold's company focused on collecting rubber, much in demand in a new phase of the industrial revolution. While rubber plantations were being set up in Southeast Asia by the British, French, and Dutch, it would be about a decade before

---

9   Edward Berenson, *Heroes of Empire: Five Charismatic Men and the Conquest of Africa* (Berkeley: University of California Press, 2010), 49–51.

the newly introduced trees matured enough to produce latex. In the meantime, Leopold realized that he could make a fortune off the Congo's wild rubber trees. Faced with this time constraint, Leopold ordered the use of as much force as necessary to amass a fortune in rubber. Some historians estimate ten million Congolese deaths. However, thanks to the brave efforts of a few witnesses, the truth about the horrifying violence came out and the Belgian state seized control of the Congo 1908. Leopold died in disgrace the following year. Belgium, however, never thought about relinquishing control of the colony. The tragedy of the Congo is the most shocking case of the violence that is inherent in the colonial system.

Germany's entry into the tropics, France's revived imperial expansion, and Belgium's bloody colonial endeavor challenged Great Britain's status as the most powerful empire. Due to its naval strength and a vibrant commercial culture, the British Empire was the largest and most profitable empire in history. While the British benefited from being the first to industrialize, they found themselves challenged by newly united Germany's unleashed potential. German naval expansion threatened England's command of the seas (a process that started with the defeat of the Spanish Armada in 1588 and reached its height with Nelson's triumph over Napoleon's fleet at Trafalgar in 1805). German industrialization and banking posed a serious economic threat. Meanwhile, France, England's traditional nemesis, returned to competing for control over land in the colonial tropics. Faced with these multiple threats to its hegemonic status, England began to seize territories lest its rivals snatch them up first. Strategic planners agitated for securing the routes to the empire's most important colony, India. Thus, to protect its maritime traffic, the empire added various ports on the west, south, and east coasts of Africa. When the French opened the Suez Canal in 1869 and it proved to be a major success in shortening the time it took to get to India, the British set about gaining control first of the canal's operating company and then of Egypt itself. Decades of seemingly relentless expansion and warfare ensured that the British Empire remained the largest. Due to its size, population, and rich resources, India was the most important British possession and was often referred to as her "jewel in the crown."

Since its declaration of independence from Britain in 1776 the United States of America had pursed a steady policy of settler colonialism in a series of genocidal wars against the indigenous people of North America but the republic only entered the New Imperialism with the Spanish–American War of 1898. Ostensibly the war was fought to liberate Cuba from Spanish rule. Cuba did gain independence from Spain, but the island was immediately tied to the United States who reserved the right to intervene as it saw fit and secured preferential treatment for Yankee investors. The United States seized other Spanish colonies in the Caribbean and the

Pacific, including Puerto Rico, Guam, and the Philippines. To oust the Spanish from the Philippine archipelago, a colonial possession since the 1500s, American representatives promised to support Filipino nationalists in an uprising. When the nationalists rebelled and Spanish rule collapsed, a new republic was declared. However, the United States quickly moved to seize the islands for itself. In the ensuing war of colonial occupation veterans of the wars against the Plains Indians were sent to fight the Filipino nationalists. As the war raged from 1899 to 1902 several hundred thousand died in the fighting, from the spread of diseases such as cholera, and due to famine. In the southern Philippines a Muslim rebellion lasted from 1904 to 1913, prolonging the misery and suffering. In the frenzy of expansion in 1898, President McKinley annexed the Republic of Hawaii, a white supremacist state established by settlers who overthrew the monarchy in 1893. In 1900, the Americans participated in the Eight Nation Alliance that brutally put down the anti-foreign Boxer Rebellion in China. In the space of a few years, the United States of America quickly became a colonial power with holdings in the Caribbean, the Pacific, and Southeast Asia. Rudyard Kipling, the poet of the British imperial adventure, dedicated "The White Man's Burden" to the United States of America. The poem was a piece of advice for the republic as it became a colonial power.

Japan was another late arrival in the competition for colonies. After a century of civil war, during which Portuguese ships brought disruptive things like guns and Catholicism, the Tokugawa Shogunate (1603–1867) decided to more or less seal off the island nation under the Sakoku laws. While trade continued with China and Korea, Westerners were only allowed to visit tiny Deshima Island in Nagasaki Bay. The Portuguese and their religion were banned and only ships from the Dutch East India Company were let in (as Calvinists and capitalists, most Dutch had little interest in spreading their faith, especially when it might interfere with profit making). Guns were outlawed and Christianity was banned. As peace prevailed through the land, many samurai warriors became bureaucrats and administrators for their feudal lords. During the nineteenth century the boom in whaling brought an increasing number of Western ships near the islands. Yet Europeans and Americans faced the threat of summary execution should they come ashore as merchants, diplomats, or even shipwrecked sailors. In 1853, an American fleet commanded by Mathew Perry flaunted the Sakoku laws by entering Edo Bay. Perry made a display of his ships' firepower and informed the authorities to open up their ports or face attack. When he returned the following year, the Shogunate begrudgingly acquiesced to the American demands. This set in motion a series of events that led to the collapse of Tokugawa rule and the rise of a modernizing faction. Under the banner of returning power to the emperor (as opposed to the

Shogun) the movement became known as the Meiji Restoration (1868–1912). During this time Japan went through a dramatic series of changes including destruction of the hereditary samurai warrior class, rapid industrialization, and adopting an aggressive foreign policy. Realizing that an industrial Japan would need access to resources and markets expansionists followed the Western example by seizing a few smaller islands in the Western Pacific and then attacking China. The Sino-Japanese War (1894–1895) resulted in Japan's colonial occupation of Taiwan (1895–1945). Japan participated with the European-led campaign against the Boxer Rebellion. Launching a surprise attack on the Russian Pacific fleet in Port Arthur, Japan started the Russo-Japanese War (1904–1905). The Japanese victory over a European power made a huge impact on the minds of many people in colonial Southeast Asia and beyond. Japan then went on to invade and occupy Korea for several brutal decades. Japan's invasion of China started the Pacific War (1931–1945), which became the Pacific Theater of World War II when it invaded the American, British, French, and Dutch colonies in Southeast Asia. While some see Japanese history as a successful example of modernization, others condemn the rise of militarism and radically aggressive imperialism. We should note that in terms of both industry and empire Japan was following precedents set by the West.

CHINA

While China was not formally colonized in this period, it was subject to a sustained imperialist intervention that induced dramatic political and socio-economic changes.[10] For centuries, China's wealth was legendary. With low labor costs due to low food prices (wet rice agriculture produces dramatically more calories per acre than wheat or maize), Chinese workshops could outproduce European manufacturers. China had access to goods from a variety of ecosystems including the Spice Islands of Southeast Asia and the tea and silk farms of Southern China. Janet Abu-Lughod has shown that its commercial connections via the famous Silk Roads or the much more active maritime trade routes of the South China Sea and the Indian Ocean brought Chinese goods to distant markets in the Islamic and European worlds.[11] They also drew merchants from around the world to China.

However, they faced a problem as the Chinese economy demanded little in the way of imports. Starting with the Ming Dynasty's decision to switch from paper currency to coinage there was an increased demand

---

10   Robert Bickers, *The Scramble for China: Foreign Devils in the Qing Empire, 1832–1914* (New York: Penguin, 2011).

11   Janet L. Abu-Lughod, *Before European Hegemony: The World System, AD 1250–1350* (New York and Oxford: Oxford University Press, 1989).

for silver. When the Emperor ordered that taxes be paid in silver coins, the demand increased dramatically. Fortunately for the Spanish monarchy, they discovered rich silver mines in their Andean and Mexican colonies. Spain's Manila galleon trade supplied China with silver for centuries and American silver allowed the Spanish to buy Chinese goods.[12] Other Europeans had difficulty figuring out how to pay for Chinese products. The British, who were increasingly addicted to tea, saw their hard currency flow towards China in an uneven balance of trade. Struggling to sell something in China, British merchants experimented with introducing a smokable and more addictive form of opium. By 1820, the British reversed the flow of silver by selling opium grown in their colonial possessions in India to markets in southern and coastal China. Despite being illegal, the opium trade was a boom for the British economy. When the Chinese Emperor tried to stop the trade, the British responded with force. The Opium War (1839–1842) resulted in the Treaty of Nanking that opened numerous coastal and river cities to foreign merchants. These so-called "treaty ports" granted special rights to British and other European merchants including "extraterritoriality" or the right not to be subject to Chinese law.[13] So, while aside from Portuguese Macao and the British lease of Hong Kong there was no direct annexation of Chinese lands and people, China experienced an insidious form of colonialism. In addition to the spread of opium use and Western penetration, Qing administrative breakdown, natural disasters, and a series of rebellions plunged China into chaos. For example, the Taiping Rebellion (1850–1864) almost overthrew the emperor and took the lives of some twenty to thirty million people.

All these factors resulted in thousands of impoverished Chinese fleeing their homeland in search of better lives in Southeast Asia, Australia, Hawai'i, California, and even Jamaica.[14] This wave of Chinese immigration provoked widespread Sinophobia and a racist backlash.[15] At the turn of the century a popular movement rose up in support of the Qing Dynasty and against foreign presence in China. The Militia United in Righteousness (Yihetuan), pejoratively known in English as the "Boxers," attacked Western

---

12   Arturo Giraldez, *The Age of Trade: The Manila Galleon and the Dawn of the Global Economy* (Lanham, MD: Rowman and Littlefield, 2015).

13   Julia Lovell, *The Opium War: Drugs, Dreams and the Making of China* (London: Picador, 2011), 223–40, and Robert Bickers and Isabella Jackson (eds.), *Treaty Ports in Modern China: Law, Land and Power* (New York: Routledge, 2016).

14   Adam M. McKeown, *Melancholy Order: Asian Immigration and the Globalization of Borders* (New York: Columbia University Press, 2008), 45–59.

15   See John Kuo Wei Tchen and Dylan Yeats, *Yellow Peril! An Archive of Anti-Asian Fear* (London and New York: Verso, 2014), for a powerful collection of Sinophobic primary sources.

missionaries and Chinese Christian converts in the countryside before laying siege to the international legations in the capital, Beijing.[16] The brutal suppression of the Boxer Rebellion (1899–1901) by an alliance of the Great Britain, France, Japan, Russia, the United States, Germany, Italy, and Austria-Hungary included the slaughter of Boxers and widespread looting. The dynasty was then forced to pay an enormous sum of silver in reparations. Historically the greatest empire on Earth, these successive disasters and insults indicated a dramatic power reversal. Nationalist Chinese historiography refers to the period from the Opium War to the Second World War as a "Century of Humiliations." China thus has a complex and central role in the history of the New Imperialism.

COLONIAL POLITICAL ECONOMIES

Colonial empires were to be profit-making enterprises. From the time the Portuguese forced their way into the Asian spice trade and the Spanish conquistadores set about looting the Aztec and Incan empires to the height of the Atlantic slave trade and the British expansion into India to the Scramble for Africa to the American annexation of Hawai'i, empire was about financial gain. Following the observations of Karl Marx, in the early twentieth century V. I. Lenin and Rosa Luxemburg argued that imperialism was the globalization of industrial capitalism.[17] They saw colonial expansion as the search for cheap labor, raw materials, opportunities for capital investment, and new markets for manufactured goods. In the Marxist perspective, economics comes first and everything else follows. On the other end of the political spectrum proponents of empire and capitalism, such as the arch-imperialist Cecil Rhodes, linked the two. Rhodes held that colonialism's economic benefits would improve the lives of the British working class and thus stave off revolution. French Prime Minister Jules Ferry made similar statements. Prefiguring Ronald Reagan's "trickle down theory," they claimed that profits made in the empire would benefit the country as a whole. A rising tide, it was said, raises all boats.

While the impact of imperialism on the colonizer's economies is still subject to debate, the impact on the colonized was almost uniformly negative. While certain collaborating elites such as landlords, entrepreneurs, and merchants benefited from empire's new economic order, most people in the colonies experienced profound disruptions in their lives. Trade monopolies, new taxation systems, and land annexations destroyed centuries-old social

---

16   Robert Bickers and R. G. Tiedemann (eds.), *The Boxers, China, and the World* (Lanham, MD: Rowman & Littlefield Publishers, 2007).

17   Vladimir Lenin, *Imperialism, the Highest Stage of Capitalism* (London: Lawrence and Wishart, 1948); Rosa Luxemburg, *The Accumulation of Capital* (New York: Routledge, 2003), 398–401 and 426–27.

relationships. Traditional social safety nets ranging from village communes that helped families in times of crisis to temple complexes that redistributed food donated as tribute collapsed under foreign rule.[18] Under the guise of modernizing colonial societies, state policies actively pulled people out of traditional subsistence agriculture and into market-oriented systems. For example, the requirement that taxes be paid in cash forced farmers to sell a portion of their crops. Elsewhere, the creation of rubber plantations in places like central Vietnam, the Malay Peninsula, and Sumatra necessitated thousands of villagers to leave their homes and travel to these relatively un-populated areas.[19] Comparable to factories in the jungle, plantation employees lived in barracks, worked according to a strict schedule, and could face brutal discipline.[20] Furthermore, employers paid their wages in cash.

As colonies were the products of conquest and were held by military occupation, the use of force was a given in most of the colonial world. Of course there were dramatic variations from case to case, with the Belgian Congo being perhaps the worst possible scenario, but the level of force used in the colonial world would have been unacceptable in Europe or the United States at the time. Colonial regimes deployed a number of different systems of un-free labor. From chattel slavery to indentured servants to corvée labor, colonized peoples were forced to work for their imperial masters. In addition to un-free labor, the colonizers benefited from very low wages paid to their native subjects. Low-cost labor made huge building projects possible. The scale of mines, plantations, railway projects, and monumental cities was impressive and only possible with colonial labor arrangements. Even in their private domestic space, colonizers benefited from the colonial political economy. White homes in the colonies were frequently spacious villas. Europeans employed numerous servants at a time when such luxuries were increasingly unaffordable in the home country. In colonial Vietnam, the lowest paid French government employee was advised to budget for a cook and at least one "boy," the catchall term for a male servant.

IMPERIAL IDEOLOGIES

To justify the various forms of colonial exploitation, the imperialist powers adopted a number of ideologies and rationalizations. The British regularly spoke of the struggle for Free Trade. Indeed, during the Opium War they claimed that it was their moral obligation to teach the Chinese that they had

18   Martin J. Murray, *The Development of Capitalism in Colonial Indochina* (Berkeley: University of California Press, 1981).

19   Stephen L. Harp, *A World History of Rubber: Empire, Industry, and the Everyday* (West Sussex: Wiley-Blackwell, 2015), 17–28.

20   Tran Bu Binh, *The Red Earth: A Vietnamese Memoir of Life on a Colonial Rubber Plantation* (Athens: Ohio University Press, 1985).

to accept drug sales in their country if there was market demand. They denigrated the Confucian argument that the emperor should intervene in the economy in the name of social harmony as backwards and ignorant. As the most progressive government in Europe the French Third Republic claimed that it had a special "civilizing mission." France would bring the values and wisdom of the Enlightenment to its subjects, whether they wanted them or not. After seizing most of Spain's remaining colonies, the Americans assured themselves that they had to protect their colonial possessions from exploitative and cynical European rule. This myth aligned nicely with Kipling's "White Man's Burden." Germans spoke of a "scientific colonialism" that would bring order to the tropics. The Dutch adopted what they called the "ethical policy" and the Belgians promoted the oxymoronic "domination to serve." Considering that the violence of military invasion, exploitative labor practices, scarcity of representative institutions, and brutalities of counter-insurgency operations characterized the colonial encounter, these slogans need to be taken with a grain of salt.

The Euro-American imperialists also made use of racism. Stemming from Enlightenment thinkers who sought to discover or impose order on the universe, Europeans were obsessed with hierarchies. Scholars used published accounts of encounters with Africans, Asians, Native Americans, and Pacific Islanders as data to develop a system of human classification. Not surprisingly, European experts consistently put Caucasians (an invented category for "white" Europeans) at the top of the list. Africans, the victims of the Atlantic slave trade for several centuries, regularly came at the bottom of the list. In the 1850s, when Charles Darwin began to publish his theories on natural selection and the origins of species, many of his ideas on evolution were perverted by racist thinking. Herbert Spencer used Darwinism as the basis for his concept of "the survival of the fittest." Soon known as Social Darwinism, this belief system held that the different races of humanity were unequal, that struggle between them was natural, and that the stronger races would vanquish the weaker, possibly exterminating them. Social Darwinism thus rationalized imperialism and what we now call genocide as the natural order of things. While not a uniform body of thought, such racist sentiment infected all aspects of the colonial encounter. Despite what apologists for empire might argue, in theory and practice, racism was inseparable from the New Imperialism.[21]

THE REALITIES OF COLONIAL RULE

Another paradox of the age of imperialism was the contradiction between the seemingly all-powerful colonial states systems and the limits of colonial rule. Despite the widespread use of military force, counter-insurgency campaigns,

---

21   Niall Ferguson, *Empire: How Britain Made the Modern World* (London: Allen Lane, 2003).

and invasive policing, the colonial state could be a surprisingly fragile system.[22] Much of this was due to the simple demographics of empire. In settler societies, where large numbers of Europeans migrated to an overseas possession, state systems could be relatively robust. North America and Australia, where epidemic diseases and acts of genocide devastated the indigenous population, saw few significant challenges to colonization. In settler colonies where the invaders did not benefit from contagious disease, they remained a minority and had to rely on the near-constant threat of violence. Algeria and South Africa, for example, where non-whites outnumbered whites by roughly ten to one, brutal systems of racial segregation provided security for the anxious settlers and ensured that the indigenous population would supply labor but not challenge colonial rule. In the majority of the colonies of the New Imperialism there were only a few white administrators and soldiers, let alone permanent residents. This was due in no small part to the difficulties faced by Europeans living in tropical environments. In these warmer and wetter climates, a host of diseases impeded white settlement. Even in colonial cities such as French Hanoi, Dutch Batavia (today's Jakarta), or British Bombay (today's Mumbai), the white population was very small. With such a weak demographic showing, the colonizers knew that they could be wiped out by a popular revolt. Memories of the widespread violence that almost brought British rule in India to its knees in 1857 surely kept many white administrators up at night.[23]

Faced with such existential threats, the colonial state invested tremendous resources in presenting itself as permanent and powerful. This was most obvious in the colonial cities. Governor Generals ruled from large colonial palaces, often built in neo-classical style with imposing Greco-Roman colonnades. Statues of conquering heroes decorated colonial streets and squares. Even office buildings and residences were oversized displays of wealth, strength, and fortitude.[24] Soldiers, be they the relatively few whites in the colony or the larger number of Asians and Africans who served their colonial masters, marched up and down wide avenues decorated with Europeans flags. All of these messages sought to dissuade potential thoughts of rebellion. The colonial state system rested on articulating white prestige.[25]

---

22   Herman Lebovics, *Imperialism and the Corruption of Democracies* (Durham and London: Duke University Press, 2006), 1–21.

23   Kim A. Wagner, *The Great Fear of 1857: Rumours, Conspiracies and the Making of the Indian Uprising* (Bern: Peter Lang, 2010).

24   Gwendolyn Wright, *The Politics of Design in French Colonial Urbanism* (Chicago: University of Chicago Press, 1991).

25   Carl Nightingale, *Segregation: A Global History of Divided Cities* (Chicago: University of Chicago Press, 2012).

Yet, in many ways the colonial regimes were similar to Potemkin villages, the fake towns built by a Russian official eager to impress Catherine the Great. The colonizers were outnumbered. The state lacked legitimacy in the eyes of the colonized. And the white population knew this. Thus, daily life was characterized by the constant threat, if not use, of physical violence against the subaltern population.[26] Any crisis could cause a panic in the fearful minds of the colonizers and lead to a brutal overreaction, revealing the violence inherent in the system. Such excesses only belied the colonial state's true fragility. As Hannah Ardent observed:

> Power and violence are opposites; where the one rules absolutely, the other is absent. Violence appears where power is in jeopardy, but left to its own course its end is the disappearance of power. This implies that it is not correct to say that the opposite of violence is nonviolence: to speak of nonviolent power is actually redundant. Violence can destroy power; it is utterly incapable of creating it.[27]

The failure of the Hanoi rat hunt illustrates the limitations faced by the colonial state.

WESTERN INDUSTRIAL CAPITALISM

The second essential historical context is the global impact of the Western industrial capitalism. If its origins were a complex process of economic development, technological innovation, and social change, it was consistently tied to the history of European colonialism. Just as the Industrial Revolution was dependent upon colonial resources and labor practices, the New Imperialism was intertwined with the maturation of industrial capitalism in the late nineteenth century.

While various forms of market mechanisms had been around since the days of the first cities and had grown with the development of long-distance trade in the ancient world, there were a series of revolutionary changes to the world economy after 1492. Living in a provincial backwater reliant on tenuous trade arrangements with the Islamic world, Western Europeans took to the seas to end their economic isolation. First, the Spanish

---

26   Martin Thomas, *Violence and the Colonial Order: Police, Workers and Protest in the European Colonial Empires, 1918–1940* (Cambridge: Cambridge University Press, 2012).

27   Hannah Arendt, "A Special Supplement: Reflections on Violence," *The New York Review of Books* (February 27, 1969): http://www.nybooks.com/articles/1969/02/27/a-special-supplement-reflections-on-violence/ (accessed January 17, 2017).

colonized islands and empires in the Americas and the Portuguese seized important ports in the Indian Ocean and Southeast Asia. But these Iberian crusaders operated under the increasingly archaic rules of feudalism. They were soon replaced by the British, Dutch, and French whose East and West Indian trading companies pioneered the practices of modern capitalism.

As maritime voyages were long (a round-trip to the Spice Islands could take over two years) and dangerous (countless ships were lost to storms and hostile navies) investors sought ways to diversify their risk. Rather than investing all of one's capital in a single ship, Dutch merchants began to divide ships into portions or shares. One might invest in 10 percent of one ship, 5 percent of another, and 8 percent of a third. If one ship sank, hopefully the other two would cover the loss. Due to the astounding profits of the trade in Southeast Asian spices, Caribbean sugar, Indian cotton, and African slaves, European investors began to amass great fortunes. However, sometimes when a ship was at sea anxiety or newly arrived information might lead a shareholder to doubt its safe return. Fearing a total loss, investors could sell shares to other speculators. Thus developed a secondary market, not in the commodity but in the investment, which began the basis of our contemporary stock markets. When the Dutch East India Company (1602–1799) sold shares not in individual ships or specific voyages but in the company as a whole, modern capitalism was born. Importantly, the investor expected the company to be around indefinitely.[28] Just as today we don't buy shares of iPhone 7 but rather shares of Apple and hope that Apple will survive long after Steve Jobs' death, seventeenth-century investors bought shares of the Dutch, British, or French East India companies. This system provided for a much more stable and predictable climate for investors and gave the merchant companies reliable sources of capital for the expensive enterprise of maintaining ships, naval bases, and plantations from Jamaica to Java. Iberian feudalism simply could not compete with Northwestern European capitalism.

For over a century, scholars, theorists, and historians have detailed capitalism's blood-soaked birth. Following Karl Marx, contemporary critics of high imperialism such as Lenin and Luxemburg stressed the violence of capitalism. In 1944, Eric Williams published a study that tied the origins of Western capitalism to Caribbean slavery.[29] In his recent history of cotton, economic historian Sven Beckert characterizes this phase of economic

---

28   Kenneth Pomeranz and Steven Topik, *The World that Trade Created: Society, Culture, and the World Economy, 1400 to the Present*, 3rd ed. (Armonk and London: M. E. Sharpe, 2013), 174–76.

29   Eric Williams, *Capitalism and Slavery* (Chapel Hill: University of North Carolina Press, 1944).

development as "war capitalism." He coined this term to call attention to the ways in which colonialism's widespread use of violence, forced labor, land expropriation, and various forms of long-distance imperial domination created Europe's dramatic economic takeoff between 1600 and 1850. Beckert also contends that many aspects of this "war capitalism" continued into the era of industrial capitalism.[30]

However, capitalism was only part of the story. Indeed, when these trading companies arrived in Asia they initially found themselves at a profound disadvantage. It seemed impossible to compete with the wealth of India and China and few Asian consumers had any interest in European goods. Militarily, Chinese and Indian armies were much larger than the forces Europeans could send halfway around the world. Economically, Asia's low-cost labor posed a serious problem for the West. It is important to note that while Asian wages were low, the standard of living was the same or higher than in much of Europe. This was due to the nature of Asian and European diets. Asia's wet rice agriculture produced substantially more calories per acre than Europe's wheat or rye fields. This meant that in Asia food was cheap. If food is cheap then labor is cheap. If labor is cheap, then it is less expensive to manufacture labor-intensive goods such as cotton fabric, porcelain, and silk. With their expensive labor cost, European manufacturers had a comparative disadvantage. However, between roughly 1750 and 1850 a series of inventions solved this problem and dramatically reversed the global power structure. Starting with the mechanization of spinning cotton into thread and the weaving of thread into fabric, British engineers created a series of labor-saving devices. Initially powered by water wheels on streams and rivers and then by coal-powered steam engines, the mechanization of production rapidly decreased the numbers of workers needed to produce larger and larger amounts of goods. Replacing humans with machines reduced labor costs. This Industrial Revolution transformed Britain, making it the greatest power in the world by the middle of the nineteenth century. Cheaper manufacturing costs allowed merchants to export items such as finished cotton textiles around the world. India, the center of global cotton production for centuries, found itself de-industrialized, importing British fabric, and producing raw cotton and opium for the British, who used the economic chaos to seize more and more land.

While Britain led the way into the industrial future, other European states were soon to follow. Belgium and the Netherlands were not far behind. France, sidelined by decades of revolutionary instability, began the process mid-century. Realizing their late start and smaller pool of accessible

---

30   Sven Beckert, *Empire of Cotton: A Global History* (London: Penguin Books, 2014).

resources, many French people resented Britain's success. Germany was not united until 1871, but it quickly became an industrial powerhouse. Industrial cities with large factories became increasingly common in Northwest Europe. While Northern Italy and parts of Spain were home to pockets of industrial manufacturing, most of Southern and Eastern Europe remained rural and agrarian.

As industrial techniques were applied to transportation, Western Europe started a new revolution in space and time. Prior to the invention of the railroad, overland travel was slow and costly. Horses could only pull or carry so much weight and moved at about the speed a human could walk. In the best of times, roads were bumpy, making for rough rides. In inclement weather they could be impassable. Heavy loads such as iron and coal were prohibitively expensive. Grain and other foodstuffs were not much better. However, as more and more powerful steam engines began to pull larger and larger wagons on reliable iron and later steel tracks transportation costs plummeted. Distances that used to be measures in weeks and days were measured in hours and minutes. People traveled further and further distances. There were direct political implications as this increased a sense of nationalism in many countries. People increasingly saw themselves not as a part of a village or regional community but as part of a larger, imagined community: the nation-state.[31] Governments, in turn, were also able to move troops quickly and efficiently to put down domestic troubles or face enemies on the border. The industrialization of maritime transportation globalized the European Industrial Revolution. Steamships were able to sail against the winds, giving them an incredible advantage over sailboats. When the British navy sent the *Nemesis* to China, many were shocked by Britain's ability to project military power around the planet. By the 1880s Western imperialists combined superior navies, rail-based troop and munitions transportation, new weapons systems such as the breech loading rifles and the machine gun, and instantaneous communications over long distances via the telegraph.[32] The radical imbalance of power turned so-called battles into outright massacres. The ability of Europeans to project power across the four major oceans and into the interiors of multiple continents was historically unprecedented. The industrialization of warfare convinced many that Europe was all-powerful.[33]

---

31   Benedict Anderson, *Imagined Communities: Reflections on the Origin and Spread of Nationalism* (London: Verso, 2006).

32   Daniel Headrick, *The Tools of Empire: Technology and European Imperialism in the Nineteenth Century* (New York: Oxford University Press, 1981).

33   Michael Adas, *Machines as the Measure of Men: Science, Technology, and Ideologies of Western Dominance* (Ithaca, NY: Cornell University Press, 1989).

Such successes had a dramatic cultural impact. European self-confidence frequently gave way to arrogance and racist disdain for what were perceived as weaker people or decadent cultures. Ignoring Europe's centuries as an under-developed backwater, many argued that the West's rise was due to its inherent superiority. Some hijacked Darwin's recently published theories on evolution and natural selection and tied them to Europe's material wealth to argue that non-whites, be they "races" or "cultures," were inferior. This supposedly scientific racism held that human inequality was natural and thus the stronger would dominate the weaker. Around the year 1900, when China floundered in chaos, Europeans divided up almost the entire continent of Africa, and tiny Britain dominated massive India, many found such ideas persuasive. Thus, the triumphs of Western industrial-capitalism bolstered imperialism and white supremacy.

When Europe's industrial achievements were paired with modern capitalism, there was a dramatic reversal in the global balance of power. These profound global changes are often understood as the birth of modernity.[34] At the time of the great Hanoi rat hunt, most French understood the West to be an advanced civilization, a bastion of progress. This could lead to a certain arrogance in the minds of colonial administrators.

THE THIRD REPUBLIC

The nature of France's government at the time of the Great Hanoi Rat Hunt is another essential historical context. When studying the colonial encounter it is always necessary to know what was going on in the society being colonized as well as in the society of the colonizer. Turn-of-the-century France was a bundle of contradictions, paradoxes, and ironies all stemming from the unresolved legacies of the French Revolution. Since the start of the revolution in 1789, France had gone through a series of dramatic political upheavals and been ruled by the Bourbon monarchy, a republic, a Napoleonic empire, the restored Bourbons, the Orleans constitutional monarchy, the Second Republic, a second Napoleonic empire, and finally another republic. The city of Paris was the site of repeated insurrections and barricades, culminating in the Paris Commune's open revolt against the newly created republic.

These radical swings of the political pendulum led few to believe that the Third Republic, founded in 1870, would survive for long. Despite challenges from the left and the right, the new regime was the longest lived French government of the nineteenth and twentieth centuries (France's current Fifth

---

34   C. A. Bayly, *The Birth of the Modern World, 1780–1914* (Malden, MA: Blackwell Publishing, 2004), 9–12.

Republic is a decade shy of the record at the time of the writing of this book). Much of the republic's success was due to the establishment of fairly conservative consensus regarding protection of property and the rights of male citizens while at the same time promoting many of the classic liberal values of the Enlightenment such as secularism, public education, and universal male suffrage. Yet the regime had many enemies. If Marxists and Anarchists hated the bourgeois republic's protection of wealth, Catholic conservatives, royalists, and aristocrats despised its rejection of tradition and inherited privilege. Republican anti-clericism, culminating in the formal separation of church and state, angered many pious French Catholics.[35] The Dreyfus Affair (1894–1906), a scandal in which a French Jewish officer was wrongly imprisoned for treason, revealed the nation's deep divisions between left and right. Internationally, the Third Republic had the most progressive constitution in Europe and was the only major republic on a continent dominated by dynastic monarchies and multi-ethnic empires. Despite the increase in representative institutions, many of the crowned heads of Europe viewed the Third Republic with suspicion if not contempt.

In order to build up popular support, the Third Republic developed a number of secular rituals celebrating the legacy of the revolution and the republic itself. These included burying national heroes such as writer Victor Hugo (1885), assassinated president Marie François Sadi Carnot (1894), and scientist Marcelin Berthelot (1907) in the Panthéon. The republic was to be associated with science, progress, and modernity and its motto of "Liberty, Equality, Brotherhood" adorned all official communication. July 14, the date of a Parisian mob's 1789 assault on the Bastille prison, became a national holiday. According to historian Edward Berenson, the anti-clerical republic sought to replace the Catholic Church's religious ceremonies and veneration of saints with celebrations of the secular state and the great men who made it.[36] Urban spaces were particularly important for the Third Republic's propaganda. The blue, white, and red of the *Tricolore* flag decorated streets from Paris to small provincial towns. Allegorical statues conveying republican values adorned public squares.[37] Public buildings such as town halls, government offices, and even train stations were symbols of the republic's modernizing mission.[38]

---

35 Theodore Zeldin, *A History of French Passions, 1848–1945, Vol. 2: Intellect, Taste, and Anxiety* (Oxford: Oxford University Press, 1973), 983–1039.

36 Edward Berenson, *Heroes of Empire: Five Charismatic Men and the Conquest of Africa* (Berkeley: University of California Press, 2010), 51–55.

37 Maurice Agulhon, *Marianne into Battle: Republican Imagery and Symbolism in France, 1789–1880* (Cambridge: Cambridge University Press, 1981).

38 Pierre Nora (ed.), *Realms of Memory: The Construction of the French Past, Vol. 3: Symbols* (New York: Columbia University Press, 1998).

The Third Republic oversaw France's rapid modernization. Continuing policies started under Napoleon III, the republic expanded railways, developed industrial and mining centers, expanded banking, and created investment opportunities for those with excess capital. Technological advances including faster printing, and telegraphs allowed for the growth of national newspapers. In a now-classic cultural history of the era, Eugene Weber argued that peasants from around the country became Frenchmen.[39] These social, cultural, and technological changes were celebrated as modernity and Paris was the capital of all that was modern.[40] This city had recently been rebuilt under the authoritarian rule of the second Napoleonic Empire and now had wide tree-lined avenues with cafés and shops. For those with money and leisure time Paris was a city of pleasures.[41] A new social phenomenon, the *flâneur*, was the archetypical urban spectator. Blending with the city's crowds, lounging in cafés and parks, the *flâneur* was a man busily doing nothing other than taking in the city. The poet Charles Baudelaire's famous discussion of the *flânuer* in his essay "The Painter of Modern Life" characterizes the figure as always at home in the city, finding energy and stimulation in all that Paris had to offer.[42] State administrators celebrated the new "science" of urbanism. Rather than allowing cities to grow in organic but haphazard ways, technocrats would plan urban growth and establish specific neighborhoods or quarters for specific functions. The state also took on the responsibility of public health, ensuring a supply of clean water and a system of waste removal. Thus, Paris' new sewer system became a point of national pride as it symbolized modernity's conquest of nature.[43] French colonists exported this exultation of urban life, so central to the culture of the Third Republic, to Hanoi at the time of the rat hunt.

Ironically, the progressive Third Republic was openly hostile to gender and racial equality. Lacking the right to vote and frequently not in complete control of their property, women were not full citizens.[44] Citizenship

---

39   Eugene Weber, *Peasants into Frenchmen: The Modernization of Rural France, 1870–1914* (Stanford, CA: Stanford University Press, 1976).

40   Tyler Stovall, *Transnational France: The Modern History of a Universal Nation* (Boulder, CO: Westview Press, 2015), 127–65.

41   David Harvey, *Paris, Capital of Modernity* (New York: Routledge, 2003), 209–24.

42   Charles Baudelaire, *The Painter of Modern Life* (New York: Da Capo Press, 1964), and Walter Benjamin, *The Writer of Modern Life: Essays on Charles Baudelaire* (Cambridge, MA: Belknap, 2006).

43   Donald Reid, *Paris Sewers and Sewermen: Realities and Representations* (Cambridge, MA: Harvard University Press, 1991).

44   Edward Berenson, *The Trail of Madame Caillaux* (Berkeley: University of California Press, 1992), 133–68.

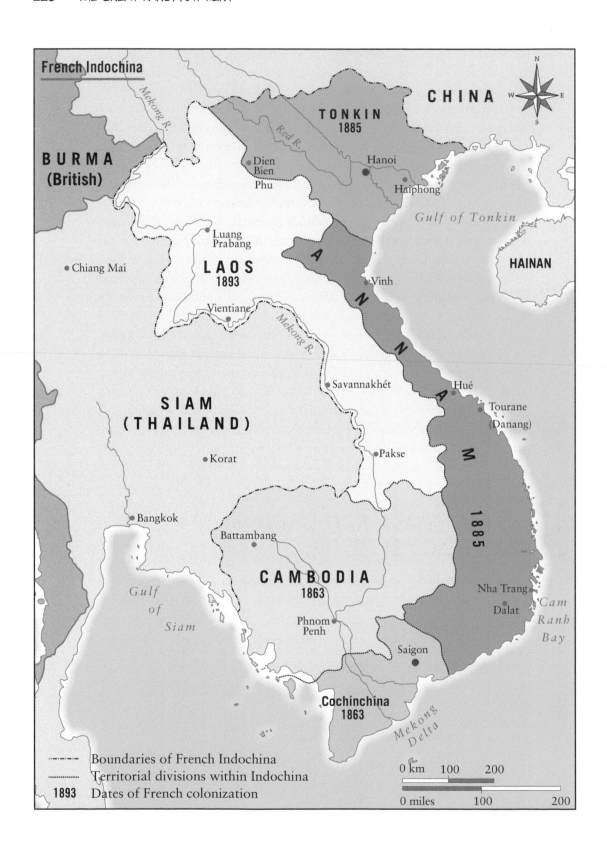

French Indochina

CHINA

TONKIN
1885

BURMA
(British)

Dien
Bien
Phu

Hanoi

Haiphong

Gulf of Tonkin

Luang
Prabang

LAOS
1893

A
N
N
A
M

Vinh

HAINAN

Chiang Mai

Vientiane

Mekong R.

Savannakhét

Hué

SIAM
(THAILAND)

Tourane
(Danang)

Korat

Pakse

1
8
8
5

Bangkok

Battambang

CAMBODIA
1863

Nha Trang

Dalat

Cam
Ranh
Bay

Gulf
of
Siam

Phnom
Penh

Saigon

Cochinchina
1863

Mekong
Delta

-··-··- Boundaries of French Indochina
············ Territorial divisions within Indochina
1893 Dates of French colonization

0 km   100   200

0 miles   100   200

was essentially a form of male supremacy, with men maintaining the right to draft laws and regulations that kept power out of the hands of women.[45] The situation was even more contradictory in the colonies where France tried to govern as a republican empire. The Third Republic paradoxically promoted the values of 1789 as it deprived national sovereignty, freedom, and equality in the lands it conquered. In the northern provinces of Algeria, which were governed as overseas *départements* equal to territory within the French mainland, Arabs and Berbers were given a path towards citizenship that required renouncing Islam. As apostasy is a capital sin, few Muslims took the French up on the offer. Elsewhere, only four municipalities in West Africa saw significant numbers of non-whites achieving citizenship. Historian Gary Wilder has called the Third Republic an "imperial-nation state," signifying the inherent contradictions in the system.[46] Others have argued that the very nature of imperialism corrupts democracies.[47]

Regardless, at the turn of the twentieth century optimistic republicans saw a moment for French greatness. Enlightenment values, liberal capitalism, and industrialization would come together to produce a new French modernity. The Third Republic would pursue its mission to civilize, spreading a colonial modernity throughout the empire. Paul Doumer's tenure as Governor-General of French Indochina serves as an example of the positivist spirit of the French colonial project. His rebuilding of Hanoi is a classic example of French colonial modernism.

VIETNAMESE RESISTANCE: NATIONALIST, COMMUNIST, AND EVERYDAY

With a history going back over two thousand years, the Vietnamese people were naturally far from pleased to have French strangers repeatedly invade their country and then occupy it for almost a century.[48] The phases of Vietnamese resistance to French imperialism form a crucial historical

---

45   Judith Surkis, *Sexing the Citizen: Morality and Masculinity in France, 1870–1920* (Ithaca: Cornell University Press, 2006).

46   Gary Wilder, *The French Imperial Nation-State: Negritude and Colonial Humanism between the Two World Wars* (Chicago: University of Chicago Press, 2005).

47   Herman Lebovics, *Imperialism and the Corruption of Democracies* (Durham and London: Duke University Press, 2006).

48   K. W. Taylor, *A History of the Vietnamese* (Cambridge: Cambridge University Press, 2013), Christopher Goscha, *Vietnam: A New History* (New York: Basic Books, 2016), and Ben Kiernan, *Việt Nam: A History from the Earliest Times to the Present* (Oxford: Oxford University Press, 2017), are the most recent and authoritative histories of Vietnam.

context to the story of the great Hanoi rat hunt.[49] In addition to resenting the French, the Vietnamese had a collective historical memory of occupation by another power, China. That said, the Vietnamese monarchy had expanded its territory through wars of imperial conquest. Historian Ben Kiernan has described the 1390–1509 conquest of Champa (central Vietnam) as genocide.[50] As the Vietnamese seized land in what was once the Khmer Empire and claimed sovereignty over the highlands, Cambodians and ethnically distinct tribal groups came under their control.

Vietnam's relationship with China has been and remains complicated. While popular memory of the various periods of Chinese occupation (111 BCE – 39 CE, 43–544, 602–938, and 1407–27) is generally bitter and to this day many Vietnamese regard China as a threat to their sovereignty, numerous aspects of Vietnamese culture, politics, and philosophy are very much the product of Chinese influence.[51] For example, since China directly governed the Tonkin region as a province of the empire, Confucian statecraft dominated Vietnamese politics for one thousand years. Developed over several centuries and based upon the teachings of Confucius (the Romanized name of Kongsi who lived 551–479 BCE), the Chinese state created a system of scholar-bureaucrats to administer the empire. Known as mandarins, these scholar-bureaucrats took a three-day imperial exam to enter the civil service. The rigorous test required applicants to show their command of Confucian philosophy by writing stylized essays, frequently the classic "Eight Legged Essay," that demonstrated their knowledge of the works of Confucius, classic texts such as *The Book of Songs* and *The Book of Rites*, and authorized interpretations of Confucianism. Based upon mastering an established canon of literature, the exams ensured that the mandarins would speak a common language and understand shared references. Confucianism promoted a system of values that placed social harmony above all. Peace and justice would be established by a clear hierarchy and the commitment to govern in accordance with firm moral rectitude. Just as it was the obligation of the civil servants to be completely loyal to the monarch, the emperor exercised absolute authority in the name of improving the people's livelihood.

Confucius taught that we are obligated to make the world a better place. This idea developed as a political tradition that required the emperor to

---

49   David Marr, *Vietnamese Anticolonialism, 1885–1925* (Berkeley: University of California Press, 1971), and *Vietnamese Tradition on Trial, 1920–1945* (Berkeley: University of California Press, 1981).

50   Ben Kiernan, *Blood and Soil: A World History of Genocide from Sparta to Darfur* (New Haven: Yale University Press, 2007): 102–12.

51   A. B. Woodside, *Vietnam and the Chinese Model: A Comparative Study of Vietnamese and Chinese Government in the First Half of the Nineteenth-Century* (Cambridge: Harvard University Press, 1971), is the classic study of the topic.

intervene in society to promote harmony and stability. As this was the exact opposite of the Western ideology of classical liberalism, which promoted *laissez-faire* or hands-off policies, the arrival of European merchants in the early nineteenth century set the stage for conflict. When the British started selling opium in China, the Daoguang Emperor saw the economic and social damage the drug was causing and demanded that the foreigners cease and desist their narco-trafficking. He famously appointed the mandarin Lin Zexu as an Imperial Commissioner tasked with halting the illegal opium trade. Devotees of Adam Smith's free-market fundamentalism and not Confucius' social interventionism, British merchants such as William Jardine and James Matheson were incensed by the Qing government's effort to hamper the free flow of goods. Three decades later the French merchant Jean Dupuis tried to enter Tonkin and local mandarins informed him that foreigners were not welcome. Nonetheless Dupuis forced his way into Vietnam, justifying his actions in the name of free trade. Both of these examples show the ways in which conflicts between Chinese or Vietnamese Confucians and British or French merchants were clashes of civilizations.[52]

When the Vietnamese expelled the Chinese and established an independent kingdom in the tenth century, the new monarchy adopted the Confucian model, complete with imperial exams and a hierarchy of mandarins.[53] While independent, a series of Vietnamese dynasties pledged their loyalty to the Chinese empire through the tribute state system. Essentially applying the Confucian principle that every relationship can be understood through the metaphor of the family, smaller neighboring kingdoms in Korea, Vietnam, and elsewhere acknowledged the Chinese emperor as the father. In return for their filial piety, demonstrated by ritualized tribute missions where kings or ambassadors would travel to the Chinese court to give the emperor presents and bow before him in the *kowtow* ceremony, the Chinese monarch agreed to give them preferential trade status and military assistance. Thus, even a sovereign and independent Vietnam was closely tied to the powerful empire to the north. Hence, when France invaded Tonkin, the Qing Dynasty went to war in defense of its tribute state.

When the French invasion force arrived in the mid-nineteenth century, the Nguyen Dynasty (1802–1945) was ruling Vietnam. While Vietnam had been governed by a series of Confucian dynasties since achieving independence in 938, the Nguyen monarchs struggled to hold their recently reunited country together. Since the 1500s, centralized dynastic power collapsed

---

52   Alexander Woodside, *Lost Modernities China, Vietnam, Korea, and the Hazards of World History* (Cambridge: Harvard University Press, 2006).

53   There is an ongoing academic debate on how important Confucianism is for understanding Vietnam; see Liam Kelley, "'Confucianism' in Vietnam: A State of the Field Essay," *Journal of Vietnamese Studies* 1, no. 1–2 (August, 2006): 314–70.

with the rise of regional noble families. The resulting three-way split saw the Le Dynasty (1428–1788) claiming authority but real power being exercised by the Trinh lords in northern Tonkin and the Nguyen lords in southern territory conquered from the neighboring Cham and Cambodian states. In the 1780s all three factions were overwhelmed by the massive Tayson Rebellion. After centuries of division and decades of civil war, the Nguyen launched a campaign of national unification. Their victory culminated in subduing Tonkin, the historic home of the Vietnamese people. During the campaign, the Nguyen established relations with France, even sending a young prince to Paris (where he converted to Catholicism, raising a few eyebrows upon his return). A handful of French military engineers assisted the Nguyen and designed Vauban-style fortresses in Saigon, Hue, and Hanoi. To govern this large and diverse land, the new monarch, Gia Long (r. 1802–1820), established a royal capital in Hue, a coastal city in the center of Vietnam. The dynasty also adopted strict neo-Confucian policies designed to cultivate obedience from Trinh, Le, and Tayson loyalists. When Catholic missionaries began to win converts in the 1820s, Emperor Minh Mang (r. 1820–1841) viewed the alien faith as a potential threat to his regime's stability. In the 1830s a series of laws persecuted Vietnamese Catholics and foreign missionaries, resulting in scores of executions (the Roman Catholic Church would later recognize them as martyrs and canonize over one hundred of them). While never entirely sealed to the outside world, the monarchy remained very suspicious of Westerners. The joint Franco-Spanish invasion to protect Catholics confirmed some of the xenophobic suspicions.

France's initial 1858 invasion of central and southern Vietnam showed the power of industrialized warfare. Steam-powered ships such as the *Némésis* with their heavy artillery devastated Vietnamese defenses as easily as the British navy had overwhelmed the Chinese fleet in the Opium War. When the Vietnamese emperor was forced to cede the southern territory around the Mekong Delta including Saigon in 1862, there was immediate resistance to the French. Some mandarins refused to acknowledge the treaty with the French and organized small bands of guerilla fighters. However, these movements lacked central organization. As the royal court pursed a policy of compromise and negotiation with the French, this early resistance suffered from weak morale. After the French seized Tonkin in 1882 and defeated China, technically Vietnam's Confucian protector, in the Sino-French War (1884–1885), the Nguyen court launched an attack on the French forces in Hue. Forced to flee to the countryside after the attack, in 1885 Emperor Ham Nghi (r. 1884–1885) issued an edict calling on all Vietnamese to support the monarchy and resist the French. The Can Vuong or "Aid the King" movement lacked central control but did inspire a number of regional leaders to take up arms against the French. While the foreign invaders were the main target, there were cases of deadly violence against thousands of Vietnamese Catholics. The resistance peaked in 1888 with Ham Nghi's capture and exile to French Algeria. As the French tried to rule through compliant puppet emperors such as Dong Khan (r. 1885–1889) and Than Thai (r. 1889–1907), many Vietnamese had conflicting loyalties. Nonetheless, the movement continued for another decade in parts of Tonkin. De Tham (1858–1913) led a popular revolt for two and a half decades, including attacks on Hanoi, until his capture and execution.

This initial phase of resistance had the fairly limited goals of sending the foreign invaders home and reestablishing an independent Confucian monarchy. Can Vuong was hardly a revolutionary movement. Historians debate whether it should even be called "nationalist" as the anti-colonial insurrection was really a traditionalist defense of the monarchy. However, its failure led to important changes within Vietnam and the subsequent development of a truly nationalist movement. One important change was an increasing dissatisfaction with the Confucian state system. In the eyes of many, both the emperor and the mandarins had failed. Worse, critics condemned the Nguyen monarchy and the scholar-officials for collaborating with the French occupiers. This is perhaps unfair, as the French removed three monarchs from the throne, exiling them in various parts of the colonial empire. In reaction to the perceived failure of the traditional Confucian system, a new generation of Vietnamese modernizers called for ejecting the French but also learning from the West. Inspired by Japan's transformation under the Meiji Restoration and by Sun Yat-Sen's Kuomintang or Chinese Nationalist Party, a movement grew in Hanoi that called for a new Vietnamese modernity. Deeming Confucianism backward, these modernizers replaced Chu Nom, the Chinese character–based script, with Quoc Ngu, a Romanized script developed in the seventeenth century. As symbols of their modernity, they cut their hair and wore European-style clothes. Politically, they sought to create a movement that would speak for all Vietnamese. In 1927, following Sun Yat-Sen's party model, the Vietnam Quoc Dan Dang (VNQDD) was founded to liberate the nation and promote social reforms. However, members were mostly drawn from the educated elite. As many activists came from wealthy families or had their own business interests, the VNQDD did not call for widespread social revolution or a challenge to the existing economic order.[54]

Meanwhile, a more radical movement developed with guidance from the Union of Socialist Soviet Republics. After successfully seizing power in 1917, Lenin and the Bolshevik Party sought to promote a world revolution along Marxist lines. In 1919, Lenin organized the Communist International

---

54   Hue-Tam Ho Tai, *Radicalism and the Origins of the Vietnamese Revolution* (Cambridge: Harvard University Press, 1992).

(Comintern) in Moscow. In order to receive Soviet support and funding, Communist Parties were required to apply for membership and obediently follow orders from the Comintern. Ho Chi Minh, who had worked for years to free his country, initially joined the French Communist Party but later founded the Vietnamese Revolutionary Youth League in 1925 and then the Indochinese Community Party (ICP) in 1930. With Comintern support, the ICP argued that both colonialism and capitalism were exploiting the Vietnamese people. Furthermore, the ICP accused traditionalists of having first failed to stand up to the French and then collaborated with the colonial occupiers.[55] Labeled "feudal," the ICP included Confucian scholars in its list of enemies. According to the party, national independence would have to be accompanied by a profound social revolution. While the ICP was intentionally vague on the details of such a program, it attracted support from the urban and rural poor who suffered so intensely under the colonial political economy. The ICP promised a new path to modernity for Vietnam.

Faced with a series of incidents starting in 1929, including the assassination of a Michelin labor "recruiter," strikes on plantations, a mutiny of Vietnamese troops, and a widespread revolt that included the formation of "Soviets," the French state responded with harsh repression against both the Nationalists and the Communists.[56] Thousands were arrested and thrown into the growing colonial prison system. Historian Peter Zinoman has described the brutal conditions in these "colonial bastilles." Members of the VNQDD, often educated elite, fared poorly in the violent jails. In contrast, the Comintern's revolutionary training gave ICP cadres the skills not only to survive incarceration but to organize and recruit new members.[57] When the French government issued a general amnesty to political prisoners in 1936, the Communists set about organizing a political-military force to defeat colonialism and start a Marxist revolution. With the Japanese invasion and occupation of Southeast Asia during World War II shattering the European and American colonial regimes, Ho Chi Minh's forces began their path to power, declaring independence in 1945 and winning it in 1954 after nearly a decade of war.

With no small amount of irony, the history of Vietnamese communism is directly tied to French rule. The exploitative colonial political economy created the conditions that convinced thousands of activists that communist revolution was the only viable solution. However, Marxism, the ideology that eventually liberated and modernized Vietnam, was initially a colonial import.

---

55   William Duiker, *The Comintern and Vietnamese Communism* (Athens: Ohio University Center for International Studies, Southeast Asia Program, 1975).

56   Michael G. Vann, "White Blood on Rue Hue: The Murder of *'le négrier'* Bazin," *Proceedings of the Western Society for French History* 34 (2006).

57   Peter Zinoman, *The Colonial Bastille: A History of Imprisonment in Vietnam, 1862–1940* (Berkeley: University of California Press, 2001).

But the rise of nationalism and communism was not the entire story. Scholars have noted that only a minority of the population was active in formal political movements. Shawn McHale has persuasively demonstrated that party activists were mostly urban elites and that Buddhism rather than Marxism was much more important to the majority of Vietnamese.[58] In a series of books, James C. Scott combines history, anthropology, and political science to argue that there were many forms of "everyday resistance" to both state power and systems of political economy. Scott terms such tactics "weapons of the weak" and notes that they might not make it into the official archival record.[59] The story of the Hanoi rat hunt and the ways in which Vietnamese citizens outsmarted French authorities illustrates the many ways in which subaltern resistance could challenge the colonial state.

While this story and many nationalist narratives focus on Vietnamese resistance, we must note that the colonial encounter created a wide variety of important economic, intellectual, and political opportunities. Many Vietnamese, while possibly resenting the French presence, were open to professional prospects. It would be a serious mistake to argue that anyone who worked with the French was a supine collaborator. Indeed, the most common complaint from Vietnamese parents about French schools was not the Eurocentric curriculum, but that there were not enough of them for their children. Nor should we assume that all who worked with the French were brainwashed traitors to their nation. One of the greatest generals in the war for national liberation and the hero of Dien Bien Phu, Vo Nguyen Giap, had taught history in a French school.

THE THIRD BUBONIC PLAGUE PANDEMIC, 1855–1959

The history of third Bubonic Plague pandemic is the final historical context necessary for the story of the great Hanoi rat hunt. Epidemic disease is an important subject in the study of world history. Germs, viruses, and bacteria

---

58   Shawn McHale, *Print and Power: Confucianism, Communism and Buddhism in the Making of Modern Vietnam* (Honolulu: University of Hawaii Press, 2004).

59   James. C. Scott, *The Moral Economy of the Peasant: Rebellion and Subsistence in Southeast Asia* (New Haven: Yale University Press, 1976), *Weapons of the Weak: Everyday Forms of Peasant Resistance* (New Haven: Yale University Press, 1985), *Domination and the Arts of Resistance: Hidden Transcripts* (New Haven: Yale University Press, 1990), and *Decoding Subaltern Politics: Ideology, Disguise, and Resistance in Agrarian Politics* (New York: Routledge, 2003). Ann Laura Stoler, *Along the Archival Grain: Epistemic Anxieties and Colonial Common Sense* (Princeton: Princeton University Press, 2009) studies the Dutch East Indies to show the ways in which much of history does not make it into the formal state archive.

move about the planet without reference to the lines men and women draw on maps. Just as world historians don't believe that the study of history should be confined within the artificial framework of the nation-state, diseases don't care about political boundaries. However, the fates of pathogens that are dependent on human hosts are directly tied to human mobility.[60] In periods with new and faster forms of travel, diseases always begin to spread. This was as true of roads and maritime routes that linked the Roman and Chinese empires to India in the Classical World, as it is today with planes, trains, and automobiles. The spread of annual strains of influenza and common colds as well as HIV/AIDS, SARS, Middle East Respiratory Coronavirus, and a host of other newly emerging diseases is facilitated by the contemporary world's network of global travel. Consider the recent hysteria in the United States of America about Ebola coming from West Africa to North America. Or the very real way in which Zika spread from Africa to Southeast Asia to Oceania to Brazil to Puerto Rico. The era of the New Imperialism, which included the movement of millions of troops, settlers, and laborers, as well as the creation of a new maritime transportation infrastructure with fast-moving steam ships, crowded port cities, and the time-saving Suez and Panama canals, naturally led to the spread of disease.[61] Indeed, imperialism created two major pandemics in the nineteenth and twentieth centuries, cholera and the bubonic plague.

But what is a pandemic? According to the Centers for Disease Control, endemic disease refers to the baseline level of an illness in a given area. An epidemic is when a disease unexpectedly begins to spread to much larger numbers, infecting a wider segment of the population. A pandemic is when an epidemic disease impacts multiple countries and continents.[62] Throughout human history, the growth of towns and cities had led to epidemics for the simple reason that people living in close proximity to each other can spread diseases among themselves. The bigger the city, the bigger the risk. Just as epidemics require urban centers, pandemics require global transportation. Historically significant developments in long-distance travel have consistently created pandemics. The faster the trip, the bigger the risk. One of the sad ironies of globalization is the spread of devastating diseases.[63]

---

60   William McNeill, *Plagues and Peoples* (New York: Doubleday, 1976), and Crosby, *The Columbian Exchange*.

61   Myron Echenberg, *Plague Ports: The Global Urban Impact of Bubonic Plague, 1894–1901* (New York: New York University Press, 2007).

62   Centers for Disease Control and Prevention, "Lesson 1: Introduction to Epidemiology," in *Principles of Epidemiology in Public Health Practice* (3rd ed.): *An Introduction to Applied Epidemiology and Biostatistics*. https://www.cdc.gov/ophss/csels/dsepd/ss1978/lesson1/section11.html (accessed January 19, 2017).

63   See Robert Peckham, *Epidemics in Modern Asia* (Cambridge: Cambridge University press, 2016), for a sustained analysis of the forces that fostered and spread epidemic diseases in Asia.

The bubonic plague is a fascinating but horrific disease whose history remains the subject of important research and debate.[64] In 2015, international headlines claimed gerbils and not rats were the cause of the Black Death in the 1300s.[65] Later in that year, the *Journal of World History* published an academic article that challenged the established consensus that the plague originated in East Africa, arguing instead for a Central Asian origin.[66] Regardless of these debates, we do know that there have been three bubonic plague pandemics. The first was the Plague of Justinian, which killed between twenty-five million and fifty million people in the late Roman Empire. At the height of the outbreak in the summer of 542, Constantinople saw a daily death rate of five thousand.[67] The second pandemic is known in the West as the Black Death for its devastation in Europe from 1346 to 1350. With somewhere between seventy million and one hundred million dead, the Black Death led to dramatic changes in Europe including the death of feudalism and the flowering of the Renaissance.[68] The disease became endemic in various locales in Europe, Asia, and Africa with periodic flare-ups such as the Great Plague of London (1665–1666) that killed one hundred thousand.[69] The third plague pandemic began with a regional outbreak in Yunnan, China, in the 1850s. Due to an increase in trade, including opium trafficking, the disease spread to Canton and Hong Kong in the 1890s.[70] From there the new global network of steamships and railways spread the disease to ports in the Pacific, Indian, and Atlantic Oceans, creating a true pandemic on six continents. Until its end after World War II, the third pandemic took some fifteen million lives. The disease remains endemic in a variety of places around the world. From Madagascar to Colorado, it lives in reservoirs of rodent population. Under the right circumstance we could see another pandemic.

As the outbreak originated in China and spread on ships coming from Chinese ports, medical experts, governments, and newspapers associated

---

64   Lester K. Little, "Plague Historians in Lab Coats," *Past and Present* 213 (2011): 267–90.

65   Rebecca Morelle, "'Gerbils Replace Rats' as Main Cause of Black Death," *BBC News*, http://www.bbc.com/news/science-environment-31588671 (accessed January 19, 2017).

66   George D. Sussman, "Scientists Doing History: Central Africa and the Origins of the First Plague Pandemic." *Journal of World History* 26, no. 2 (June 2015): 325–54.

67   William Rosen, *Justinian's Flea: Plague, Empire, and the Birth of Europe* (New York: Viking, 2007).

68   Ole J. Benedictow, *The Black Death, 1346–1353: The Complete History* (Rochester, NY: The Boydell Press, 2004).

69   Daniel Defoe, *A Visitation of the Plague* (New York: Penguin, 1996).

70   Carol Benedict, *Bubonic Plague in Nineteenth-Century China* (Stanford, CA: Stanford University Press, 1994), 17–71.

the disease with Chinese bodies. Hysteria over the plague fused with existing Sinophobia, resulting in openly racist policies against members of the Chinese diaspora.[71] When considering the Sinophobic response, we must keep in mind that the bubonic plague was still poorly understood at the turn of the century. Working in Hong Kong in 1894, the Swiss researcher Alexandre Yersin of the French Institut Pasteur identified the bacterium that spread the disease; although his rival, the German-trained Japanese doctor Kitasato Shibasaburo initially claimed credit. Four years later, another Pasteurian, Paul Simond, identified rat fleas as the vector that spread the plague. Understanding the transmission mechanisms led to public health measures to control rat populations. In cities such as Hanoi, Rio de Janeiro, and San Francisco public health officials experimented with various rat eradication programs. Meanwhile, research scientists at the Institut Pasteur field-tested a variety of vaccines.

The bubonic plague is a terrifying and fast-moving disease. While we currently have extremely effective treatments, for most of human history it was a death sentence. After being bit by an infected flea, the bacillus enters the victim's lymphatic system. Within a few days to a week, patients show a variety of flu-like symptoms including dizziness, nausea, and fatigue. Infected lymph nodes in the neck, armpits, and groin swell to a painful size. These are known as "buboes," giving the malady its name. Fingers and toes can turn black and victim's faces can become discolored. Without treatment death occurs in the majority of cases within ten days. The disease can also take two other forms. Exposure to contaminated flesh or fluids can lead to septicemia, a blood infection. There is also a pneumatic form, a lung infection, in which the disease is spread from person to person in droplets coughed out by a carrier. These two forms kill even faster and bear a higher mortality rate. There are stories of people feeling fine at bedtime but dying in their sleep as the infection rapidly spread through their body in the night. The horrors of the symptoms, the speed with which the disease can move, and the staggering numbers of dead have created panics over the centuries. Memories of the Black Death still resonate in Western culture. Knowledge that rats play a crucial role has only increased our feelings of repulsion and fear of the bubonic plague.[72]

Ironically, both plague and rat are closely associated with modernity. While we might think of the bubonic plague as a medieval malady, an anachronism in the modern age, and a disease that should be banished to

---

71   This is the premise of the essays in Robert Peckham (ed.), *Empires of Panic: Epidemics and Colonial Anxieties* (Hong Kong: Hong Kong University Press, 2015).

72   Hans Zinsser, *Rats, Lice, and History: A Chronicle of Pestilence and Plague* (New York: Black Dog & Leventhal Publishers, 1934), 189–211.

history, the Third Plague Pandemic was a direct consequence of Western industrial capitalism's creation of a global system. Both plague and cholera were diseases of imperial modernity. Tied to the opium trade and the British penetration of China, plague spread through colonial ports of call before it infected Europe and North America. The rat, which carried the infected fleas, traveled the world on steamships and populated the growing port cities of New York, San Francisco, Singapore, Bombay, Dakar, and Rio de Janeiro.[73] Since industrialized transportation moved the rat around the world and sprawling urban centers led to rat population booms, Jonathan Burt suggested that the rat is a "totem animal for modernity."[74]

---

73   Robert Sullivan, *Rats: Observations on the History and Habitat of the City's Most Unwanted Inhabitants* (New York: Bloomsbury, 2004), 5–14.

74   Jonathan Burt, *Rat* (London: Reaktion Books, 2006), 18.

PART IV
MAKING
THE GREAT HANOI
RAT HUNT

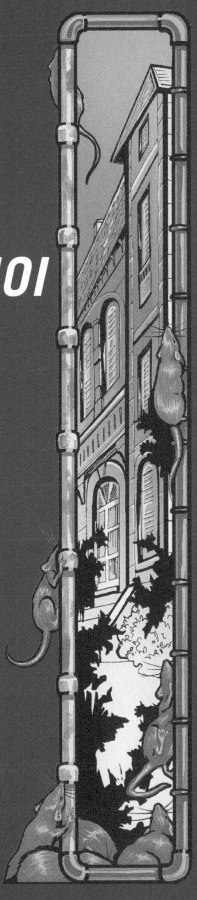

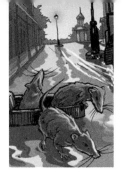

I did not start my career planning to publish a comic version of the morbid tale of the killing of thousands of sewer rats in French colonial Vietnam. On the contrary, I began with writing a rather conventional urban history of Hanoi. But a chance encounter with a forgotten dossier, the influence of cultural anthropology, my efforts to find engaging teaching sources, and inspiration from the success of Trevor Getz's *Abina and the Important Men* led me to this project.[1] Each step of the process forced me to think about important questions regarding history. How did we make it? How do we write it? How do we read it? How do we tell it?

ADVENTURES AND BOREDOM IN THE ARCHIVES

My path to this graphic or comic history started two decades ago. As a graduate student, I was fortunate enough to receive a generous Fulbright grant for doctoral research. I was also very lucky that my archives were located in beautiful Aix-en-Provence in southern France. Initially, my project was a fairly conventional urban history of Hanoi under French colonial rule. My doctoral advisor, Tyler Stovall, had recently written *The Rise of the Paris Red Belt*, a study of the city's working-class suburbs, and suggested the kinds of sources I could use.[2] In the Centre des Archives Section d'Outre-Mer, the archives of the French colonial empire, there were all sorts of official documents for an urban historian: maps, population charts, taxation reports, official orders, construction expense reports, building statistics, and first-hand accounts of the city.

To be honest, charting Hanoi's transformation from traditional Vietnamese to French colonial was rather easy. It fit the classic pattern of a colonial dual city. French rule dramatically altered urban space, destroying existing structures and practices such as pagodas, gated streets, and open-air markets and creating new urban forms such as monumental office buildings,

---

1   Trevor Getz and Liz Clarke, *Abina and the Important Men* (New York: Oxford University Press, 2012).

2   Tyler Stovall, *The Rise of the Paris Red Belt* (Berkeley: University of California Press, 1990).

spacious villas, and wide boulevards lined with sidewalk cafés. Administrative maps showed how French urbanists created a quarter system that functioned as a form of racial segregation. The minority white population enjoyed access to most of the city. The commercial district around rue Paul Bert, the administrative and military compounds to the west, and the neighborhood of comfortable homes to the south were the French domain. The Vietnamese and Chinese communities, which made up roughly 90 to 95 per cent of the city, lived in the Old Quarter. Composed of thirty-six winding streets, each devoted to a craft or commodity, the Asian population was crammed into about a third of the city's space. When I looked at the reports on urban infrastructure, Hanoi's roads, gas and electrical lighting, and fresh water distribution and waste removal systems, it was clear that colonial rule meant unequal access to the benefits of modernity. The sewer system, a point of pride for the French administration, was very well developed and sophisticated for the white neighborhoods but only rudimentary in the Old Quarter. Based on my reading of Donald Reid's and Alain Corbin's analyses of Parisian sewers, I decided to highlight this aspect of French colonial Hanoi.[3]

Now while I had a nice and tidy case study of colonial urbanization and racial inequality, I began to get a little discouraged with my sources. Surprisingly, files on tax collection, dossiers on land use, and reports on how many kilometers of pipes were laid in a given year could be somewhat dry and often dull. I worried that my traditional urban history approach lacked the drama of a good narrative that the average reader finds engaging. More seriously, I was frustrated that the official documents did not really give a feel for what was going on in the city. Many reports painted a rosy view of French efforts in Hanoi, downplaying or ignoring conflicts that could raise concerns in Paris. I felt that I was reading half-truths and propaganda. I saw that I was gaining few insights into the nature of daily life in colonial Hanoi. Yes, I could write one version of history, but it was the narrative that government officials wanted me to write. After several months of digging through boxes of documents I felt like a prisoner of the archives.

HISTORY IN THE FUNNIEST OF PLACES

While I would like to say that creative methodology inspired me to search for unusual primary source material, the truth is that I got bored in the archives. To amuse myself I started to look for entertaining material. When reading articles on city building in old French newspapers on the microfilm

---

3   Donald Reid, *Paris Sewers and Sewermen: Realities and Representations* (Cambridge, MA: Harvard University Press, 1991) and Alain Corbin, *The Foul and the Fragrant: Odor and the French Social Imagination* (Cambridge, MA.: Harvard University Press, 1986).

machine, I spent far too much time looking at cartoons and caricatures, hoping for a good laugh. When researching hospital construction, I spent far too many hours looking at accounts of epidemics out of morbid curiosity. When flipping through the decades-old card catalogue for material on municipal regulations, I came across a card for a dossier on "Destruction of Hazardous Animals." Thinking that it would be amusing, I ordered the file. When it came, I was stunned to discover the contents. There were dozens of dated, signed, and stamped forms informing the colonial administration of the capture and killing of thousands of rats. The numbers were startling. In one day, over twenty thousand furry creatures met their death. As I dug deeper in the box I found a series of other documents detailing the various debates among French bureaucrats in the colonial city. Not for public dissemination, these reports, memos, and dispatches revealed not a united and orderly colonial regime engaged in a clear program for modernity but rather a chaotic situation full of anxiety, bitter feuds, and exasperation at the limits of French power in Hanoi.

While I initially opened the dossier for my personal entertainment, I began to think I might have the making of a micro-history. Micro-histories use an interesting historic event to demonstrate a number of larger and much more significant processes at work. For example, Edward Berenson used the trial of Madame Caillaux, the ex-wife of a former Prime Minister who murdered the editor of *Le Figaro*, as a vehicle to explore gender, class, politics, and psychiatry in *Belle* Époque France.[4] Elsewhere, Carlo Ginzburg published a famous study of an Italian miller burned at the stake for heresy, and Robert Darnton wrote on essay on printing apprentices who expressed their work frustrations by putting their bosses' cats on trial and murdering them.[5] Micro-histories use their quirky and unusual case studies to explore their social, cultural, and economic contexts. Often, they draw from methodologies associated with cultural anthropology. For example, Clifford Geertz's famous article "Deep Play: Notes on a Balinese Cockfight" uses "thick description" to tease out the significance and meaning of social rituals at a village gathering.[6]

Tyler Stovall suggested that the rat killing dossiers could be the basis of a cultural history of the colonial encounter. I included the story as a subsection of one of my dissertation chapters and then expanded it into a

---

4   Edward Berenson, *The Trial of Madame Caillaux* (Berkeley: University of California Press, 1992).

5   Carlo Ginzburg, *The Cheese and the Worms: The Cosmos of a Sixteenth-Century* Miller (Baltimore: Johns Hopkins University Press, 2013) and Robert Darnton, *The Great Cat Massacre and Other Episodes in French Cultural History* (New York: Basic Books, 1984).

6   Clifford Geertz, "Deep Play: Notes on the Balinese Cockfight," *Daedalus* vol. 101, no. 1 (Winter).

conference paper and then an academic journal article in *French Colonial History*. Following a similar influence from cultural anthropology, I then moved on to take a serious look at some of the visual sources from the colonial era. I studied postcards and cartoons from the period to understand power relationships in the colonial encounter. When I found a surprising number of postcards of executions I published another article on the creation of these commercial images of colonial state violence. I also wrote an article and a short book on cartoons and caricatures produced by French men living in colonial Vietnam. Both literally and metaphorically, these visual artifacts opened up new ways of seeing the colonial encounter that were far richer than the documents in the state-curated archives.

My research directly impacted my approach to teaching. While lecturing on imperialism, students responded well to stories drawn from these unusual sources. With the arrival of digital photography and PowerPoint, I was able to integrate images from my research into my lectures. This led to some very interesting conversations about how to do history, including stretching our understanding of what a "document" could be. Our discussions often wrestled with the problem of how to find the history that did not make it into the archives.

I was increasingly convinced that we can find history in the funniest and strangest of places. We don't have to be prisoners of the archives.

HISTORY OUTSIDE OF THE IVORY TOWER

My article on the Hanoi rat massacre came out in 2003. Like many scholars in the Humanities I thought that my work would be read by a few colleagues and then disappear into a black hole. But that was not the case. Like Hanoi's resilient rodents, the article kept coming back to me in surprising and startling ways. Over the next few years a number of professors mentioned that they were including the piece on their course syllabi. Then, while googling something related to Hanoi and rats, I found that the article was being taught in a few high schools. I was happy that young students were working with the curious event which I found so thought-provoking.

But things took an interesting turn in 2012 when a producer from WNYC sent me an email. He wanted to know if I'd be willing to speak on the *Freakonomics* radio show about how my research illustrated the concept of "perverse incentive." Being a public radio nerd, I immediately said yes and then got off the phone to google "perverse incentive." It turned out that my discovery of the French bounty on rats ironically leading to the breeding of rats for profit demonstrated this concept. Evidently various economists had cited my case study in their work. *Freakonomics* led to interviews with the Canadian Broadcasting Corporation, a regional National Public Radio affiliate in Santa Cruz, California, and a popular magazine in Ho Chi Minh City, Vietnam. In the fall of 2016, as I was finishing the graphic history version of the rat hunt, Indonesia's capital faced a rat crisis. When municipal officials in Jakarta proposed a bounty on rats, newspapers from the United Kingdom's *The Guardian* to Australia's *Sydney Morning Herald* cited my article in their reports. Recently it has come to my attention that the National Council of Education and Research Training, India's largest English language curriculum developer, used my research on rat hunting as a major section of a Class 10 history textbook and the Central Board of Secondary Education included questions on the significance of Hanoi's sewers on the annual national exam.[7]

Despite gaining a reputation as "the rat guy," I've been delighted by the diverse uses of my research both inside and outside of the classroom. That this research project stemmed from an accidental discovery of an unusual window into history makes it even more rewarding. Now, with the story in graphic format, I hope an even larger audience will learn lessons from the experiences in Hanoi over a century ago.

WHY A GRAPHIC HISTORY?

The decision to pitch the great Hanoi rat hunt as a graphic history came to me in an epiphany. I was in my office at Sacramento State, watching the final edit of a short documentary that I made with my colleague Jeff Dym, when I started to daydream about other non-traditional ways to present history. Our 29-minute film, *Cambodia's Other Lost City: French Colonial Phnom Penh*, was an effort to present history in a medium other than an academic article or a monograph.[8] I was returning to work on Hanoi and was unsure on how to start my new project. My eyes came to rest on a section of my bookshelf that held several graphic novels, memoirs, and histories, including Trevor Getz's award-winning and path-breaking *Abina and the Important Men*. I realized that the genre was perfect for illustrating some of the complex ideas that I wanted to discuss in my work on colonial urbanism. The rat hunt could be a compelling hook to explore a theoretical discussion of empire, white privilege, modernity, disease, and

---

7   National Council of Educational Research and Training, *India and the Contemporary World*, vol. 2 (New Delhi: NCERT, 2014), 37–38. Sadly, NCERT failed to properly cite my article.

8   Jeffrey Dym and Michael G. Vann, "Cambodia's Other Lost City: French Colonial Phnom Penh". Filmed July, 2013. YouTube video, 29:02. Posted June, 2014. https://www.youtube.com/watch?v=j5gKeQFMVw4.

the environment. I grabbed my copy of *Abina* to look for the editor. Realizing that I had previously worked with Charles Cavaliere, I sent him an email pitching my idea. After a few exchanges and phone conversations, I sold him on the idea and I began my collaboration with the incredibly talented Liz Clarke.

Nothing in my education or career had formally prepared me to write a graphic history. Professional historians are trained to write journal articles, research monographs, and works of synthesis drawn from secondary sources, and we sometimes write about teaching in pieces on pedagogy. Fortunately, I had worked with comic images in a number of ways. In addition to my research that used cartoons from colonial Vietnam as a primary source, I had been teaching with graphic histories for years. When I first started to teach a course on twentieth-century Europe, which soon became the twentieth-century world, I used Art Spiegelman's *Maus*.[9] This brilliant Pulitzer Prize–winning book tells how the author's parents survived the Nazi genocide known as the Shoah or the Holocaust. Recreating his father's oral history, Spiegelman provocatively drew Jews as mice, Germans as cats, Poles as pigs, French as frogs, and Americans as slobbering happy dogs. While some readers were initially skeptical and even offended at such a treatment of the Shoah, the power of the story and the visual metaphor of mice hiding from bloodthirsty cats captures the horrifying inhumanity of occupied Poland. Coming from the underground comic scene, Spiegelman referred to his work as "comix" to set it apart from work designed to amuse. In a course on comparative genocide, I used *Safe Area Goražde*, a work of graphic journalism by Joe Sacco, author of the award-winning *Palestine*.[10] Spiegelman's and Sacco's works modeled the power of images to depict social conflict.

As I started to storyboard the chapters, I went on a comic and graphic novel binge. Truth be told, I was never a comic book nerd. I was a history nerd. As a child I read more serious comics, such as *Doonesbury*, not tales of superheroes. But as I was trying to figure out how to storyboard a graphic history, a number of people told me to read Alan Moore's *Watchmen*.[11] This brilliant deconstruction of the superhero genre demonstrates a variety of ways in which the graphic format can enhance narrative. In particular, comic storytelling, be it fact or fiction, can utilize the art form's self-referential or "meta" opportunities. For example, in *Maus*,

---

9   Art Spiegelman, *Maus* (New York: Pantheon Books, 1991).

10   Joe Sacco, *Palestine* (Seattle: Fantagraphics Books, 1997) and *Safe Area Gorazde: The War in Eastern Bosnia 1992–1995* (Seattle: Fantagraphics Books, 200).

11   Alan Moore, *Watchmen* (New York: D.C. Comics, 1986).

Spiegelman uses animal imagery to communicate the terror and dehumanization of the Nazi genocide. Elsewhere, he depicts himself wearing a mouse mask, to question his Jewish-American identity. In *Watchmen*, Moore uses the graphic novel to insert subtle philosophical reflections on simultaneity and scale. Jeff Dym, who teaches a course on the history of Japanese Manga, suggested I read Nick Sousanis' *Unflattening*.[12] Originally his doctoral dissertation in education at Columbia University, the book carefully explains how comics can convey multiple concepts at the same time. I realized that this was the perfect medium for capturing the cultural history of a colonial city where French and Vietnamese lived among each other but in two very different worlds. To demonstrate colonial Hanoi's nature as a "dual city," we used different shapes and colors for people speaking either Vietnamese or French. This clue shows how two communities could share the same physical space yet remain culturally apart. The graphic format was also useful to visually demonstrate that Hanoi's urban history was nestled in larger world historical contexts. In other words, graphic history could convey the story of the Hanoi rat hunt as "glocal" history, where it is necessary to simultaneously understand the global and the local.

The graphic genre works well for the story of the rat hunt as visual sources from my research could serve as the basis for the book. Because the French colonized Hanoi in the early age of photography, there is a rich archive of images of the city. With a long tradition of grand tableaux paintings, turn-of-the-century French society celebrated photography as the new art form of modernity, a creative science. Throughout the colonial empire, photographers played an important role in documenting indigenous societies and celebrating imperial triumphs. Thus, there are excellent images of how the Vietnamese lived in Hanoi as well as of French construction projects such as the Pont Doumer. Working with the incredibly talented Liz Clarke, I was able to set events from my research on specific streets or in front of specific buildings. This was especially useful in recreating the feeling of Hanoi as a colonial dual city where white and nonwhite have access to separate and unequal urban infrastructure.

The graphic genre presented me with an unusual opportunity. In constructing the scenes and the narrative, I realized that I could insert characters that would personify crucial aspects of the urban experience. Obviously, the pages are filled with Vietnamese and Chinese people from Hanoi's various classes, ranging from prisoners to mandarins. I worked with Liz to insert street vendors, rickshaw pullers, and laborers to convey

12   Nick Sousanis, *Unflattening* (Cambridge, MA: Harvard University Press, 2015).

the street's social dynamism. I was also able to insert two characters, French *flâneurs*, who roam the city as they would have done in Hanoi or in Paris. As they enjoy the urban spectacle before them, the *flâneurs* discuss what they see, playing the role of a Greek chorus in the narrative.

Finally, the meta nature of the genre presents the ability to insert the author (in this case myself) into the narrative. Art Spiegelman does this in *Maus* in a very sophisticated way that shows his interactions with his father as he records his oral history. I decided to use comic format to present my personal interaction with Hanoi and its history. My aim is to show that while historical research involves searching through old documents, there are real-world connections and implications. For me, living in Hanoi in 1997 and subsequent visits to the city are like stepping into history, into my research. It was very surreal to encounter buildings I'd studied and to see the subsequent layers of history that have been laid upon them. As I watched Hanoi's changes between 1997 and 2015, I realized that it was comparable to the city's transformation exactly a century earlier. I wrote the graphic history's framing devices, a prologue and an afterword, to highlight the layers of history that I personally experienced. The meta conceit of inserting myself into the narrative also highlights the fact that historians are storytellers. Far too many of us forget that history should be a good tale, something that enlightens and educates but also entertains.

FINALLY, VIETNAM

One of the last comments I want to make about writing the story is the obligation American citizens have to understand Vietnam's history. Up until the 1960s few Americans had heard of Vietnam. Then, because of Washington's Cold War military interventions, Americans suddenly talked about Vietnam. However, for many Americans, Vietnam is a war and not a country. I'm regularly frustrated with how little of the nation's history my fellow citizens know. I constantly surprise people when I tell them it was a French colonial possession for almost a century. Because of America's destructive history in Southeast Asia, its citizens have a moral obligation to learn more about the people and cultures of the region. That America is home to large communities of diasporic Vietnamese, known as Viet Kieu, reinforces this point. Considering that the United States of America repeatedly bombed the city of Hanoi, causing tremendous collateral damage, I hope that this book is a small contribution toward dispelling ignorance about Vietnam's past.

I am surprisingly optimistic about this task. Two events in 2016 gave me hope. While I was writing this book, Viet Thanh Nguyen became the first Vietnamese-American to win the Pulitzer Prize. His brilliant novel, *The Sympathizer*, is opening many readers' consciousness to an unfamiliar Vietnamese reality that includes the traumas of war and exile but also a joyous celebration of centuries-old cultural traditions.[13] Later in the year, celebrity chef Anthony Bourdain lured Barack Obama to a small restaurant in Vietnam's capital. The American president sat on a tiny plastic chair, drank local beer, and ate bun cha, one of city's many delicious culinary offerings. It is difficult not to smile at this quintessentially Hanoi moment.

---

13   Viet Thanh Nguyen, *The Sympathizer* (New York: Grove Press, 2015).

PART V
THE GREAT HANOI RAT HUNT IN THE CLASSROOM

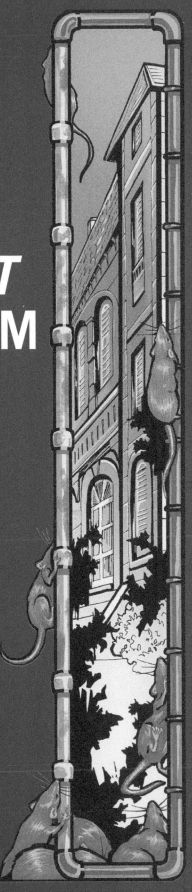

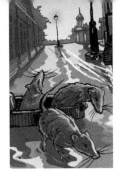

DISCUSSION QUESTIONS

THE GREAT HANOI RAT HUNT

1. What were the most important features of Paul Doumer's rebuilding of Hanoi?

2. Why were sewers so important to Paul Doumer?

3. How did rats take advantage of industrialized transportation and Hanoi's new environment?

4. Why were rats such a threat to the city?

5. What challenges did the French authorities face in trying to remove Hanoi's rat population?

6. How did the Vietnamese outsmart the French colonial government?

7. How does *The Great Hanoi Rat Hunt* illustrate the economic principle of "perverse incentive?"

COLONIAL HISTORY

1. What were some of the forces behind imperialist expansion in Asia?

2. How was industrialization linked to imperialism?

3. What were the power differentials in the era of imperialism?

4. How did cultural attitudes, including racism, justify colonial expansion and rule?

5. How did colonial racial inequality structure economic relationships?

6. What were the daily realities of white supremacy in colonial Vietnam?

7. What benefits did colonial rule offer to the Vietnamese?

8. What did the Vietnamese find particularly unjust or insulting about colonial rule?

URBAN HISTORY

1. Why was urbanization so important to the French?

2. How did Westerners view non-French Hanoi? What did they comment upon regarding the people of Hanoi?

3. What aspects of French culture did the colonizers export to Vietnam?

4. How did the French see their colonial empire as a "mission to civilize"?

5. What did French city building improve in Hanoi?

6. What did French city building make worse in Hanoi?

7. What was the symbolic value of French buildings and statues in Hanoi?

8. How would you describe colonial Hanoi in terms of social justice?

9. How were social inequalities in colonial cities different from those in European cities?

10. How did the people of Hanoi enjoy its public space? What were the similarities and differences between the Vietnamese and French experiences of the city?

VIETNAMESE HISTORY

1. What role did the Vietnamese people play in the colonial economic system?

2. How did French medical policies impact the Vietnamese and Chinese population?

3. What were the various ways that Vietnamese citizens challenged or resisted the French colonial order?

4. How did Vietnamese nationalism and communism develop in reaction to French rule?

HISTORY OF MEDICINE AND DISEASE

1. How are epidemics linked to globalization?

2. How did industrialization and imperialism impact the spread of disease?

3. Why was the bubonic plague such a terrifying disease?

4. What racial and ethnic assumptions do the primary source documents reveal?

5. Why was racism, and specifically Sinophobia, intertwined with the fear of disease?

6. How did French and other Western public health measures show the power of the state over individual bodies?

7. Why did the Vietnamese try to hide plague victims, both dying and dead, from the French authorities?

CHINA IN WORLD HISTORY

1. What has been China's historical role in global economic history?

2. What were the roles of Chinese labor and Chinese capital in Tonkin?

3. Why did Europeans want to get to China?

4. What problems did Europeans face trading with China?

5. How did the British solve their trade deficit with China?

6. How did Western trade destabilize China?

7. What was the global impact of the Chinese diaspora?

8. What are some of the attitudes toward the Chinese seen in the primary source documents?

METHOD AND HISTORIOGRAPHY

1. How does a world historical perspective challenge the tradition historical writing based upon the nation-state?

2. What does a world historical perspective offer to historical narratives?

3. How can cultural anthropology be used to enrich our understanding of history?

4. What are the benefits of using a micro-history to study global phenomena?

ESSAY TOPICS

These questions are designed to be answered with reference to the graphic history, the historical contexts essay, and the primary sources.

1. How did French colonization illustrate some of the processes of globalization in the era of the New Imperialism?

2. Why was Hanoi such an important symbol for the French colonial empire?

3. In what ways were Vietnamese reactions to the French medical policies demonstrations of resistance to colonial rule?

4. How did international fear of the plague align with anti-Chinese sentiment in Hanoi, Honolulu, San Francisco, and elsewhere?

5. How was Hanoi a classic colonial dual city? What were the structural inequalities of the colonial urban environment? Did the French, Vietnamese, and Chinese live within the same city, or were they really in two different worlds?

6. Consider the concept of white privilege. How was it manifest in French Hanoi? How did whites and non-whites have unequal access to power?

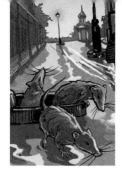

TIMELINE OF EVENTS IN VIETNAM, FRANCE, AND THE WORLD

3000 BCE

2879 BCE–258 BCE —— Hồng Bàng dynasty

257–179 —— Thục dynasty

207–111 —— Triệu dynasty

0 CE

111 BCE – 40 CE —— First Chinese occupation: Han Dynasty

40–43 —— Trưng Sisters lead rebellion against Chinese rule

43–544 —— Second Chinese occupation: Han, Jin, and Chen Dynasties

500 CE

544–602 —— Early Lý dynasty

602–938 —— Third Chinese occupation: Tang Dynasty

939–967 —— Ngô dynasty

968–980 —— Đinh dynasty

980–1009 —— Early Lê dynasty

1000 CE

1009–1225 —— Later Lý dynasty

1225–1400 —— Trần dynasty

1400–1407 —— Hồ dynasty

1407–1427 —— Fourth Chinese occupation: Ming Dynasty

1407–1413 —— Later Trần dynasty

1428–1788 —— Later Lê dynasty

1500 CE

1527–1592 —— Mạc dynasty

1545–1787 —— Trịnh lords (North)

1558–1777 —— Nguyễn lords (South)

1760–1840 —— British Industrial Revolution

1770–1802 —— Tây Sơn rebellion and dynasty

1789–1795 —— French Revolution

1800 CE

1801–1814	——	Napoleonic France
1802–1945	——	Nguyễn dynasty
1839–1842	——	First Opium War

1850 CE

1855–1959	——	Third Plague Pandemic
1856–1860	——	Second Opium War
1858	——	French attack Da Nang
1859	——	French seize Saigon
1862	——	Cochinchine becomes a French Colony
1863	——	Cambodia becomes a French Protectorate
1870–1940	——	French Third Republic
1871–1939		New Imperialism
1882	——	French seize Hanoi
1883	——	Annam and Tonkin become French Protectorates
1883–1886	——	Tonkin Campaign
1884–1885	——	Sino-French War

1886 —— Paul Bert in Hanoi

1894 —— Plague in Canton and Hong Kong

1896–1898 —— Plague in Bombay

1897–1902 —— Paul Doumer Governor-General of Indochine

1899 —— Plague in Honolulu

1900 CE

1900 —— Plague in San Francisco

1901 —— Plague in Hanoi

1902 —— The Great Hanoi Rat Hunt

1931–1945 —— Pacific War (World War II in Asia)

1945 CE

1945 —— Japanese Occupy Hanoi; Declaration of Vietnamese Independence by Ho Chi Minh in Ba Dinh Square

1945–1976 —— North Vietnam: Democratic Republic of Vietnam

1946–1954 —— French Indochina War (First Indochina War)

1954 —— French evacuate Hanoi

1955–1975 —— South Vietnam: Republic of Vietnam

1963–1973 —— American War in Vietnam (Second Indochina War)

1972 ——— Christmas Bombing of Hanoi

1973 ——— End of American War

1975 ——— Invasion of South Vietnam, culminating in the fall/ liberation of Saigon

1976 ——— Formal unification of Vietnam and establishment of Socialist Republic of Vietnam

1986 ——— Start of Doi Moi Reforms in Vietnam

1995 ——— Diplomatic relations between Vietnam and the United States reestablished

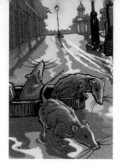

FURTHER RESOURCES

This reading list is limited to English-language books. Obviously, there are more relevant titles in French and Vietnamese.

SUGGESTED HISTORIES OF VIETNAM

For many years the books in English on Vietnam focused far too much on the American War (1963–1973). Now there are a number of books that take a much longer view of Vietnam's history. Recent historical surveys of Vietnam include Ben Kiernan, *Việt Nam: A History from the Earliest Times to the Present* (Oxford: Oxford University Press, 2017); Christopher Goscha, *Vietnam: A New History* (New York: Basic Books, 2016); and Keith W. Taylor, *A History of the Vietnamese* (Cambridge: Cambridge University Press, 2013). William S. Logan's, *Hanoi: Biography of a City* (Seattle: University of Washington Press, 2000) remains the best history of Hanoi's thousand-year history.

Neil L. Jamieson's *Understanding Vietnam* (Berkeley: University of California Press, 1993) offers an interesting, yet arguably essentialist, cultural history of Vietnam. Alexander Woodside's now classic *Vietnam and the Chinese Model: A Comparative Study of Vietnamese and Chinese Government in the First Half of the Nineteenth-Century* (Cambridge: Harvard University Press, 1971) and his more recent *Lost Modernities: China, Vietnam, Korea, and the Hazards of World History* (Cambridge: Harvard University Press, 2006) discuss Vietnam as a Chinese-style Confucian state. Keith Taylor's *The Birth of Vietnam* (Berkeley: University of California Press, 1983) argues for Vietnam's connections to Southeast Asia.

Translated from its original French, Pierre Brocheux and Daniel Hémery's *Indochina: An Ambiguous Colonization, 1858–1954* (Berkeley: University of California Press, 2009) is the most authoritative survey of the French colonial era. Nicola Cooper's *France in Indochina: Colonial Encounters* (New York: Berg, 2001) and Panivong Norinder's *Phantasmatic Indochina: French Colonial Ideology in Architecture, Film, and Literature* (Durham: Duke University Press, 1996) are both wide-ranging cultural studies of French colonialism in Southeast Asia. Milton E. Osbourne's *River Road to China: The Mekong River Expedition 1866–1873* (New York: Liveright, 1975) is a very readable discussion of French colonial explorers. While its heavy-handed Marxist methodology may seem dated, the content of Martin J. Murray's *The Development of Capitalism in Colonial Indochina* (Berkeley: University of California Press, 1981) is still crucial information for under-standing French colonialism as a system of economic exploitation. Using the French prisons as a case study for imperialism, Peter Zinoman's *The Colonial Bastille: A History of Imprisonment in Vietnam, 1862–1940* (Berkeley: University of California Press, 2001) is an enlightening study of French rule.

David Marr's *Vietnamese Anticolonialism, 1885–1925* (Berkeley: University of California Press, 1971) and *Vietnamese Tradition on Trial, 1920–1945* (Berkeley: University of California Press, 1981) are founda-tional studies of the Vietnamese response to French occupation. Hue-Tam Ho Tai's *Radicalism and the Origins of the Vietnamese Revolution* (Cambridge: Harvard University Press, 1992) is an essential history of the non-Communist anti-colonial activists in the interwar era. Shawn McHale, in *Print and Power: Confucianism, Communism, and Buddhism in the Making of Modern Vietnam* (Honolulu: University of Hawaii Press, 2004) discusses the various ways the Vietnamese made their own modernity.

Truong Buu Lam's *Patterns of Vietnamese Response to Foreign Intervention: 1859–1900* (New Haven: Yale University Press, 1967) and *Colonialism Experienced: Vietnamese Writings on Colonialism, 1900–1931* (Ann Arbor: University of Michigan Press, 2000) are two ex-cellent anthologies of Vietnamese voices during French rule. The introduc-tory essays in *Colonialism Experienced* are highly recommended. Editor Huynh Sanh Thong's *An Anthology of Vietnamese Poems: From the Eleventh Century through the Twentieth* (New Haven: Yale University Press, 1996) contains scores of poems with beautiful images of Vietnam's history. Greg Lockhart and Monique Lockhart's *The Light of the Capital: Three Modern Vietnamese Classics* (Kuala Lumpur: Oxford University Press, 1996) offers translations of local journalism from early twentieth-century Hanoi and opens important windows into the Vietnamese per-spective on colonialism. Peter Zinoman and Nguyen Nguyet Cam's graceful and humorous translation of Vu Trong Phung's satirical novel *Dumb Luck* (Ann Arbor: University of Michigan Press, 2002) is a fun portrait of cul-tural confusion during colonial modernization. Written by a communist activist and veteran of the anti-colonial struggle, Tran Bu Binh, *The Red Earth: A Vietnamese Memoir of Life on a Colonial Rubber Plantation* (Athens, OH: Ohio University Press, 1985) is a shocking memoir of the horrors of the colonial economy.

Brocheux, Pierre, and Daniel Hémery. *Indochina: An Ambiguous Colonization, 1858–1954* (Berkeley: University of California Press, 2009).

Cooper, Nicola. *France in Indochina: Colonial Encounters* (New York: Berg, 2001).

Goscha, Christopher. *Vietnam: A New History* (New York: Basic Books, 2016).

Jamieson, Neil L. *Understanding Vietnam* (Berkeley: University of California Press, 1993).

Kiernan, Ben. *Việt Nam: A History from the Earliest Times to the Present* (Oxford: Oxford University Press, 2017).

Lam, Truong Buu. *Patterns of Vietnamese Response to Foreign Intervention: 1859–1900* (New Haven: Yale University Press, 1967).

Lam, Truong Buu. *Colonialism Experienced: Vietnamese Writings on Colonialism, 1900–1931* (Ann Arbor: University of Michigan Press, 2000).

Lockhart, Greg, and Monique Lockhart. *The Light of the Capital: Three Modern Vietnamese Classics* (Kuala Lumpur: Oxford University Press, 1996).

Logan, William S. *Hanoi: Biography of a City* (Seattle: University of Washington Press, 2000).

Marr, David. *Vietnamese Anticolonialism, 1885–1925* (Berkeley: University of California Press, 1971).

Marr, David. *Vietnamese Tradition on Trial, 1920–1945* (Berkeley: University of California Press, 1981).

McHale, Shawn. *Print and Power: Confucianism, Communism and Buddhism in the Making of Modern Vietnam* (Honolulu: University of Hawaii Press, 2004).

Murray, Martin J. *The Development of Capitalism in Colonial Indochina* (Berkeley: University of California Press, 1981).

Osbourne, Milton E. *River Road to China: The Mekong River Expedition 1866–1873* (New York: Liveright, 1975).

Tai, Hue-Tam Ho. *Radicalism and the Origins of the Vietnamese Revolution* (Cambridge: Harvard University Press, 1992).

Taylor, Keith W. *A History of the Vietnamese* (Cambridge: Cambridge University Press, 2013).

Thong, Huynh Sanh Thong (ed.). *An Anthology of Vietnamese Poems: From the Eleventh Century through the Twentieth* (New Haven: Yale University Press, 1996).

Tran Bu Binh, *The Red Earth: A Vietnamese Memoir of Life on a Colonial Rubber Plantation* (Athens, OH: Ohio University Press, 1985).

Woodside, Alexander. *Vietnam and the Chinese Model: A Comparative Study of Vietnamese and Chinese Government in the First Half of the Nineteenth Century* (Cambridge; Harvard University Press, 1971).

Woodside, Alexander. *Lost Modernities: China, Vietnam, Korea, and the Hazards of World History* (Cambridge: Harvard University Press, 2006).

Zinoman, Peter. *The Colonial Bastille: A History of Imprisonment in Vietnam, 1862–1940* (Berkeley: University of California Press, 2001).

FRENCH HISTORY

Obviously, there is a massive literature on the history of France. Here are some of my favorites that cover the era of the great Hanoi rat hunt. Tyler Stovall's, *Transnational France: The Modern History of a Universal Nation* (Boulder, CO: Westview Press, 2015) gives French national history a much-needed world historical context. Theodore Zeldin's massive *A History of French Passions, 1848–1945, Volume 1: Ambition, Love, and*

Politics and *Volume 2: Intellect, Taste, and Anxiety* (Oxford: Oxford University Press, 1973), stands the test of time and remains an insightful, wide-ranging, and comprehensive cultural history. Edward Berenson's *The Trail of Madame Caillaux* (Berkeley: University of California Press, 1992) is a micro-history of a famous murder that sheds insights into gender, power, and culture in early twentieth-century France. Maurice Agulhon's *Marianne into Battle: Republican Imagery and Symbolism in France, 1789–1880* (Cambridge: Cambridge University Press, 1981) is an important discussion of monuments and political representations.

David Harvey's, *Paris, Capital of Modernity* (New York: Routledge, 2003) is one of the greatest studies of the world's most studied city. Donald Reid's *Paris Sewers and Sewermen: Realities and Representations* (Cambridge, MA: Harvard University Press, 1991) takes the study of Paris underground—literally underground.

Eugene Weber's *Peasants into Frenchmen: The Modernization of Rural France, 1870–1914* (Stanford: Stanford University Press, 1976) is essential for any student of modernization under the Third Republic. The essays in Herman Lebovics's *Imperialism and the Corruption of Democracies* (Durham and London: Duke University Press, 2006) shows the impact of the empire on the colonizing power. Judith Surkis's *Sexing the Citizen: Morality and Masculinity in France, 1870–1920* (Ithaca: Cornell University Press, 2006) is one of several new studies that genders French history.

Agulhon, Maurice. *Marianne into Battle: Republican Imagery and Symbolism in France, 1789–1880* (Cambridge: Cambridge University Press, 1981).

Berenson, Edward. *The Trail of Madame Caillaux* (Berkeley: University of California Press, 1992).

Harvey, David. *Paris, Capital of Modernity* (New York: Routledge, 2003).

Lebovics, Herman. *Imperialism and the Corruption of Democracies* (Durham and London: Duke University Press, 2006).

Reid, Donald. *Paris Sewers and Sewermen: Realities and Representations* (Cambridge, MA: Harvard University Press, 1991).

Stovall, Tyler. *Transnational France: The Modern History of a Universal Nation* (Boulder, CO, Westview Press, 2015).

Surkis, Judith. *Sexing the Citizen: Morality and Masculinity in France, 1870–1920* (Ithaca, NY: Cornell University Press, 2006).

Weber, Eugene. *Peasants into Frenchmen: The Modernization of Rural France, 1870–1914* (Stanford: Stanford University Press, 1976).

Zeldin, Theodore. *A History of French Passions, 1848–1945, Volume 1: Ambition, Love, and Politics* and *Volume 2: Intellect, Taste, and Anxiety* (Oxford: Oxford University Press, 1973).

IMPERIALISM

For a survey of the history of colonialism read Heather Streets-Salter and Trevor R. Getz's *Empires and Colonies in the Modern World: A Global Perspective* (New York: Oxford University Press, 2016). C. A. Bayly's magnum opus, *The Birth of the Modern World, 1780–1914* (Malden, MA: Blackwell Publishing, 2004), situates imperialism in a larger global context. Tracey Rizzo and Steven Gerontakis bring us *Intimate Empires: Body, Race, and Gender in the Modern World* (New York: Oxford University press, 2017), which surveys the intersections of race, class, and gender in colonial history, as does Marie-Paule Ha's *French Women and the Empire: The Case of Indochina* (New York: Oxford University Press, 2014). While often dismissed as an apologist for empire, Niall Ferguson has written books, including *Empire: How Britain Made the Modern World* (London: Allen Lane, 2003), which are not without merit and are, at the very least, refreshingly retro in their positive assessment of colonialism. Robert Bickers's *The Scramble for China: Foreign Devils in the Qing Empire, 1832–1914* (New York: Penguin, 2011) is excellent context for Western imperialism in Asia. Edward Berenson's *Heroes of Empire: Five Charismatic Men and the Conquest of Africa* (Berkeley: University of California Press, 2010) is an engaging and informative cultural history of Europe's imperial madness. Edward Said's *Culture and Imperialism* (New York: Random House, 1993) connects Western literature to the era of high imperialism.

Students of technology and empire should consult Michael Adas's *Machines as the Measure of Men: Science, Technology, and Ideologies of Western Dominance* (Ithaca: Cornell University Press, 1989) and Daniel Headrick's *The Tools of Empire: Technology and European Imperialism in the Nineteenth Century* (New York: Oxford University Press, 1981) and *The Tentacles of Progress: Technology Transfer in the Age of Imperialism, 1850–1940* (New York: Oxford University Press, 1988).

Carl Nightingale's *Segregation: A Global History of Divided Cities* (Chicago: University of Chicago Press, 2012) and Gwendolyn Wright's *The Politics of Design in French Colonial Urbanism* (Chicago: University of Chicago Press, 1991) are both first-rate discussions of colonial dual cities.

While focused on two very different subjects, Mike Davis's *Late Victorian Holocausts: El Niño Famines and the Making of the Third World* (London: Verso, 2001) and Sven Beckert's *Empire of Cotton: A Global History* (London: Penguin Books, 2014) reveal imperialism as an abusive economic system. Martin Thomas's *Violence and the Colonial Order: Police, Workers and Protest in the European Colonial Empires, 1918–1940* (Cambridge: Cambridge University Press, 2012) covers the physical abuses of empire.

Adas, Michael. *Machines as the Measure of Men: Science, Technology, and Ideologies of Western Dominance* (Ithaca, NY: Cornell University Press, 1989).

Bayly, C. A. *The Birth of the Modern World, 1780–1914* (Malden, MA: Blackwell Publishing, 2004).

Beckert, Sven. *Empire of Cotton: A Global History* (London: Penguin Books, 2014).

Berenson, Edward. *Heroes of Empire: Five Charismatic Men and the Conquest of Africa* (Berkeley: University of California Press, 2010).

Bickers, Robert. *The Scramble for China: Foreign Devils in the Qing Empire, 1832–1914* (New York: Penguin, 2011).

Crosby, Alfred. *Ecological Imperialism: The Biological Expansion of Europe, 900–1900* (New York: Cambridge University Press, 1986).

Crosby, Alfred. *The Columbian Exchange: Biological and Cultural Consequences of 1492* (Westport, CT: Greenwood Publishing Co., 1972).

Davis, Mike. *Late Victorian Holocausts: El Niño Famines and the Making of the Third World* (London: Verso, 2001).

Ferguson, Niall. *Empire: How Britain Made the Modern World* (London: Allen Lane, 2003).

Ha, Marie-Paule. *French Women and the Empire: The Case of Indochina* (New York: Oxford University Press, 2014).

Headrick, Daniel. *The Tools of Empire: Technology and European Imperialism in the Nineteenth Century* (New York: Oxford University Press, 1981).

Headrick, Daniel. *The Tentacles of Progress: Technology Transfer in the Age of Imperialism, 1850–1940* (New York: Oxford University Press, 1988)

Lebovics, Herman. *Imperialism and the Corruption of Democracies* (Durham and London: Duke University Press, 2006).

Nightingale, Carl. *Segregation: A Global History of Divided Cities* (Chicago: University of Chicago Press, 2012).

Rizzo, Tracey, and Steven Gerontakis, *Intimate Empires: Body, Race, and Gender in the Modern World* (New York: Oxford University Press, 2017).

Said, Edward. *Culture and Imperialism* (New York: Random House, 1993).

Streets-Salter, Heather, and Trevor R. Getz, *Empires and Colonies in the Modern World: A Global Perspective* (New York: Oxford University Press, 2016).

Thomas, Martin. *Violence and the Colonial Order: Police, Workers and Protest in the European Colonial Empires, 1918–1940* (Cambridge: Cambridge University Press, 2012).

Wright, Gwendolyn. *The Politics of Design in French Colonial Urbanism* (Chicago; University of Chicago Press, 1991).

DISEASE

Mark Harrison's *Disease and the Modern World: 1500 to the Present Day* (Cambridge: Polity, 2004) is an excellent starting point for the history of illness. The paradigm-setting studies of disease and European expansion are Alfred Crosby's *The Columbian Exchange: Biological and Cultural Consequences of 1492* (Westport, CT: Greenwood Publishing Co., 1972) and *Ecological Imperialism: The Biological Expansion of Europe, 900–1900* (New York: Cambridge University Press, 1986).

The horrors of the bubonic plague ensure that there will always be a number of books to satisfy readers' morbid curiosity. Recent popular histories include Edward Marriott's *Plague: A Story of Scientists, Rivalry, and the Scourge that Won't Go Away* (New York: Metropolitan Books, 2002), Wendy Orent's *Plague: The Mysterious Past and the Terrifying Future of the World's Most Dangerous Disease* (New York: Free Press, 2004), and

Ole J. Benedictow's *The Black Death, 1346–1353: The Complete History* (Rochester, NY: The Boydell Press, 2004). For plague in the ancient world, see William Rosen's *Justinian's Flea: Plague, Empire, and the Birth of Europe* (New York: Viking, 2007) and the revisionist history of George D. Sussman's "Scientists Doing History: Central Africa and the Origins of the First Plague Pandemic" (*Journal of World History,* June 2015).

For the plague in Asia, consult Carol Benedict's *Bubonic Plague in Nineteenth-Century China* (Stanford: Stanford University Press, 1994), William C. Summers' *The Great Manchurian Plague of 1910–1911: The Geopolitics of an Epidemic Disease* (New Haven: Yale University Press, 2012), and Robert Peckham's *Epidemics in Modern Asia* (Cambridge: Cambridge University press, 2016).

For studies of disease and colonialism/imperialism, these books are essential: Philip D. Curtin, *Death by Migration: Europe's Encounter with the Tropical World in the Nineteenth Century* (Cambridge: Cambridge University Press, 1989), Myron Echenberg, *Plague Ports: The Global Urban Impact of Bubonic Plague, 1894–1901* (New York: New York University Press, 2007), Robert Peckham (ed.), *Empires of Panic: Epidemics and Colonial Anxieties* (Hong Kong: Hong Kong University Press, 2015), and Robert Peckham and David Pomfret (eds.), *Imperial Contagions: Medicine, Hygiene, and Cultures of Planning in Asia* (Hong Kong: Hong Kong University Press, 2013).

Patrick Deville's critically acclaimed novel *Plague and Cholera* (London: Abacus, 2012) is a heavily researched but rather quirky recreation of Alexandre Yersin's life. While it offers many insights, it leans toward a hagiography of this troubled genius.

Benedict, Carol. *Bubonic Plague in Nineteenth-Century China* (Stanford: Stanford University Press, 1994).

Benedictow, Ole J. *The Black Death, 1346–1353: The Complete History* (Rochester, NY: The Boydell Press, 2004).

Curtin, Philip D. *Death by Migration: Europe's Encounter with the Tropical World in the Nineteenth Century* (Cambridge: Cambridge University Press, 1989).

Deville, Patrick. *Plague and Cholera* (London: Abacus, 2012).

Echenberg, Myron. *Plague Ports: The Global Urban Impact of Bubonic Plague, 1894–1901* (New York: New York University Press, 2007).

Harrison, Mark. *Disease and the Modern World: 1500 to the Present Day* (Cambridge: Polity, 2004).

Marriott, Edward. *Plague: A Story of Scientists, Rivalry, and the Scourge that Won't Go Away* (New York: Metropolitan Books, 2002).

Orent, Wendy. *Plague: The Mysterious Past and the Terrifying Future of the World's Most Dangerous Disease* (New York: Free Press, 2004).

Peckham, Robert (ed.). *Empires of Panic: Epidemics and Colonial Anxieties* (Hong Kong: Hong Kong University Press, 2015).

Peckham, Robert. *Epidemics in Modern Asia* (Cambridge: Cambridge University Press, 2016).

Peckham, Robert, and David Pomfret (ed.). *Imperial Contagions: Medicine, Hygiene, and Cultures of Planning in Asia* (Hong Kong: Hong Kong University Press, 2013).

Rosen, William. *Justinian's Flea: Plague, Empire, and the Birth of Europe* (New York: Viking, 2007).

Summers, William C. *The Great Manchurian Plague of 1910–1911: The Geopolitics of an Epidemic Disease* (New Haven: Yale University Press, 2012).

Sussman, George D. "Scientists Doing History: Central Africa and the Origins of the First Plague Pandemic." *Journal of World History* 26, no. 2 (June 2015): 325–354.

RATS

Jonathan Burt's *Rat* (London: Reaktion Books, 2006) and Robert Sullivan's *Rats: Observations on the History and Habitat of the City's Most Unwanted Inhabitants* (New York: Bloomsbury, 2004) are delightful and empathetic studies of our much-maligned fellow urbanites. Hans Zinsser's classic *Rats, Lice, and History: A Chronicle of Pestilence and Plague* (New York: Black Dog & Leventhal Publishers, 1934) explains why so many of us harbor deep prejudices toward these little furry beasts.

Burt, Jonathan. *Rat* (London: Reaktion Books, 2006).

Sullivan, Robert *Rats: Observations on the History and Habitat of the City's Most Unwanted Inhabitants* (New York: Bloomsbury, 2004).

Zinsser, Hans. *Rats, Lice, and History: A Chronicle of Pestilence and Plague* (New York: Black Dog & Leventhal Publishers, 1934).